CARDIOLOGY

REVIEW 2018

DEV B. PAHLAJANI

M.D., F.A.C.C., F.I.S.E., F.I.C.P.
Head, Department of Cardiology
Breach Candy Hospital
Mumbai

AKSHAY MEHTA

M.D., D.M.
Consultant Cardiologist
Department of Cardiology
Nanavati Superspeciality Hospital
Mumbai

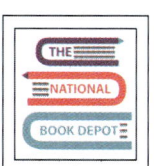

www.nationalbookdepot.com

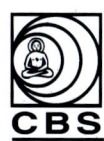

CBS

CBS Publishers & Distributors Pvt Ltd

Published by

Raju Shah for

THE NATIONAL BOOK DEPOT

Opp. Wadia Children's Hospital, Parel, Mumbai - 400 012.

Tel : 2416 5274 / 2413 1362 / 24132411 | Fax : 2413 0877

E-mail : nationalbook55@gmail.com

Website : nationalbookdepot.com

and

Satish Kumar Jain for

CBS Publishers & Distributors Pvt Ltd

4819/XI Prahlad Street, 24 Ansari Road, Daryaganj, New Delhi - 110 002, India.

Ph: 23289259, 23266861, 23266867 | Fax: 011-23243014

Website: www.cbspd.com | e-mail: delhi@cbspd.com; cbspubs@airtelmail.in.

Corporate Office: 204 FIE, Industrial Area, Patparganj, Delhi - 110 092.

Ph: 4934 4934 | Fax: 4934 4935 | E-mail: publishing@cbspd.com; publicity@cbspd.com

ISBN : 978-93-80206-94-3

Printed by : Neel Graphics

PREFACE

What would interest a practicing cardiologist or a physician that could benefit his or her patients - the ultimate beneficiary?

That is the question that dominated our minds when we set out to scan important articles from prominent cardiology journals of 2017 to produce this compilation, our third in last three years.

The criteria for selection were that they should be well conducted trials and research studies, published during 2017 that have relevance to patient care in our day-to-day practice, though it may be possible that some important studies may have missed our attention and not been included in this compendium.

The book is divided into 3 parts:

First, The Top Ten : From the wealth of research data published during the previous year we have carefully selected ten important research publications that are likely to impact or alter the pattern of our cardiology practice

Second is Critical Journal Review, in which, besides rewritten abstracts of research articles, critical analyses of these articles are also presented along with their strengths, weaknesses and clinical relevance for day to day practice. These appraisals are purely ours and readers and the authors have full freedom to disagree and arrive at different conclusions.

Thirdly, we present discussions in the format of Cardiology Currents which is an attempt to dissect a topic that has appeared in more than one journals with its varied nuances.

In an era of information explosion on the computer or phone screen, this book offers a paper reading experience that, sitting back, one can savor in the comfort of one's lap. We hope it serves the purpose for which it was created.

We gratefully acknowledge the secretarial assistance so ably provided by Mrs. Rajkumari Jethani and the technical assistance of Mr. Ravi Bhatt for uploading these articles onto our website "cardiositeindia.com".

Wish you all, happy reading!

Dev Pahlajani
Akshay Mehta

FOREWORD

As the time goes by, plethora of information accumulates at such galloping speed that it becomes increasingly difficult for a practicing cardiologist to be able to deliver evidence based health care as expected on the basis of published literature.

The medical science is largely the science of probabilities and obviously every conclusion drawn at the end of any study will have the other side of the story too. Not uncommonly there are studies in the literature with cintradirectory conclusion leading to confusion.

While going through this book, I had profound sense of clarity on many topics, which have significant bearing on hte way we practice. Both the authors have dealt with contemporary isuues with succinctness and clarity.

Importantly, the reading is very lucid, and rapid. Every topic is dealt with total crystalization of plethora of data and the final conclusions or we may say even the guidline has been outlined so precisely that the reader understands its application in clinical practice without any ambiguity in mind.

The book is divided into three sections and every section is independent of the other. I am going to make this book as my compendium and a "ready reference book", as each question is answered precisely, which can help one to apply it in his day to day practice.

This book is a testimony of remarkable skill that these two authors possess. From existing jargon of medical facts and figures they have provided crystalized decantation for a practicing Cardiologist, who then can breathe a respite of practicing eveidence based medicine after reading this book.

I, would read this book again and again and refer to it every time as and when. I face the question on my related subjects and seek the answer from the book.

It has been pleasure to write a forward to this unique book, which is meeting with the needs of a practising cardiologist. Surely a great addition to any library!

Dr A B Mehta

- International Cardiologist

MD, F.A.C.C., F.I.S.E., F.I.C.P

Director Cardiology

Jaslok Hospital & Research Centre, Mumbai

CONTENTS

SECTION 3 - CARDIO CURRENTS

SECTION 1 - TOP TEN CARDIOLOGY STORIES THAT WILL REDEFINE CARDIOLOGY PRACTICE

1

"Coronary Angioplasty - Not for Stable Angina ?"

Dev Pahlajani

Percutaneous coronary intervention (PCI) was expected to improve the quality of life by reducing angina and in some sub set of patients to prevent myocardial infarction (MI) and possibly decrease cardiovascular death. However several earlier studies indicated that while PCI improved quality of life by relieving symptoms, it did not prevent MI or decrease mortality as compared to medical treatment. The procedure continued to be performed with an "occulo-stenotic reflex". However, recently data from ORBITA trial was published in the Lancet November 02, 2017 issue that indicated PCI did not offer benefit of relieving angina as expected, when compared to optimum medical treatment. The study enrolled 200 patients with stable angina who were randomized to placebo or "sham" PCI procedure or actual PCI. Patients with sham procedure were given optimal medical treatment. All patients had significant coronary artery disease as measured by FFR with a mean reading of 0.69. The primary end point was exercise time increment between groups. There was no significant difference in exercise time increment between 2 groups (p=0.2). Thus concluding patients with stable angina subjected to PCI did not achieve significant relief of symptoms as compared to patients treated with optimum medical treatment. While the study involved small number of patients the results are very striking and have great therapeutic relevance. This is perhaps the first trial that has compared the results of PCI with that of a sham procedure. They cannot be ignored lightly. They are also in consonance with those of COURAGE trial which found that the patients of stable ischemic heart disease (SIHD) had similar rates of death, MI or hospitalization for acute coronary syndrome and stroke with optimum medical treatment as compared to PCI.

The impact of COURAGE trial was significant after it was published in 2007. There was 25% decrease in the over-all PCI numbers in USA. This was particularly driven by SIHD patients. Will data of ORBITA trial further impact the PCI volume particularly in developing countries like India with restricted health care resources? The number of PCI so far is largely driven by SIHD patients. This trial has already generated high powered discussion among the cardiology community as regards to the therapeutic value of PCI in SIHD. In the light of the results of ORBITA and COURAGE perhaps one will have to adhere to the guideline recommended optimum medical treatment as the first line of management for SIHD and reserve PCI for patients who continue to be symptomatic with optimum medical treatment.

Suggested Readings

1. Percutaneous Coronary Intervention in Stable Angina (ORBITA): A double-blind, randomised controlled trial. Rasha Al-Lamee, MRCP, David Thompson, MRCPI, Hakim-MoulayDehbi, PhD, Sayan Sen, MRCP, Kare Tang, FRCP, John Davies, MRCP, Thomas Keeble, MRCP, Michael Mielewczik, PhD, Raffi Kaprielian, FRCP, Iqbal S Malik, FRCP, Sukhjinder S Nijjer, MRCP, Ricardo Petraco, MRCP, Christopher Cook, MRCP, Yousif Ahmad, MRCP, James Howard, MRCP, Christopher Baker, FRCP, Andrew Sharp, FRCP, Robert Gerber, FRCP, Suneel Talwar, MRCP, Ravi Assomull, MRCP, Prof Jamil Mayet, FRCP, Roland Wensel, MRCP, David Collier, PhD, Matthew Shun-Shin, MRCP, Prof Simon A Thom, FRCP, Dr Justin E Davies, MRCP. The Lancet 2017. DOI: http://dx.doi.org/10.1016/S0140-6736(17)32714-9.

Post PCI DAPT duration - Impact of PRECISE-DAPT

Akshay Mehta

The delicate balance to be achieved between ischemic and bleeding risks after coronary stenting is well recognized.

Shortening the DAPT duration to 6 or even 3 months has been shown to significantly reduce bleeding in patients with drug-eluting stents. At the other extreme, prolonging DAPT treatment in selected patients who tolerate 12 months of DAPT without bleeding events can reduce ischemic events.

Hence the need is for an algorithm that can be tailored to individual patients at the time of stent implantation.

The limitations of a previously described DAPT score are that its generalizability is limited as it has not been well validated in trials and that it omits baseline variables such as anemia, important in predicting risk of bleeding with DAPT.

In a recent paper, Costa F et al describe a bedside risk scoring tool that was devised using patient-level data pooled from 14,963 patients on DAPT with aspirin and a P2Y12 inhibitor after coronary stenting in eight randomized trials.

They found five predictors of out-of-hospital TIMI major or minor bleeding occurring at least 7 days after stenting and assigned points to each factor (table). A nomogram to calculate the score is available online.

Out-of-Hospital TIMI Bleeding Risk Predictors*

Risk	Hazard Ratio (95% CI) P
Previous bleeding	4.14 (1.22-14.02) 0.023
Age (per 10-year increase)	1.34 (1.11-1.48) 0.005
White blood cell count (per increase of 103 cells/μL)	1.06 (0.99-1.13) 0.078
Baseline hemoglobin (per increase of 1 g/dL)	0.67 (0.53-0.84) 0.001
Creatinine clearance (per increase of 10 mL/min)	0.90 (0.82-0.99) 0.004

Based on this and the earlier DAPT trials, The European Society of Cardiology has issued a new "focused update" on its guidelines on dual antiplatelet therapy (DAPT) in coronary artery disease (CAD).

Announced at the European Society of Cardiology (ESC) 2017 Congress and published online in the European Heart Journal on August 26, 2017, and developed in collaboration with the European Association for Cardio-Thoracic Surgery (EACTS), the following were the key messages that can be utilized in clinical practice:

1. For ACS patients, the default DAPT duration should be 12 months, irrespective of the revascularization strategy (medical therapy, PCI, or CABG surgery).

2. Six months of DAPT should be considered in patients at high bleeding risk (PRECISE-DAPT score ≥ 25).

3. Therapy longer than 12 months may be considered in ACS patients who have tolerated DAPT without a bleeding complication.

4. As far as the need for a short DAPT regimen goes, newer-generation drug-eluting stents are as good as bare-metal stents.

5. Hence DAPT duration should be guided by an assessment of the individual patient's ischemic vs bleeding risks and not by the stent type.

6. In stable CAD patients treated with PCI, the duration of DAPT should be 1 to 6 months depending on the bleeding risk, irrespective of the type of metallic stent implanted.

7. A longer DAPT duration may be considered in patients whose ischemic risk is greater than the risk of bleeding.

8. There are insufficient data to recommend DAPT in stable CAD patients treated with CABG.

▌ Suggested Readings

1. Costa F, van Klaveren D, James S, et al. Derivation and validation of the predicting bleeding complications in patients undergoing stent implantation and subsequent dual antiplatelet therapy (PRECISE-DAPT) score: a pooled analysis of individual-patient datasets from clinical trials. Lancet 2017; 389:1025-1034.

2. Valgimigli M, Bueno H, Byrne R A et al. 2017 ESC focused update on dual antiplatelet therapy in coronary artery disease developed in collaboration with EACTS: The Task Force for dual antiplatelet therapy in coronary artery disease of the European Society of Cardiology (ESC) and of the European Association for Cardio-Thoracic Surgery (EACTS). Eur Heart J 2017; DOI:10.1093/eurheartj/ehx419.

3

Whither BVS

Dev Pahlajani

It was about 5 years back that bioresorbable stent - BVS was introduced into the market by Abbot to treat obstructive coronary artery disease. The initial animal and human data indicated that BVS could replace metallic drug eluting stents which were made of either stainless steel or cobalt chromium. The BVS was made from polylactide - PLLA and coated with everolimus drug. The stent was designed to get absorbed from the vessel wall over a period of about 2 years with some of the OCT images showing faint persistence up to 4 years. The term "scaffold" was coined for BVS and the metallic stents were compared to a "cage". It was expected that with absorption of PLLA the vasomotor tone would be restored and endothelial function would be preserved. Further the need for antiplatelets would be greatly reduced. While the early data published was encouraging for the BVS, the 3 years data from ABSORB II which was presented in the later part of 2016 at TCT and subsequently published in Lancet were disappointing. Target vessel myocardial infarction (MI occurred in 7% of ABSORB patients as opposed to 1% in Xience (metallic stents) treated patients (p=0.006). There was two fold increase in stent thrombosis in BVS treated patients versus Xience treated patients. ABSORB was a prospective randomized multi-centre trial which randomized 501 patients to BVS or Xience V metallic stent. The most disappointing was the failure of concept of preservation of vasomotor tone. The study revealed there was no vasomotor tone preservation in BVS treated versus Xience treated patients. The clinical events of composite of death, TV failure, MI and clinically indicated TLR was twice the number in BVS versus Xience patients. In an individual patient data meta-analysis ABSORB randomized trials published in October 2017 in Circulation the authors confirmed the conclusions arrived at in the earlier ABSORB II data. The meta-analysis concluded that BVS was associated with increased rates of target lesion failure and device thrombosis when compared with everolimus eluting stent.

Subsequently the ABBOT company has withdrawn the device from the market.

However, in the ever evolving field of stent technology,one should be optimistic that a refined version of the absorbable polymer or metallic based stent would meet the expectations of interventional cardiologists version of the absorbable polymer or metallic based stent would meet the expectations of interventional cardiologists.

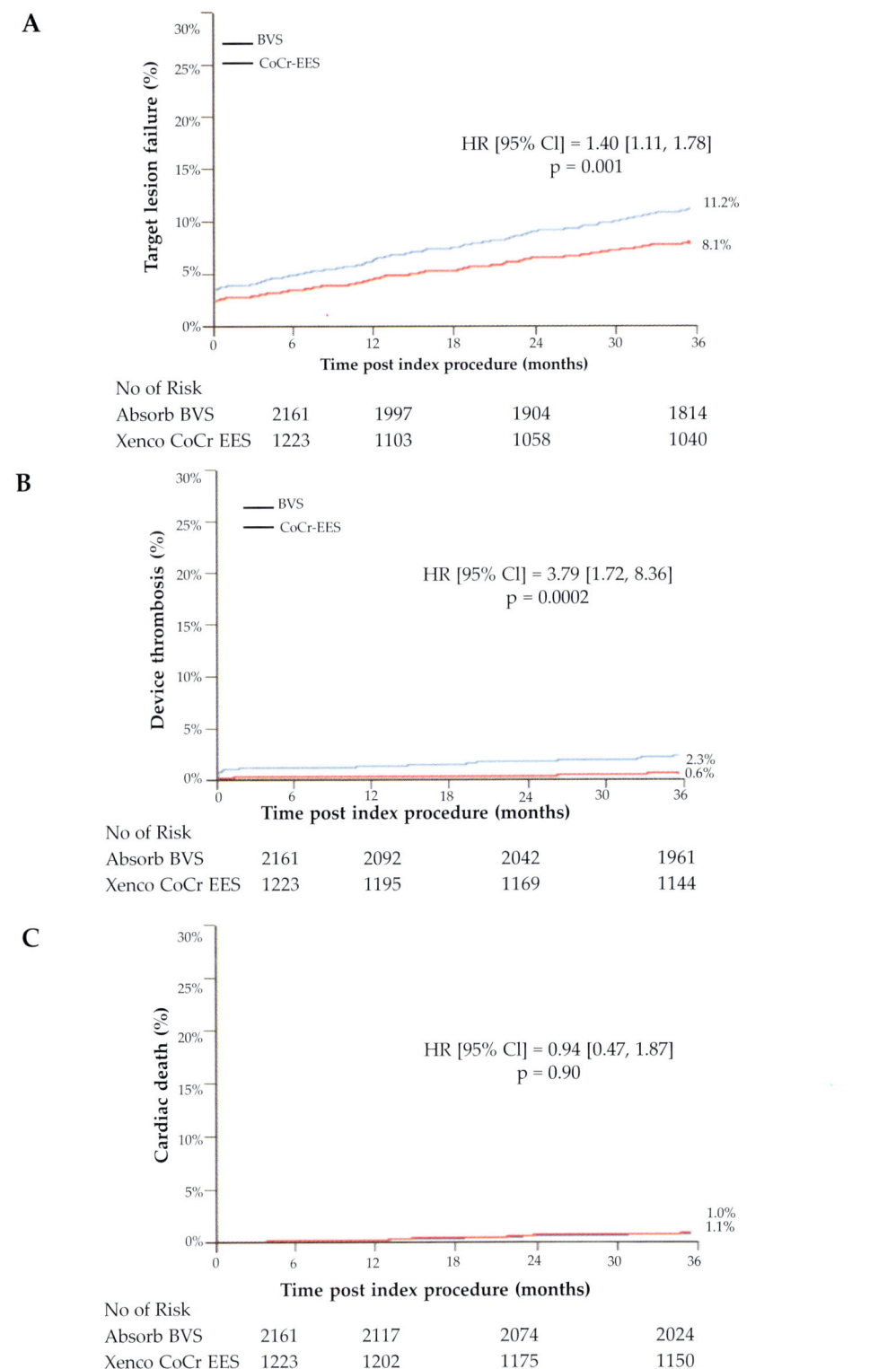

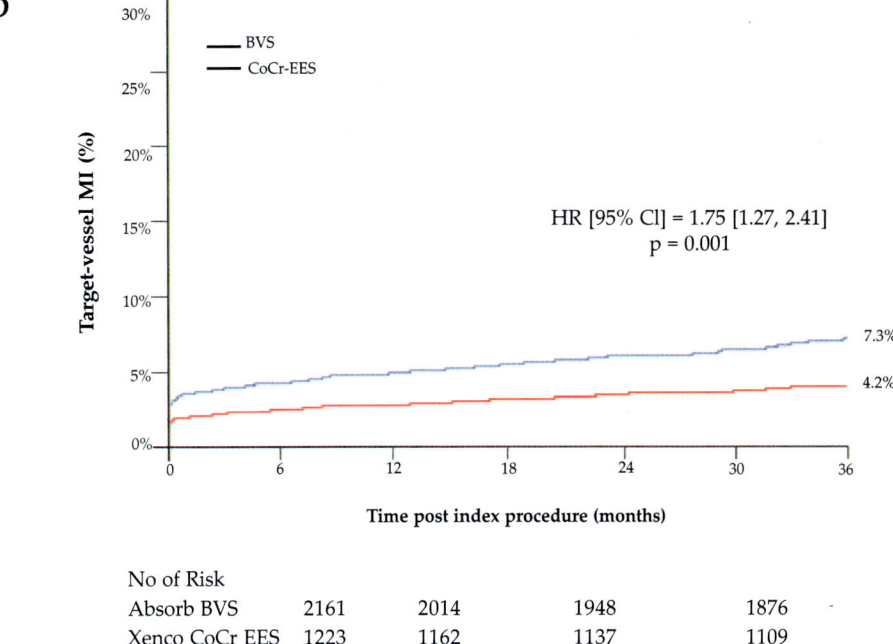

D

No of Risk

Absorb BVS	2161	2014	1948	1876
Xenco CoCr EES	1223	1162	1137	1109

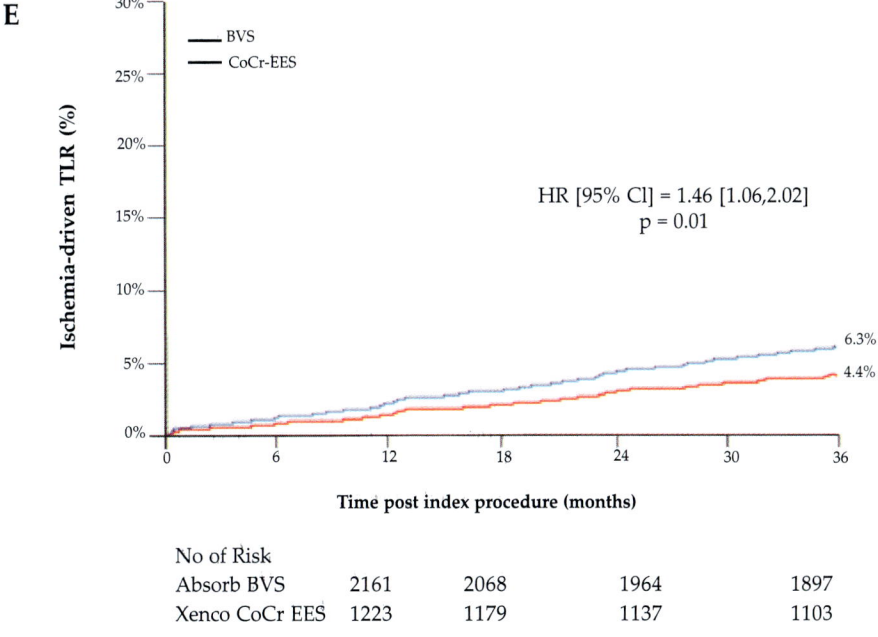

E

No of Risk

Absorb BVS	2161	2068	1964	1897
Xenco CoCr EES	1223	1179	1137	1103

▮ Suggested Readings

1. Three-Year Outcomes With the Absorb Bioresorbable Scaffold Individual-Patient-Data Meta-Analysis From the ABSORB Randomized Trial. Circulation 2017;136:1-16.

2. Comparison of an everolimus-eluting bioresorbable scaffold with an everolimus-eluting metallic stent for the treatment of coronary artery stenosis (ABSORB II): a 3 year, randomised, controlled, single-blind, multicentre clinical trial. The Lancet 2016;388(10059):2479-2491.

4

The (Saturated) Fat Debate

Akshay Mehta

Randomized clinical trials, prospective observational studies in many populations and atherosclerosis regression studies in nonhuman primates over last decades have strengthened the long-standing AHA recommendations (since 1961) to replace saturated fat with polyunsaturated and monounsaturated fat to lower the incidence of CVD.

The recent 2017 Presidential Advisory from the American Heart Association reiterated the danger of saturated fat.

However, there have always been arguments favoring saturated fats.

Latest amongst these is a large study which made headlines recently. Called the PURE (Prospective Urban Rural Epidemiology) study, it observed the dietary patterns of 135335 people from 18 countries for about of 7·4 years, to find a correlation between fat and carbohydrate intake and cardiovascular disease.

It found that those people with the highest intake of dietary fat (35% of daily calories) had 23% lesser mortality than those with the lowest intake of fat (10% of daily calories). Both total fat and individual types of fat were related to lower total mortality. On the other hand, those with the highest intake (77% of daily calories) of carbohydrates were 28% more likely to have died than those with the lowest intake (46% of daily calories).

Neither total fat nor types of fat were associated with cardiovascular disease, myocardial infarction, or cardiovascular disease mortality, whereas saturated fat had an inverse association with stroke.

So, now should we change our opinion about fats in food?

Before we do that, it do well to remind ourselves that an observational study such as the PURE study suffers from major weaknesses:

1. Diet records of patients are dependent on memory- people either may not remember or may slightly misrepresent what they have been eating.

2. It is almost impossible to disentangle the large number of confounding factors, such as income, education and life style. One of the most important risk factors for poor health is poverty, which not only impacts food selection but also access to proper health care.

3. The study was unable to distinguish the type of carbohydrates a person was eating, and thus a carbohydrate from whole grains was considered the same as one from heavily processed

foods or soft drinks. Most study participants located in low-income countries subsisted almost entirely on carbohydrates, especially from refined sources.

4. The study did not assess trans- fat intake (particularly high in South Asian diets), which may have confounded associations for other types of fat.

On the other hand, consider the following from the 2017 presidential advisory:

1. Randomized clinical trials as well as prospective observational studies in many populations have showed that lower intake of saturated fat coupled with higher intake of polyunsaturated and monounsaturated fat is associated with lower rates of CVD and all-cause mortality.

2. A dietary strategy of reducing intake of total dietary fat, including saturated fat, and replacing the fats mainly with unspecified carbohydrates does not prevent CHD.

3. Saturated fat increases LDL cholesterol, a major cause of atherosclerosis and CVD, and replacing it with polyunsaturated or monounsaturated fat decreases LDL cholesterol.

4. Replacing saturated with polyunsaturated or monounsaturated fat lowers blood triglyceride levels, an independent biomarker of risk for CVD.

5. Replacing saturated with polyunsaturated fat prevents and regresses atherosclerosis in nonhuman primates.

Thus, one study (that too with all the pitfalls of being observational in design) should not steer us away from the long-standing AHA recommendations to replace saturated fat with polyunsaturated and monounsaturated fat to lower the incidence of CVD. This shift from saturated to unsaturated fats should occur simultaneously in an overall healthful dietary pattern such as the DASH or Mediterranean diet as emphasized by the 2013 AHA/American College of Cardiology lifestyle guidelines and the 2015 to 2020 Dietary Guidelines for Americans.

▌ Suggested Readings

1. Dr Mahshid Dehghan, PhD' Correspondence information about the author Dr Mahshid Dehghan Email the author Dr Mahshid Dehghan, Andrew Mente, PhD, Xiaohe Zhang, MSc, Sumathi Swaminathan, PhD, Prof Wei Li, PhD, Prof Viswanathan Mohan, MD, Romaina Iqbal, PhD, Prof Rajesh Kumar, MD, Edelweiss Wentzel-Viljoen, PhD, Prof Annika Rosengren, MD, Leela Itty Amma, MD, Prof Alvaro Avezum, MD, Jephat Chifamba, DPhil, Rafael Diaz, MD, Rasha Khatib, PhD, Prof Scott Lear, PhD, Prof Patricio Lopez-Jaramillo, MD, Xiaoyun Liu, PhD, Prof Rajeev Gupta, MD, Noushin.

   Associations of fats and carbohydrate intake with cardiovascular disease and mortality in 18 countries from five continents (PURE): a prospective cohort study.

   THE LANCET, Volume 390, No. 10107, p2050-2062, 4 November 2017.

5

PCI in Atrial Fibrillation : Good Bye to Triple Therapy

Dev Pahlajani

Approximately 30% patients with atrial fibrillation (AF) have atherosclerotic coronary artery disease while 8-10% patients who undergo PCI have AF. Currently these patients are advised triple drug therapy consisting of vitamin K antagonist (VKA) or NOAC with aspirin and P2Y12 inhibitor clopidogrel or ticagrelor for a brief period of time ranging from one month to 3 months. However, triple drug therapy carries the risk of extensive major bleeding. Several earlier trials have shown that bleeding is a major and independent risk factor for increased mortality. Whether dual therapy with clopidogrel or ticagrelor with VKA or currently available NOACs would have reduced risk of bleeding has been a matter of several studies. Of late two important trials viz. PIONEER AF and REDUAL- PCI were undertaken to see if small dose rivaroxaban or dabigatran with P2Y12 inhibitor will be superior to triple drug therapy. In PIONEER AF trial 2124 patients with AF who had undergone PCI with stent were randomized to receive 1) standard triple therapy with DAPT with VKA 2) dual therapy with rivaroxaban 15 mg once a day with P2Y12 inhibitor 3) very low dose rivaroxaban 2.5 mg twice daily plus DAPT. The risk of clinically significant bleeding was lower in the double therapy than in standard triple therapy (Fig. 1).

In a recently published REDUAL - PCI trial 2725 patients with AF who had undergone PCI were randomized to two different doses of

a) 110 mg twice a day with clopidogrel or ticagrelor

b) 150 mg twice a day with clopidogrel or ticagrelor

c) Standard triple therapy with VKA plus DAPT. The risk of bleeding was lower who received dual therapy with dabigatran plus P2Y12 inhibitor. The primary end point of major or clinically relevant non major bleeding occurred in 4% in 110 mg dabigatran with P2Y12 inhibitor therapy versus 26.9% in triple therapy group. With the 150 mg b.i.d dose with dabigatran the primary end point occurred in 20.2% when compared to 25.7% in the triple therapy group (Fig. 2). Similarly in the earlier WOEST trial, dual therapy with VKA with clopidogrel proved to be superior to triple therapy group.

The message from the 3 trials is clear. Dual therapy either with warfarin or rivaroxaban or dabigatran with clopidogrel/ticagrelor is associated with reduced risk of bleeding and may become default strategy in the coming years. Perhaps time has come to say "good bye" to triple therapy.

PIONEER AF

A   Primary safety end point

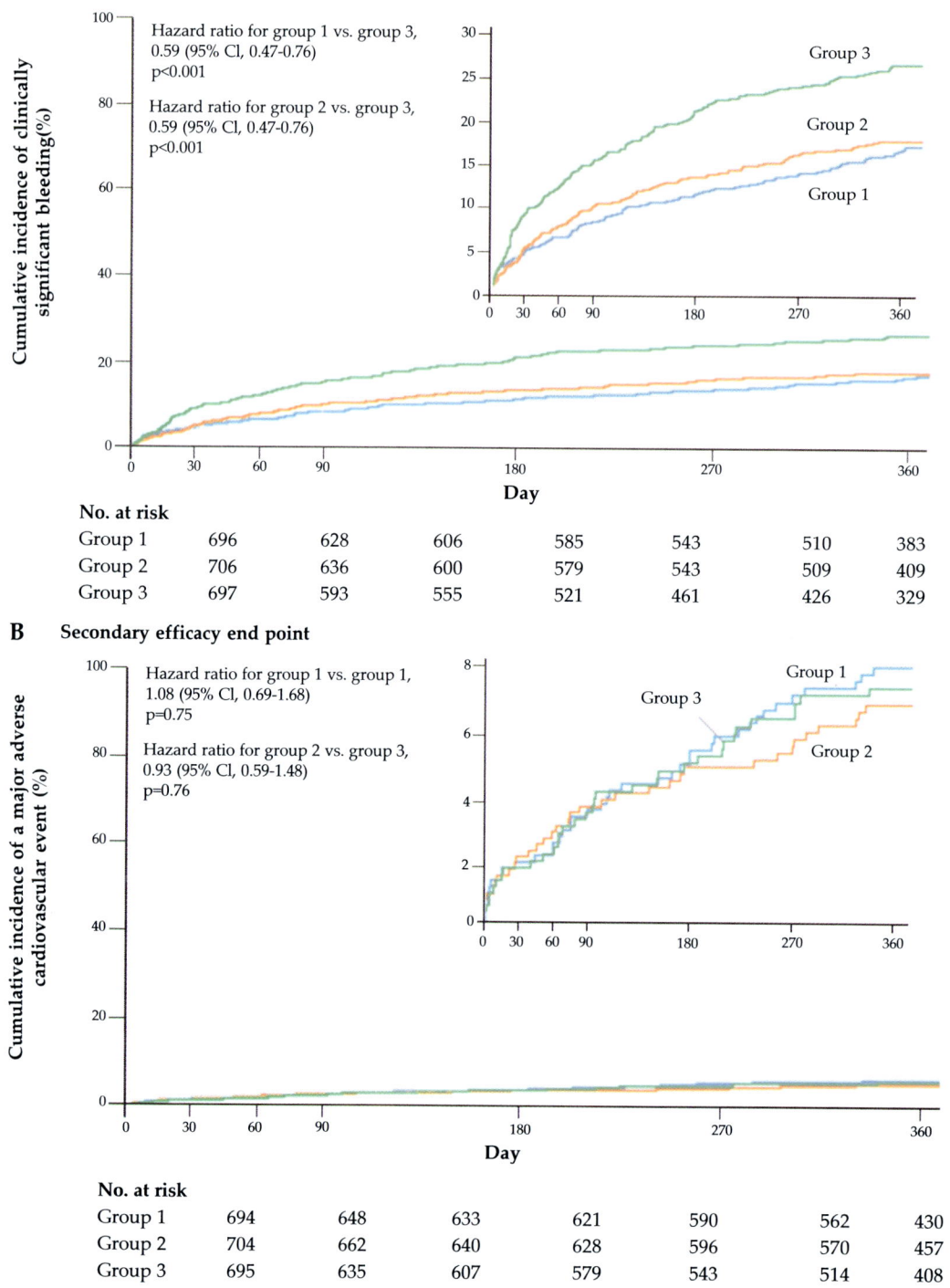

Hazard ratio for group 1 vs. group 3,
0.59 (95% Cl, 0.47-0.76)
p<0.001

Hazard ratio for group 2 vs. group 3,
0.59 (95% Cl, 0.47-0.76)
p<0.001

Cumulative incidence of clinically significant bleeding(%)

Day

No. at risk

Group 1	696	628	606	585	543	510	383
Group 2	706	636	600	579	543	509	409
Group 3	697	593	555	521	461	426	329

B   Secondary efficacy end point

Hazard ratio for group 1 vs. group 1,
1.08 (95% Cl, 0.69-1.68)
p=0.75

Hazard ratio for group 2 vs. group 3,
0.93 (95% Cl, 0.59-1.48)
p=0.76

Cumulative incidence of a major adverse cardiovascular event (%)

Day

No. at risk

Group 1	694	648	633	621	590	562	430
Group 2	704	662	640	628	596	570	457
Group 3	695	635	607	579	543	514	408

A. Primary end point dual therapy group (110mg) vs. Triple therapy group

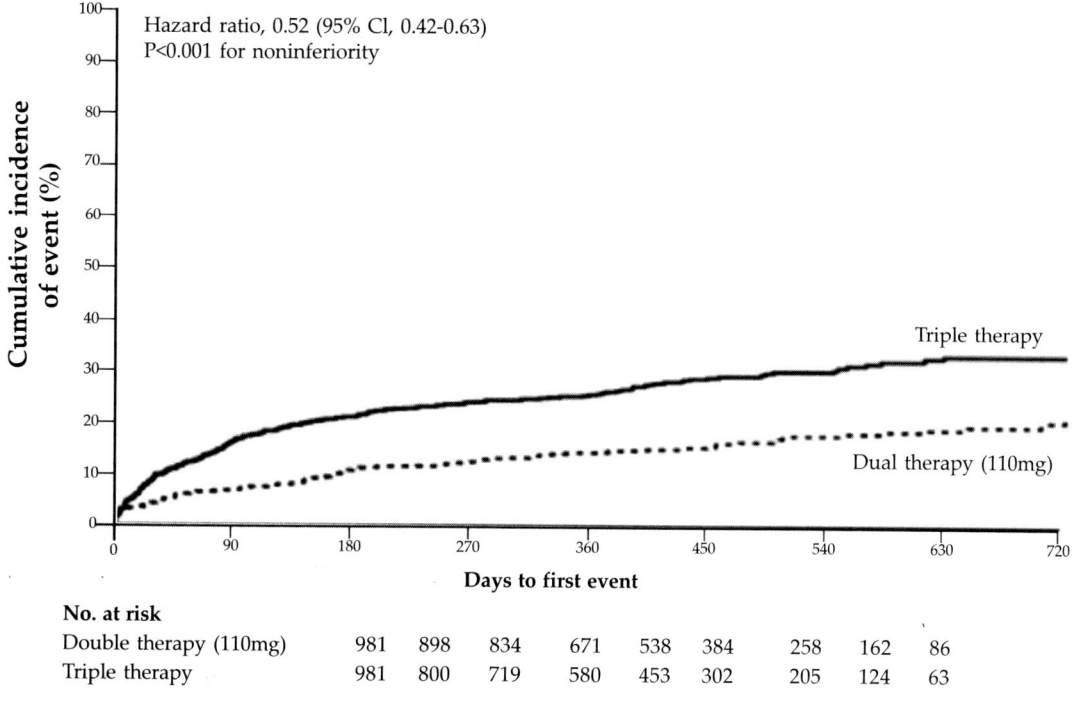

Hazard ratio, 0.52 (95% CI, 0.42-0.63)
P<0.001 for noninferiority

Triple therapy

Dual therapy (110mg)

No. at risk

Double therapy (110mg)	981	898	834	671	538	384	258	162	86
Triple therapy	981	800	719	580	453	302	205	124	63

B. Primary end point dual therapy group (150mg) vs. Triple therapy group

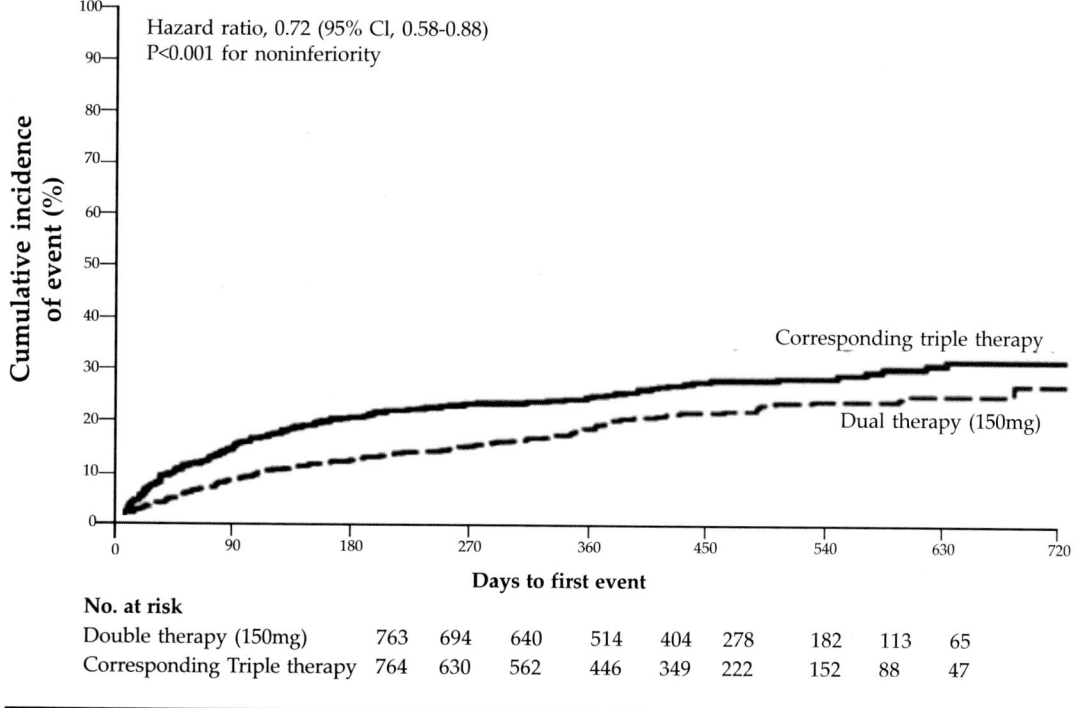

Hazard ratio, 0.72 (95% CI, 0.58-0.88)
P<0.001 for noninferiority

Corresponding triple therapy

Dual therapy (150mg)

No. at risk

Double therapy (150mg)	763	694	640	514	404	278	182	113	65
Corresponding Triple therapy	764	630	562	446	349	222	152	88	47

C. Secondary efficacy end point in dual therapy group (combined) vs. Triple therapy group

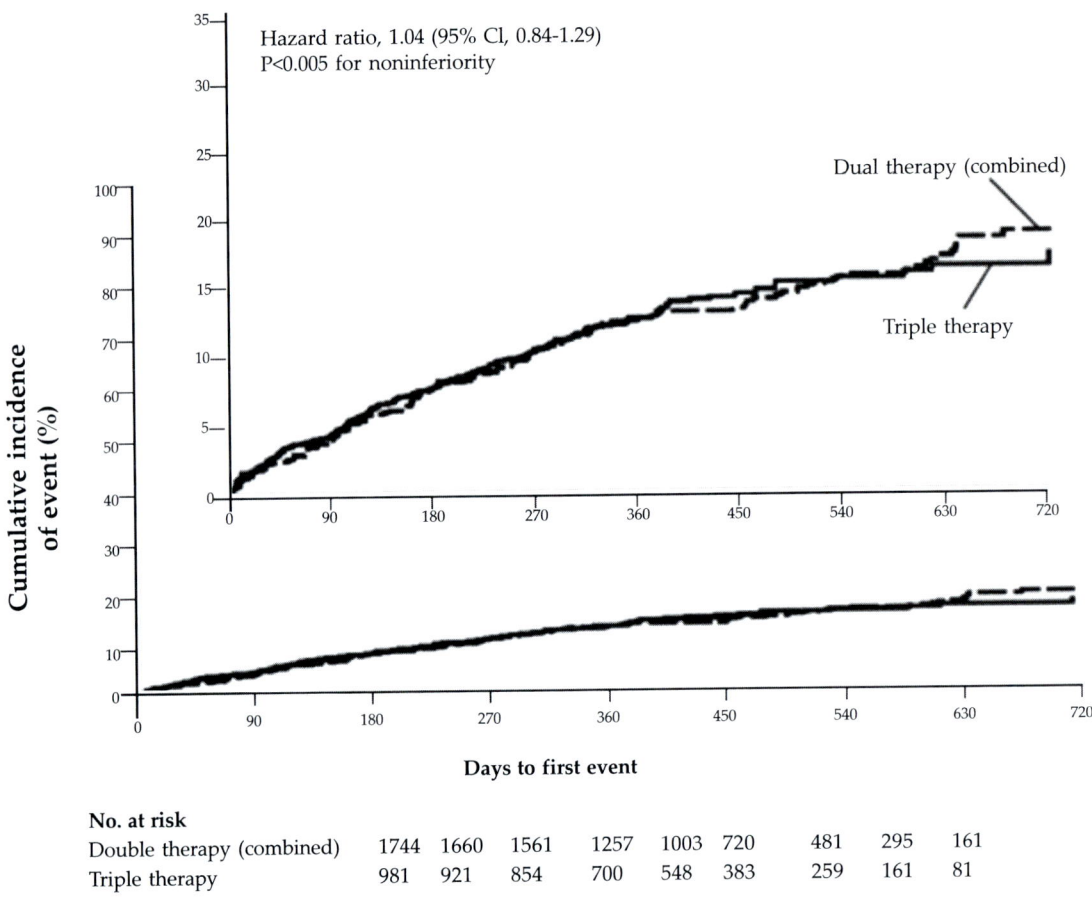

Hazard ratio, 1.04 (95% CI, 0.84-1.29)
P<0.005 for noninferiority

Dual therapy (combined)

Triple therapy

Cumulative incidence of event (%)

Days to first event

No. at risk									
Double therapy (combined)	1744	1660	1561	1257	1003	720	481	295	161
Triple therapy	981	921	854	700	548	383	259	161	81

▌ **Suggested Readings**

1. RE-DUAL PCI Dual Therapy Vs. Triple Therapy in AFib Patients Undergoing PCI; August 08, 2017.

6

Clot Sucking Not Attractive in Veins

Akshay Mehta

Postthrombotic syndrome, occurs in about half of patients with proximal DVT despite use of standard blood-thinning drugs.

Hence, to assess in a randomized trial whether the addition of pharmaco-mechanical catheter-directed thrombolysis (along with thrombus aspiration or maceration) to anticoagulation results in a lower risk of the post-thrombotic syndrome, 692 patients with acute proximal deep-vein thrombosis were randomly assigned to receive either anticoagulation alone (control group) or anticoagulation plus pharmacomechanical thrombolysis (catheter-mediated or device-mediated intrathrombus delivery of recombinant tissue plasminogen activator and thrombus aspiration or maceration, with or without stenting).

There were no significant between-group difference in the percentage of patients with the post-thrombotic syndrome or in recurrent venous thromboembolism seen over the 24-month follow-up period. (47% versus 48% with a risk ratio (RR) of 0.96 : 95% CI 0.82-1.11; P=0.56).

Pharmacomechanical thrombolysis led to more major bleeding events within 10 days.

Moderate-to-severe post-thrombotic syndrome occurred 27% lower in the pharmaco mechanical thrombolysis group as compared to the control group. However there was no difference in quality of life from baseline to 24 months between the treatment groups.

Thus, in patients with acute proximal deep-vein thrombosis, the addition of pharmaco mechanical catheter-directed thrombolysis to usual anticoagulation did not result in a lower incidence of the post-thrombotic syndrome but had a higher risk of major bleeding.

Although improvement in quality of life from baseline to 24 months did not differ significantly between the treatment groups, the severity scores for the post-thrombotic syndrome were lower in the pharmaco mechanical-thrombolysis group than in the control group at 6, 12, 18, and 24 months of follow-up.

Hence, most patients can avoid an unnecessary procedure that would confer some bleeding risk and significant cost.

It could be of value in carefully selected patients, for instance in a young patient with a very extensive high proximal DVT who is very symptomatic but who is at low risk for bleeding.

Suggested Readings

1. Suresh Vedantham, M.D., Samuel Z. Goldhaber, M.D., Jim A. Julian, M.Math., Susan R. Kahn, M.D., Michael R. Jaff, D.O., David J. Cohen, M.D., Elizabeth Magnuson, Sc.D., Mahmood K. Razavi, M.D., Anthony J. Comerota, M.D., Heather L. Gornik, M.D., Timothy P. Murphy, M.D., Lawrence Lewis, M.D., James R. Duncan, M.D., Ph.D., Patricia Nieters, B.S.N., Mary C. Derfler, M.S.N., Marc Filion, M.Sc., Chu-Shu Gu, Ph.D., Stephen Kee, M.D., Joseph Schneider, M.D., Ph.D., NaelSaad, M.D., Morey Blinder, M.D., Stephan Moll, M.D., David Sacks, M.D., Judith Lin, M.D., John Rundback, M.D., Mark Garcia, M.D., Rahul Razdan, M.D., Eric VanderWoude, M.D., Vasco Marques, M.D., and Clive Kearon, M.B., Ph.D., for the ATTRACT Trial Investigators*.

Pharmacomechanical Catheter-Directed Thrombolysis for Deep-Vein Thrombosis.

N Engl J Med 2017; 377:2240-2252December 7, 2017DOI: 10.1056/NEJMoa1615066.

7

Transcatheter Aortic Valve Replacement in Intermediate Risk Patients-Widening the Net

Dev Pahlajani

Patients with critical aortic stenosis with mean gradient of > 40 mmHg or 4 mtrs/sec velocity carry ominous prognosis with more than 50% mortality at the end of 2 years.

In patients with high EURO or STS (Society of Thoracic Surgeons) score the risk of surgical aortic valve replacement (SAVR) is extremely high. Recently in last 10 years patients with severe aortic stenosis with high surgical risk have been subjected to transcatheter aortic valve replacement (TAVR) either by balloon expanding or self expanding aortic valves. According to current guidelines TAVR is restricted to patients with high surgical risk score. Earlier devices and lack of operator experience were responsible for high complication rate including high mortality of TAVR leading to such stringent recommendations. Therefore the procedure was restricted only to high risk patients. However, with the refinement and variety of the devices available with improved operator experience the results of TAVR have become comparable to those of SAVR. Recently two important studies were published which compared the results of TAVR to SAVR in patients with intermediate risk score.

In PARTNER 2 cohort randomized second generation balloon expandable valve to compare the results of TAVR with SAVR in the intermediate risk clinical profiles. Over 2000 patients from 57 centers were randomized to undergo TAVR or SAVR. The rate of death from any cause or disabling stroke at 2 years was 19.3% in TAVR group and 21.1% in the SAVR group (p=0.25). Patients treated with TAVR had larger aortic valve area as compared to SAVR. Rates of acute kidney injury, severe bleeding and newer onset atrial fibrillation were also lower in TAVR group as compared to SAVR group. Patients with SAVR had lower rates of major vascular complications, and aortic regurgitation.

In another trial - SURTAVI, 1746 patients with intermediate STS clinical risk score with predicted risk of mortality $4.5 \pm 1.6\%$ were enrolled. The patients were randomized at 87 centers to undergo TAVR or SAVR.

At 24 months, the primary end point of composite of death from any cause or disabling stroke occurred in 12.6% in TAVR group and 14% in SAVR (non inferiority > 0.999). There were higher rates of acute kidney injury, AF in the SAVR group. TAVR patients had lower mean gradient, larger aortic valve areas as compared to SAVR treated patients. However, greater number of TAVR patients had aortic regurgitation and need for placement.

Larger number of patients of severe aortic stenosis fall in the intermediate risk group particularly those in the younger age group. With these encouraging results which are comparable, and to a certain extent better than those achieved with SAVR it is quite possible that the next few years will see big surge in the number of TAVR treated with either balloon expandable or self-expanding aortic valve. Lower morbidity, better new designs of the device, wider operator experience and earlier return to work would be compelling factors to choose TAVR over SAVR.

B. Primary outcome

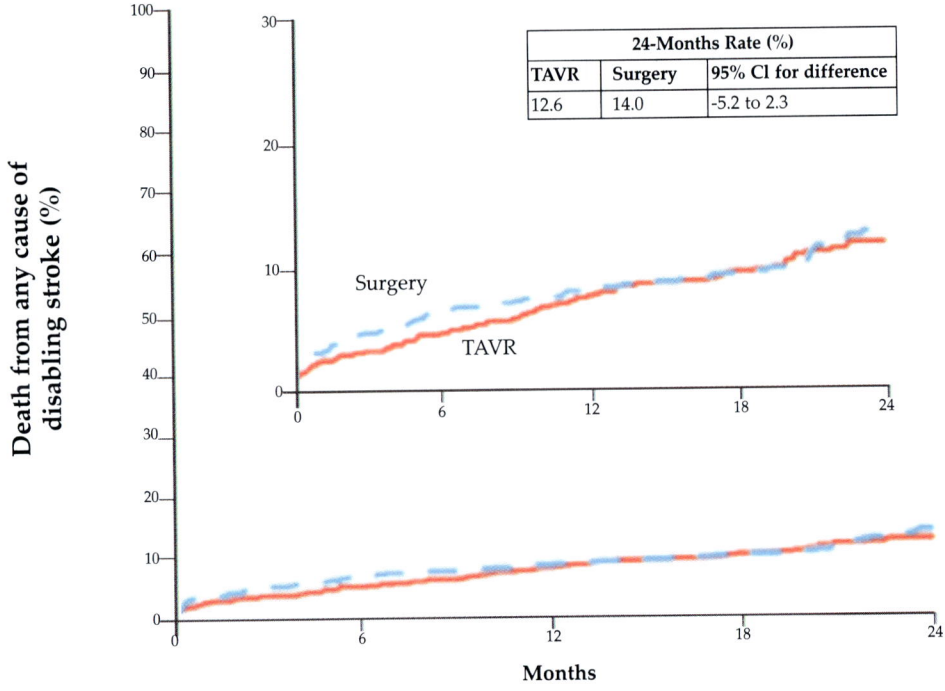

	24-Months Rate (%)		
	TAVR	Surgery	95% CI for difference
	12.6	14.0	-5.2 to 2.3

No. at risk

TAVR	864	755	612	456	272
Surgery	796	674	555	407	241

C. Death from any cause

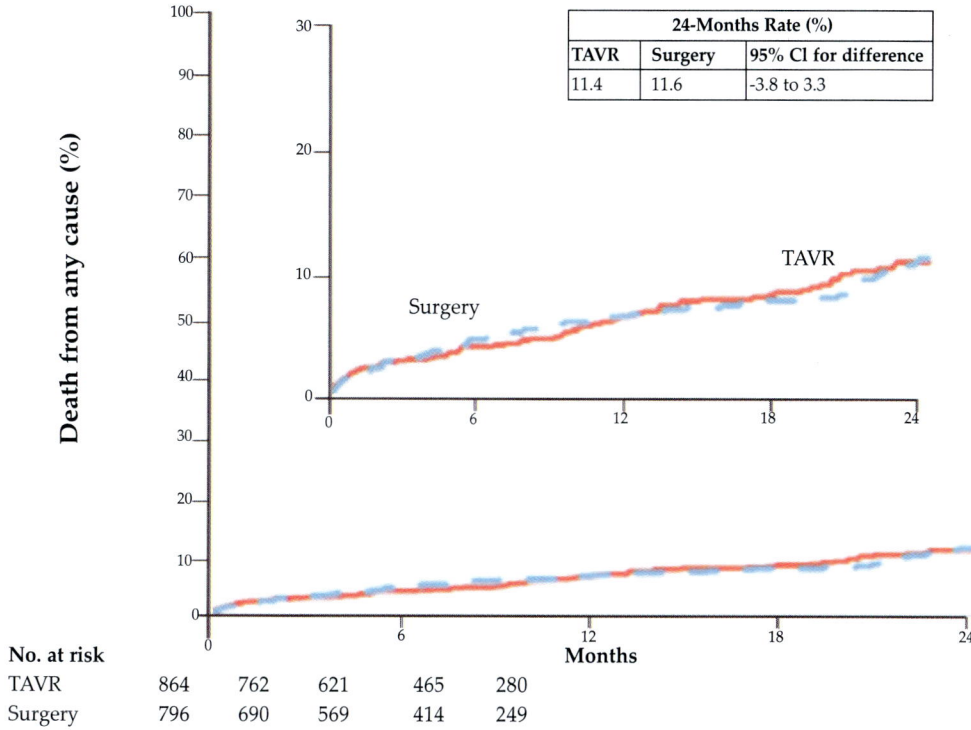

24-Months Rate (%)		
TAVR	Surgery	95% CI for difference
11.4	11.6	-3.8 to 3.3

No. at risk

TAVR	864	762	621	465	280
Surgery	796	690	569	414	249

D. Disabling stroke

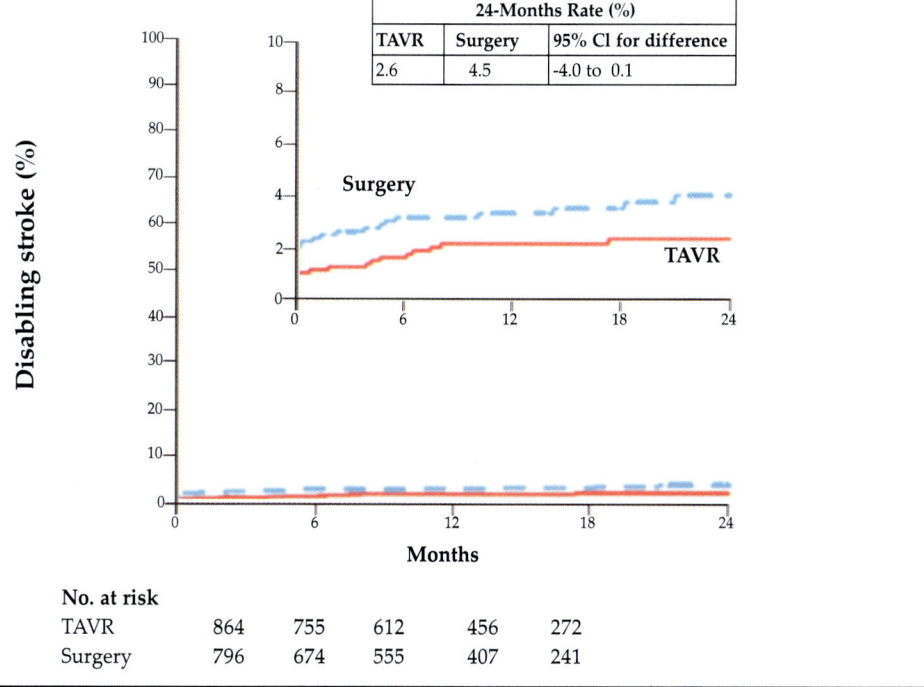

24-Months Rate (%)		
TAVR	Surgery	95% CI for difference
2.6	4.5	-4.0 to 0.1

No. at risk

TAVR	864	755	612	456	272
Surgery	796	674	555	407	241

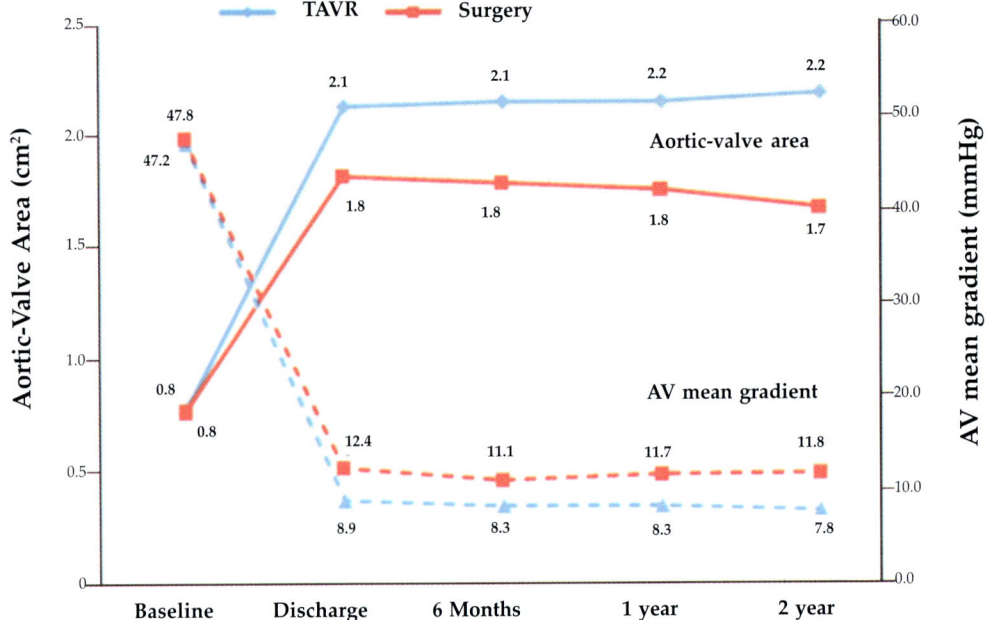

A. Intention to treat population

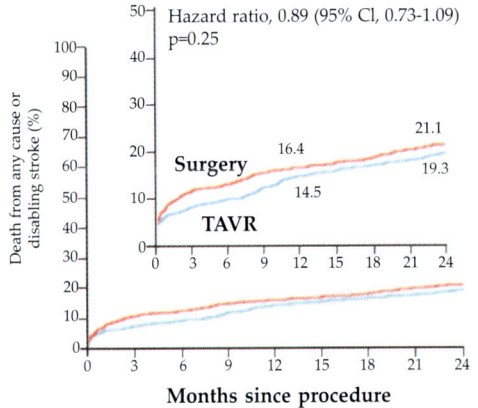

Hazard ratio, 0.89 (95% CI, 0.73-1.09)
p=0.25

Death from any cause or disabling stroke (%)

Months since procedure

No of Risk

TAVR	1001	918	901	870	842	825	811	801	774
Surgery	1021	838	812	783	770	747	735	717	695

B. As treated population

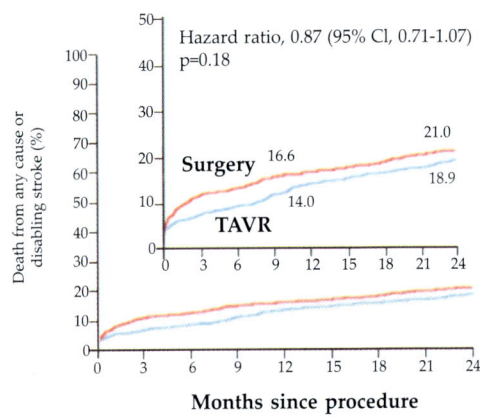

Hazard ratio, 0.87 (95% CI, 0.71-1.07)
p=0.18

Death from any cause or disabling stroke (%)

Months since procedure

No of Risk

TAVR	994	917	900	870	942	825	811	801	774
Surgery	944	826	807	779	766	743	731	715	694

C. Transfemoral access Cohort, Intention to treat analysis

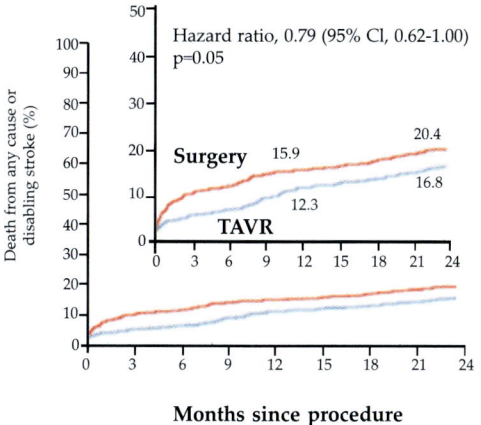

Hazard ratio, 0.79 (95% Cl, 0.62-1.00)
p=0.05

D. Transfemoral access Cohort, As treated analysis

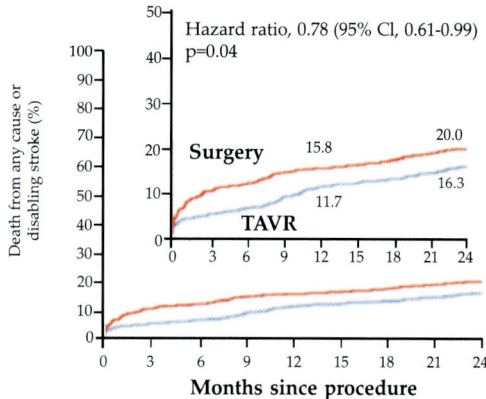

Hazard ratio, 0.78 (95% Cl, 0.61-0.99)
p=0.04

No of Risk									
TAVR	775	718	709	685	663	652	644	634	612
Surgery	775	643	628	604	595	577	569	557	538

No of Risk									
TAVR	762	717	708	685	663	652	644	634	612
Surgery	722	636	624	600	591	573	565	555	537

▮ Suggested Readings

Surgical or Transcatheter Aortic-Valve Replacement in Intermediate-Risk Patients.

1. M.J. Reardon, N.M. Van Mieghem, J.J. Popma, N.S. Kleiman, L. Sondergaard, M. Mumtaz, D.H. Adams, G.M. Deeb, B. Maini, H. Gada, S. Chetcuti, T. Gleason,J. Heiser, R. Lange, W. Merhi, J.K. Oh, P.S. Olsen, N. Piazza, M. Williams, S. Windecker, S.J. Yakubov, E. Grube, R. Makkar, J.S. Lee, J. Conte, E. Vang, H. Nguyen, Y. Chang, A.S. Mugglin, P.W.J.C. Serruys, and A.P. Kappetein,for the SURTAVI Investigators* NEJM 2017;376(14):1321-1331.

Transcatheter or Surgical Aortic-Valve Replacement in Intermediate-Risk Patients.

2. Martin B. Leon, M.D., Craig R. Smith, M.D., Michael J. Mack, M.D., Raj R. Makkar, M.D., Lars G. Svensson, M.D., Ph.D., Susheel K. Kodali, M.D., Vinod H. Thourani, M.D., E. Murat Tuzcu, M.D., D. Craig Miller, M.D., Howard C. Herrmann, M.D., DarshanDoshi, M.D., David J. Cohen, M.D., Augusto D. Pichard, M.D., Samir Kapadia, M.D., Todd Dewey, M.D., Vasilis Babaliaros, M.D., Wilson Y. Szeto, M.D., Mathew R. Williams, M.D., Dean Kereiakes, M.D., Alan Zajarias, M.D., Kevin L. Greason, M.D., Brian K. Whisenant, M.D., Robert W. Hodson, M.D., Jeffrey W. Moses, M.D., Alfredo Trento, M.D., David L. Brown, M.D., William F. Fearon, M.D., Philippe Pibarot, D.V.M., Ph.D., Rebecca T. Hahn, M.D., Wael A. Jaber, M.D., William N. Anderson, Ph.D., Maria C. Alu, M.M., and John G. Webb, M.D., for the PARTNER 2 Investigators* NEJM 2016;374(17):1609-1620.

8

New Hypertension Guidelines

Akshay Mehta

The 2017 ACC/AHA hypertension guidelines were released at the American Heart Association (AHA) 2017 Scientific Sessions and published simultaneously in the Journal of the American College of Cardiology and in the AHA journal Hypertension.

The key changes in the new guidelines were as follows :

1. A strong emphasis on blood-pressure measurement, especially on out-of-office blood-pressure measurements, using the average of measures over several visits.

2. A new blood-pressure classification system: Adults with an average systolic pressure of 130 to 139 mm Hg or diastolic pressure of 80 to 89 mm Hg are now categorized as having stage 1 hypertension (who would have previously been considered as having "prehypertension").

3. Lower targets for blood pressure during the management of hypertension. These are reductions in blood pressure to less than 130 mm Hg systolic and less than 80 mm Hg diastolic in most adults (down from previous 140/90 mm Hg).

4. Incorporation of underlying cardiovascular risk in decision-making for treatment with an emphasis on lifestyle approaches. For stage 1 hypertension at low atherosclerotic risk (10-year risk < 10%), lifestyle changes alone are recommended, whereas for patients at high risk (including those with diabetes and kidney disease), lifestyle changes plus drug therapy is advised.

5. New stage 2 hypertension: This is average systolic pressure higher than 140 mm Hg or diastolic above 90 mm Hg. As before, drug therapy is recommended for all these patients irrespective of atherosclerotic risk.

6. Older adults have the same treatment target as younger patients, and drug therapy is recommended for all older adults (age >65 years) with an average systolic pressure of 130 mm Hg or greater.

7. Initiating treatment with two drugs : Most adults (especially those with stage 2 hypertension or blacks) should be treated initially with two agents,

A lot of debate is and will be generated regarding the pros and cons of the guidelines, and coming months will tell us more.

Suggested Readings

1. Paul K. Whelton, Robert M. Carey, Wilbert S. Aronow, Donald E. Casey, Karen J. Collins, Cheryl Dennison Himmelfarb, Sondra M. DePalma, Samuel Gidding, Kenneth A. Jamerson, Daniel W. Jones, Eric J. MacLaughlin, Paul Muntner, Bruce Ovbiagele, Sidney C. Smith, Crystal C. Spencer, Randall S. Stafford, Sandra J. Taler, Randal J. Thomas, Kim A. Williams, Jeff D. Williamson, Jackson T. Wright.

    2017 ACC/AHA/AAPA/ABC/ACPM/AGS/APhA/ASH/ASPC/NMA/PCNA Guideline for the Prevention, Detection, Evaluation, and Management of High Blood Pressure in Adults: Executive Summary.

    A Report of the American College of Cardiology/American Heart Association Task Force on Clinical Practice Guidelines.

    Hypertension. 2017;HYP.0000000000000066. Originally published November 13, 2017.

9

Left Main Coronary Artery Disease: No More Exclusive Domain for CABG?

Dev Pahlajani

Coronary artery bypass graft surgery (CABG) is considered as a Class I indication for patients with left main coronary artery disease (LMCAD). However, there have been several recent trials particularly the EXCEL trial that compared percutaneous coronary intervention (PCI) with CABG for patients with left main coronary artery disease. The results of majority of them have indicated that in a large number of selected patients LMCAD, PCI can be a viable and an acceptable alternative to CABG. In EXCEL trial 2905 patients were screened and randomized 1095 to PCI with everolimus eluting stent (EES)or CABG. Patients had Syntax score of 32 or lower and significant obstruction of left main as measured by IVUS or FFR. The primary end point of composite of death from any cause, stroke or MI occurred in 15.4% in the PCI arm versus 14.7% in the CABG arm. The secondary outcome of death, stroke, MI at 30 days occurred in 4.9% patients in the PCI arm versus 7.9% in the CABG arm. The trials results perhaps could change the pattern of practice of performing CABG in as the only strategy of revascularization in each and every patient with LMCAD.

In a meta analysis of 4 randomized controlled trials involving 4394 patients with LMCAD there was similar risk of adverse events with PCI when compared to CABG in low to intermediate complexity coronary artery disease patients. Incidence of all cause death, myocardial infarction, or stroke over 5 years was noted in 18.3% patients with PCI and 16.9% in patients who were treated with CABG.

At least patients with low and intermediate SYNTAX score could be treated with PCI with acceptable risk.

Fig. 1. *Time to event curves for the primary compositeend point and its component*

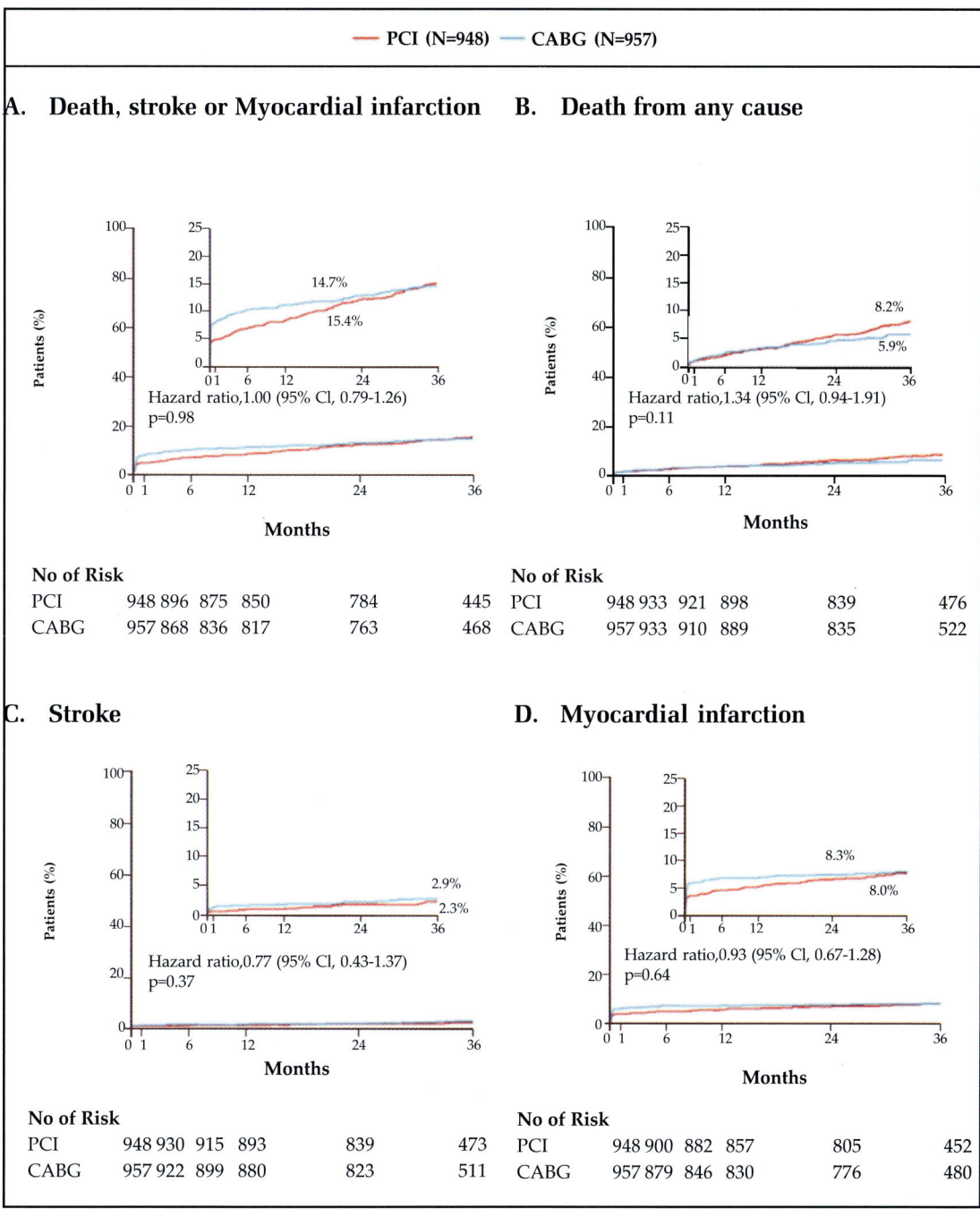

Suggested Readings

1. Percutaneous Coronary Intervention vs Coronary Artery Bypass Grafting in Patients With Left Main Coronary Artery Stenosis A Systematic Review and Meta-analysis.

2. Daniele Giacoppo, MD1; Roisin Colleran, MB, BCh1; Salvatore Cassese, MD, PhD1; et al.

3. JAMA Cardiol. 2017;2(10):1079-1088. doi:10.1001/jamacardio.2017.2895.

4. Everolimus Eluting Stents or Bypass Surgery for Left Main Coronary Artery Disease. G.W. Stone, J.F. Sabik, P.W. Serruys, C.A. Simonton, P. Généreux, J. Puskas, D.E. Kandzari, M.-C. Morice, N. Lembo, W.M. Brown III, D.P. Taggart, A. Banning, B. Merkely, F. Horkay, P.W. Boonstra, A.J. van Boven, I. Ungi, G. Bogáts, S. Mansour, N. Noiseux, M. Sabaté, J. Pomar, M. Hickey, A. Gershlick, P. Buszman, A. Bochenek, E. Schampaert, P. Pagé, O. Dressler, I. Kosmidou, R. Mehran, S.J. Pocock and A.P. Kappetein for the EXCEL Trial Investigators* NEJM 2016;375(23):2223-2235.

Noninvasive Cardiac Radiation for Ablation of Ventricular Tachycardia

Akshay Mehta

Cuculich PS et al from Washington University in Saint Louis recently reported the first series of noninvasive mapping combined with external radiation to reduce ventricular tachycardia burden in five patients.

Noninvasive mapping of cardiac arrhythmias with electrocardiographic imaging and noninvasive delivery of precise ablative radiation with stereotactic body radiation therapy (SBRT) were combined to perform catheter-free, electrophysiology-guided, noninvasive cardiac radioablation for ventricular tachycardia.

After the 6-week blanking period, there were four episodes of VT over the next 46 patient-months, representing a reduction of 99.9% from baseline and reduction in episodes of VT in all five patients. The mean left ventricular ejection fraction did not decrease with treatment. At 3 months, adjacent lung showed opacities consistent with inflammatory changes, which resolved by 1 year.

The successful procedure lasted only an average of 14 minutes, required no sedation, and resulted in no obvious complications.

If its success is replicated in larger number of patients, it would herald a new era in ablation treatment for arrhythmias, especially for those invasively-difficult-to-access myocardial scars.

Future studies will also throw light on the potential long-term effects of radiation including degree of collateral damage to the healthy tissue especially the arterial and conduction systems.

▌ Suggested Readings

1. Cuculich PS, Schill MR, Kashani R, et al. Noninvasive cardiac radiation for ablation of ventricular tachycardia. N Engl J Med 2017; 377:2325-2336.

2. Lehmann HI, Graeff C, Simoniello P, et al. Feasibility study on cardiac arrhythmia ablation using high-energy heavy ion beams. Sci Rep 2016; 6:38895.

Critical Journal Review

11

The Association between Alcohol Abuse and Cardiac Disease

Ref.: Isaac R. Whitman, Vratika Agarwal, Gregory Nah, Jonathan W. Dukes, Eric Vittinghoff, Thomas A. Dewland, Gregory M. Marcus. Journal of the American College of Cardiology 69:13-24 2017.

Key Point:

Alcohol abuse is associated with increased risk of atrial fibrillation, myocardial infarction and congestive heart failure

Dev Pahlajani

▌ Background:

Cardiovascular disease is the most prevalent threat to health and survival. Myocardial infarction (MI) and incident congestive heart failure (CHF) and atrial fibrillation (AF) are on the rise along with the aging population. Therefore, understanding modifiable risk factors for cardiovascular disease is very important. There are conflicting reports of the effect of alcohol on cardiovascular disease. According to some studies, moderate levels of alcohol consumption may help prevent incident MI and CHF. Some studies have demonstrated that low to moderate levels of alcohol consumption increase the incidence of AF. The cardiovascular effects of alcohol abuse are not well characterized because majority of epidemiological studies rely on self-reported alcohol consumption which can be faulty.

▌ Objectives:

This study aimed to investigate the associations between alcohol abuse and AF, MI and CHF.

▌ Methods:

The Healthcare Cost and Utilization Project database was used to collect information about all Californian residents ≥ 21 years of age who received ambulatory surgery, emergency, or inpatient medical care in between 2005 and 2009. The risk of an alcohol abuse diagnosis on incident AF, MI, and CHF was noted. All demographic data including age, sex, race, and income was recorded. Those with Hispanic ethnicity were treated as a distinct group. AF was not recorded if a patient had undergone cardiothoracic surgery as post-operative AF after cardiothoracic surgery may have a different underlying mechanism. A sensitivity analysis was performed using heart failure without systolic dysfunction alone. MI diagnoses were limited to acute MI. Comorbidities assumed to confuse or mediate the association among alcohol abuse and AF, MI, or CHF were recorded.

❚ Results:

14,727,591 patients were included in the final analysis. Out of these, 268,084 (1.8%) had alcohol abuse. Alcohol abuse was associated with an increased risk of incident AF (hazard ratio [HR]: 2.14; 95% confidence interval [CI]: 2.08 to 2.19; p < 0.0001), MI (HR: 1.45; 95% CI: 1.40 to 1.51; p < 0.0001), and CHF (HR: 2.34; 95% CI: 2.29 to 2.39; p < 0.0001). Patients with alcohol abuse had a > 2-fold higher risk of AF, (figure 1). Presence of alcohol abuse increased the risk of acute MI. Alcohol abuse was linked to a 3-fold higher risk of heart failure with preserved systolic function (adjusted HR: 3.2; 95% CI: 1.86 to 5.51). Individuals without conventional risk factors for cardiovascular disease exhibited an unreasonable enhanced risk of each outcome. The risk of alcohol abuse on each outcome was similar to other modifiable risk factors.

❚ Conclusions:

The findings suggested that alcohol abuse increased the risk of AF, MI and CHF to a similar degree as other well-established risk factors. People without traditional cardiovascular risk factors were extremely prone to cardiac diseases in the presence of alcohol abuse. Reduction in alcohol abuse might cause meaningful reductions of cardiovascular disease.

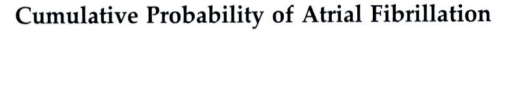

Fig. 1: *Cumulative Probability of Atrial Fibrillation Myocardial Infarction and Congestive Heart Failure by presence or absence of Alcohol Abuse*

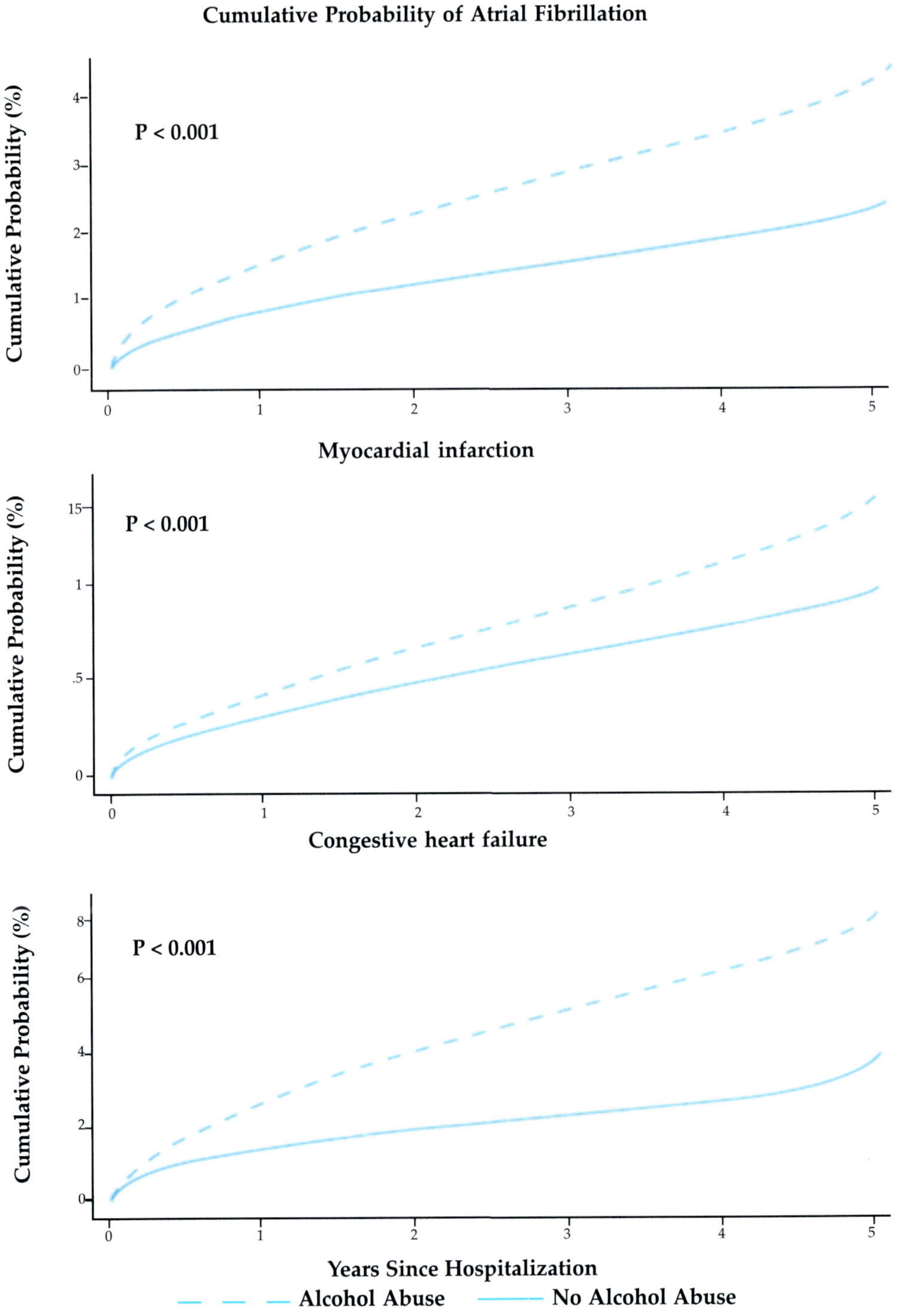

Cumulative Probability of Atrial Fibrillation

P < 0.001

Myocardial infarction

P < 0.001

Congestive heart failure

P < 0.001

Years Since Hospitalization

– – – Alcohol Abuse   ——— No Alcohol Abuse

Suggested Readings

1. Go AS, Mozaffarian D, Roger VL, et al. Heart disease and stroke statistics-2014 update: a report from the American Heart Association. Circulation 2014;129:e28-292.

2. World Health Organization. Non Communicable Diseases. Country Profiles. Geneva, Switzerland: WHO, 2014. Available at: http://www.who.int/nmh/publications/ncd-profiles-2014/en/. Accessed November 1, 2016.

3. Isaac R. Whitman et al. Alcohol Abuse and Cardiac Disease. J Am Coll Cardiol 2017;69:13-24.

4. Abramson JL, Williams SA, Krumholz HM, Vaccarino V. Moderate alcohol consumption and risk of heart failure among older persons. JAMA 2001;285:1971-7.

5. Bryson CL, Mukamal KJ, Mittleman MA, et al. The association of alcohol consumption and incident heart failure: the Cardiovascular Health Study. J Am Coll Cardiol 2006;48:305-11.

6. Djousse L, Gaziano JM. Alcohol consumption and risk of heart failure in the Physicians' Health Study I. Circulation 2007;115:34-9.

7. Djousse L, Gaziano JM. Alcohol consumption and heart failure: a systematic review. Curr Atherscler Rep 2008;10:117-20.

8. Camargo CA Jr., Stampfer MJ, Glynn RJ, et al. Moderate alcohol consumption and risk for angina pectoris or myocardial infarction in U.S. male physicians. Ann Intern Med 1997;126:372-5.

9. Maclure M. Demonstration of deductive metaanalysis: ethanol intake and risk of myocardial infarction. Epidemiol Rev 1993;15:328-51.

10. Yano K, Rhoads GG, Kagan A. Coffee, alcohol and risk of coronary heart disease among Japanese men living in Hawaii. N Engl J Med 1977;297: 405-9.

11. Mukamal KJ, Chung H, Jenny NS, et al. Alcohol consumption and risk of coronary heart disease in older adults: the Cardiovascular Health Study. J Am Geriatr Soc 2006;54:30-7.

12. Tavani A, Bertuzzi M, Negri E, Sorbara L, La Vecchia C. Alcohol, smoking, coffee and risk of non-fatal acute myocardial infarction in Italy. Eur J Epidemiol 2001;17:1131-7.

13. Conen D, Tedrow UB, Cook NR, et al. Alcohol consumption and risk of incident atrial fibrillation in women. JAMA 2008;300:2489-96.

14. Kodama S, Saito K, Tanaka S, et al. Alcohol consumption and risk of atrial fibrillation: a meta analysis. J Am Coll Cardiol 2011;57:427-36.

15. Larsson SC, Drca N, Wolk A. Alcohol consumption and risk of atrial fibrillation: a prospective study and dose-response meta-analysis. J Am Coll Cardiol 2014;64:281-9.

Troponin Concentration Change at 1 year is Associated with Future Coronary Risk Independent of Cholesterol Lowering

High-Sensitivity Cardiac Troponin, Statin Therapy, and Risk of Coronary Heart Disease.

Ref.: Ford I, Shah AS, Zhang R, McAllister DA, Strachan FE, Caslake M, Newby DE, Packard CJ, Mills NL. Journal of the American College of Cardiology. 2016;68(25):2719-2728. doi:10.1016/j.jacc.2016.10.020.

Akshay Mehta

▮ Study Objectives:

Long term studies have established the significance of benefits of intervention in asymptomatic high-risk subjects but debate over the merits of drug therapy in the wider primary prevention setting, still continues. A study of biomarkers that enhance the risk predication may be the answer to this controversy. Cardiac troponin is a specific marker of myocardial injury and an independent predictor of cardiovascular mortality in asymptomatic individuals with possible cardiovascular disease (CVD). Higher troponin concentrations may reflect subclinical coronary artery disease and identify those at greatest risk who could benefit from targeted preventive therapies. The present study determined whether cardiac troponin I concentrations could predict future coronary events, be modified by statins, and assess response to therapy in WOSCOPS.

▮ Protocol of the Study:

West of Scotland Coronary Prevention Study (WOSCOPS) was a randomized primary prevention trial involving men aged 45-64 yr with raised plasma cholesterol levels.

- Total no. of patients: 6595
- No. of participants identified for this analysis: 3318/6595 with sufficient stored plasma before randomization and at 1 year

Primary Outcome: a composite of nonfatal myocardial infarction (including non-hospitalized silent myocardial infarction) and death from coronary heart disease.

Participants who had a coronary event before the 1-year visit were excluded for the purpose of this analysis.

▮ Results:

The median troponin concentration at baseline was 4.0 ng/l (IQR: 3.1 to 5.2 ng/l).

Primary Outcome:

a. Baseline troponin and CVD risk:

Higher troponin concentrations at baseline were associated with increased risk of CHD at both 5- and 15-year follow-up.

5 year: Lowest quarter (≤ 3.1 ng/l), vs. highest quarter (≥ 5.2 ng/l) of troponin
Hazard ratio: 2.27; 95% confidence interval: 1.42 to 3.65; $p < 0.001$

15 year: Lowest quarter (≤ 3.1 ng/l), vs. highest quarter (≥ 5.2 ng/l) of troponin
Hazard ratio: 1.54; 95% confidence interval: 1.16 to 2.05; $p < 0.001$

All-cause mortality and cardiovascular death was also associated with baseline troponin concentration ($p < 0.001$), but non-cardiovascular death was not ($p = 0.890$).

b. 1-year reduction in troponin:

The absolute change in troponin concentration from baseline with pravastatin was 2.0 ng/l (IQR: 1.2 to 2.8 ng/l; $p < 0.001$). Change in troponin concentration on treatment correlated weakly with change in LDL cholesterol ($r = 0.20$; $p < 0.001$).

c. Change in troponin and CVD risk:

After adjustment for baseline troponin concentration, and baseline and change in LDL cholesterol; change in troponin concentration at 1 year was an independent predictor of nonfatal myocardial infarction or death from coronary heart disease at both 5 and 15 years in both treatment arms.

▌ Conclusions:

There was a strong, specific, and independent association between baseline and 1-year change in plasma troponin I concentration and the onset of coronary heart disease over 5 and 15 years in WOSCOPS trial. Cardiac troponin I was found to be an independent predictor of CHD events in middle-aged hypercholesterolemic men without prior myocardial infarction. Statin therapy reduces the troponin concentrations, and these reductions are associated with better outcomes independent of LDL cholesterol lowering.

▌ Review:

The study evaluated plasma troponin concentration in a primary prevention setting rather than in populations that included patients with established coronary heart disease and suggested that high-sensitivity cardiac troponin has major potential to identify those at greatest risk. It also proposed that cardiac troponin can assess the response to interventions that were used for the prevention of coronary heart disease. The study also showed that troponin predicted fatal and nonfatal myocardial infarction rather than heart failure events. There is a nonlinear association between troponin and coronary heart disease risk, with an apparent threshold at 5.2 ng/l; identifying those 2 to 3 times more likely to have a coronary event over 15 years. Therefore cardiac troponin may help to better stratify those healthy individuals at risk for CHD who would benefit most from statin therapies.

The study limitations were mainly confined to the parent trial. It recruited middle-aged men with raised cholesterol levels, and therefore the findings cannot be generalised to the wider population including women.

∎ Clinical Relevance:

A biomarker that can dynamically track the risk of CHD over time would be a major step forward in management of this fatal disease. Serial high-sensitivity troponin concentrations may represent a new paradigm in the assessment of the efficacy and safety of novel cardiovascular and non-cardiovascular therapies.

∎ Suggested Readings

1. Ford I, Murray H, Packard CJ, Shepherd J, Macfarlane PW, Cobbe SM. Long-term follow-up of the West of Scotland Coronary Prevention Study. N Engl J Med 2007;357:1477-86.

2. Pencina MJ, Navar-Boggan AM, D'Agostino RB Sr., et al. Application of new cholesterol guidelines to a population-based sample. N Engl J Med 2014;370: 1422-31.

3. Omland T, de Lemos JA, Sabatine MS, et al. A sensitive cardiac troponin T assay in stable coronary artery disease. N Engl J Med 2009;361: 2538-47.

4. de Lemos JA, Drazner MH, Omland T, et al. Association of troponin T detected with a highly sensitive assay and cardiac structure and mortality risk in the general population. JAMA 2010;304:2503-12.

5. Zeller T, Tunstall-Pedoe H, Saarela O, et al. High population prevalence of cardiac troponin I measured by a high-sensitivity assay and cardiovascular risk estimation: the MORGAM Biomarker Project Scottish Cohort. Eur Heart J 2014;35:271-81.

13

Timing of Coronary Invasive strategy in Non-ST-Segment elevation acute coronary syndrome and clinical outcomes

Ref.: Laurent Bonello, MD, PHD,a,b,c Marc Laine, MD,a,c Etienne Puymirat, MD, PHD,d,e Gilles Lemesle, MD, PHD,f Franck Thuny, MD, PHD,a,c Franck Paganelli, MD,a Pierre Michelet, MD, PHD,c,g Antoine Roch, MD, PHD,c,h François Kerbaul, MD, PHD,c,i Laurent Boyer, MD, PHD.
JACC: Cardiovascular Interventions 2016; 9:2267-276.

Key Point:
Early invasive treatment is not associated with decreased risk of death or myocardial infarction when compared with delayed strategy.
However there is reduced risk of recurrent ischemia and duration of hospital stay.

Dev Pahlajani

▌ Study Objectives:

To compare the benefits of early versus delayed invasive strategy in patients with non-ST-segment elevation acute coronary syndrome (NSTEMI-ACS).

▌ Protocol:

The current study is a meta-analysis of 10 randomized control trials (RCT). There were 6397 patients enrolled in these RCTs. Out of 6397 patients 3313 were randomized to early and 3084 to delayed invasive strategy. The primary end point was mortality rate, myocardial infarction (MI), reduction in recurrent ischemia, refractory angina and length of hospital stay.

▌ Results:

The median time between randomization and angiography in the early invasive treatment patients was 0.5-14 hours and 18.3-86 hours in delayed group. There was no significant difference in mortality between the two strategies (4% versus 4.7% OR 0.85). The rate of MI was 6.7% in early invasive versus 7.7% in delayed invasive (p=0.62) (Fig. 1,2). However, the risk of recurrent ischemia or refractory angina was lower in patients with early invasive versus delayed (3.8% versus 5.8% p = < 0.01). The median hospital stay in early invasive was 112 hours whereas it was 168 hours in delayed invasive. The rate of major bleeding was similar in both the groups (Ref Fig).

▌ Conclusion:

Thus the meta-analysis indicates that there is no significant difference in the hard end points of MI with early versus delayed invasive treatment except that the duration of hospital stay and recurrent ischemia, refractory angina is lower with early invasive strategy.

▊ Reviewer's Comments:

Several studies in the past have shown the benefit of invasive strategy as compared to conservative strategy in managing patients with ACS. However, it has been a matter of debate how soon after admission to hospital one should perform coronary angiography coronary intervention. Initial treatment with antiplatelet drugs like aspirin, P2Y12 inhibitors or GP2B3A inhibitors along with statins have been shown to stabilize the plaques and the patient. Also in patients with ACS there are plaques which may be unstable but not culprit. Initial treatment during first few hours with medical treatment would stablize these plaques. If clinical and hemodynamic state of the patient permits, delayed intervention could offer better outcomes. It could also make the procedure safer. European guidelines recommend early invasive strategy immediately after admission in those patients who sustained cardiac arrest or very high risk patients with GRACE score of more than 140. Early invasive is defined as performing coronary angiography within < 24 hours after admission to the hospital. Some of the earlier RCTs have shown benefit of early invasive only in reducing the number of hospitalization days and recurrent ischemia. However, there has been no impact on the death and MI. In a meta-analysis that enrolled 5370 patients from RCTs and 77499 from 4 observational studies, performing early coronary angiography within < 24 hours of admission did not provide any statistically significant benefit in death and MI. However the number of hospital days and recurrence ischemia was lower in early invasive group.

▊ Clinical Relevance:

Results of the current meta-analysis suggest that performing coronary angiography immediately after admission is not indicated in all patients with NSTEMI-MI except those with very high risk score. Stablizing the patient with antiplatelet drugs for several hours before taking them to the cath lab is associated with similar death and MI rates.

Fig. 1: *Individual and summery odds ratio for mortality trials comparing early and delayed invasive strategies*

Study name	Events / total		Statistics for each study					Odds ratio and 95% CI
	Early stretegy	Delayed stretegy	Odds ratio	Lower limit	Upper limit	p-value	Relative weight	
ISAR-Cool	0/203	3/207	0.14	0.01	2.80	0.20	0.7	
ELISA	3/109	5/111	0.60	0.14	2.57	0.40	2.8	
TMACS	76//1593	85/1433	0.80	0.53	1.10	0.16	58.7	
ABOARD	5/175	2/177	2.57	0.49	13.45	0.26	2.2	
OPTIMA	1/73	0/69	2.88	0.12	71.80	0.52	0.6	
Zhang et al, 2010	16/446	12/369	1.11	0.52	2.37	0.79	10.2	
LPSIA-NSTEM	9/200	12/200	0.74	0.30	1.79	0.50	7.5	
ELISA 3	3/269	3/265	0.98	0.20	4.92	0.99	2.3	
SSCA	13/83	14/86	0.96	0.42	2.18	0.91	8.8	
RDDLE-NSTEM	8/162	9/161	0.88	0.33	2.33	0.79	6.2	
			0.85	0.67	1.09	0.20		

0.01 0.1 1 10 100

Favors early   Favors delayed

Fig. 2: *Individual and summery odds ratio for myocardial infarction in randomized trials comparing early and delayed invasive strategies*

Study name	Events / total		Statistics for each study					Odds ratio and 95% CI
	Early stretegy	Delayed stretegy	Odds ratio	Lower limit	Upper limit	p-value	Relative weight	
ISAR-Cool	12/203	21/207	0.56	0.27	1.16	0.12	11.3	
ELISA	7/109	6/111	1.20	0.39	3.70	0.75	8.5	
TMACS	76//1593	82/1433	0.83	0.60	1.14	0.25	14.0	
ABOARD	16/175	8/177	2.13	0.89	5.10	0.09	10.2	
OPTIMA	44/73	27/69	2.36	1.20	4.60	0.01	11.7	
Zhang et al, 2010	23/446	40/369	0.45	0.26	0.76	0.00	12.7	
LPSIA-NSTEM	33/200	20/200	1.78	0.98	3.22	0.06	12.3	
ELISA 3	5/269	2/265	2.49	0.48	12.95	0.28	5.7	
SSCA	1/83	10/86	0.09	0.01	0.74	0.02	4.2	
RDDLE-NSTEM	5/162	22/161	0.20	0.07	0.55	0.00	9.4	
			0.88	0.53	1.45	0.62		

Favors early   Favors delayed

Fig. 3: *Individual and summery odds ratio for recurrent ischemia or refractory angina randomized trials comparing early and delayed invasive strategies*

Study name	Events / total		Statistics for each study					Odds ratio and 95% CI
	Early stretegy	Delayed stretegy	Odds ratio	Lower limit	Upper limit	p-value	Relative weight	
ISAR-Cool	27/203	39/207	0.66	0.39	1.13	0.13	20.0	
ELISA	13/109	14/111	0.94	0.42	2.10	0.88	11.2	
TMACS	16//1593	14/1433	0.30	0.17	0.53	0.00	18.3	
ABOARD	21/175	33/177	0.60	0.33	1.08	0.09	17.5	
LPSIA-NSTEM	0/200	13/200	0.01	0.00	3.64	0.12	0.2	
ELISA 3	20/269	33/265	0.56	0.32	1.01	0.05	17.8	
RDDLE-NSTEM	16/162	27/161	0.54	0.28	1.05	0.07	15.0	
			0.55	0.40	0.74	0.00		

Favors early   Favors delayed

CI = confidence interval; other abbreviation as in **Table 1.**

▌ Suggested Readings

1. 2015 ESC guidelines for the management of acute coronary syndromes in patients presenting without persistent ST-segment elevation: Task Force for the Management of Acute Coronary Syndromes in Patients Presenting Without Persistent ST-Segment Elevation of the European Society of Cardiology (ESC). Eur Heart J 2016;37:267-315.

2. O'Donoghue M, Boden WE, Braunwald E, et al. Early invasive vs conservative treatment strategies in women and men with unstable angina and non-ST-segment elevation myocardial infarction: a meta-analysis. JAMA 2008;300:71-80.

3. Navarese EP, Gurbel PA, Andreotti F, et al. Optimal timing of coronary invasive strategy in non-ST-segment elevation acute coronary syndromes: a systematic review and meta-analysis. Ann Intern Med 2013;158:261-70.

4. Riezebos RK, Ronner E, Ter Bals E, et al., OPTIMA trial. Immediate versus deferred coronary angioplasty in non-ST-segment elevation acute coronary syndromes. Heart 2009;95:807-12.

5. Milosevic A, Vasiljevic-Pokrajcic Z, Milasinovic D, et al. Immediate versus delayed invasive intervention for non-ST-segment elevation myocardial infarction patients: the RIDDLE-NSTEMI study (Randomized Study of Immediate Versus Delayed.

6. Invasive Intervention in Patients With Non-ST-Segment Elevation Myocardial Infarction). J Am Coll Cardiol Intv 2016;9:541-9.

7. Neumann FJ, Kastrati A, Pogatsa-Murray G, et al. Evaluation of prolonged antithrombotic pretreatment ("cooling-off" strategy) before intervention in patients with unstable coronary syndromes: a randomized controlled trial. JAMA 2003;290:1593-9.

8. Montalescot G, Cayla G, Collet JP, et al., for the ABOARD Investigators. Immediate vs delayed intervention for acute coronary syndromes: a randomized clinical trial. JAMA 2009;302:947-54.

9. Higgins JP, Altman DG, Gøtzsche PC, et al. The Cochrane Collaboration's tool for assessing risk of bias in randomized trials. BMJ 2011;343:5928.

10. Wan X, Wan W, Liu J, et al. Estimating the sample mean and standard deviation from the sample size, median range and/or interquartile range. BMC Med Res Methodol 2014;14:135.

11. Der Simonian R, Laird N. Meta-analysis in clinical trials. Control Clin Trials 1986;7:177-88.

14

Death in Atrial Fibrillation Patients: Known and Unknown Culprits

Causes of Death in Anticoagulated Patients with Atrial Fibrillation

Ref.: Gómez-Outes A, Lagunar-Ruíz J, Terleira-Fernández AI, Calvo-Rojas G, Suárez-Gea ML, Vargas-Castrillón E

J Am Coll Cardiol. 2016 Dec 13;68(23):2508-2521. doi: 10.1016/j.jacc.2016.09.944.

Akshay Mehta

Atrial fibrillation (AF) is the commonest arrhythmia globally and is associated with an increased mortality rate. Oral anticoagulation reduces the risk of mortality in these patients however other causes of death also need to be investigated so that newer strategies can be developed to combat these. In the present study, the authors analyzed and compared causes of death in patients receiving direct oral anticoagulants (DOAC) or warfarin for prevention of stroke and systemic embolism (SE) in AF.

▋ Protocol of the Study:

Data from randomized controlled trials of the DOACs for prophylaxis against stroke and systemic embolism (SE) in patients with AF was systematically reviewed and meta-analyzed.

- Total no. of patients: 71683 AF patients

- Period: Upto May 2016

- Databases: CENTRAL and MEDLINE

Data pooled from following trials:

- RE-LY [Randomized Evaluation of Long-Term Anticoagulation Therapy]

- ROCKET AF [An Efficacy and Safety Study of Rivaroxaban With Warfarin for the Prevention of Stroke and Non-Central Nervous System Systemic Embolism in Patients With Non-Valvular Atrial Fibrillation]

- ARISTOTLE [Apixaban for the Prevention of Stroke in Subjects With Atrial Fibrillation]

- ENGAGE AF-TIMI 48 [Effective Anticoagulation With Factor Xa Next Generation in Atrial Fibrillation-Thrombolysis In Myocardial Infarction 48]

▋ Primary Outcome:

All-cause death and adjudicated specific causes of death.

Results:

There was a predominance of men (range 60% to 65%) and permanent/persistent AF (range 67% to 83%).

Primary Outcome:

64% of all deaths were attributed to vascular causes, whereas 30% of deaths were of nonvascular cause, and 6% of deaths were due to unknown causes. The more frequent causes of death were cardiac death, in 46% of cases (28% sudden cardiac deaths/dysrhythmia, 15% heart failure, and 3% myocardial infarction), followed by malignancies (11%), infections (9%), ischemic stroke/SE (6%), and bleeding (6%).

Secondary Outcomes:

Average annual mortality rate by anticoagulant type:

- DOACs: 4.46%/year (95% CI: 3.85% to 5.12%/year)

- Warfarin: 4.87%/year (4.15% to 5.64%/year)

All-cause mortality difference between the 2 therapies: RR: 0.90; 95% CI: 0.86 to 0.95; favored DOACs.

Conclusions:

This meta-analysis concluded that about 46% deaths in AF patients are cardiac deaths (sudden cardiac death, heart failure, and myocardial infarction), whereas stroke and bleeding only account for approximately 6% of all deaths. DOACs prove to be beneficial however that is not the only remedy. An improvement in current management of comorbidities and associated risk factors is essential to reduce mortality rates in AF beyond anticoagulation.

Review:

This systematic review and meta-analysis indicates that the main cause of death in anticoagulated AF patient is heart-related mortality, including sudden cardiac death, heart failure, and myocardial infarction, whereas ischemic stroke and fatal bleedings only account for very minimal percentage. Heart failure, decreased creatinine clearance, diabetes, advanced age, and male sex were also found to be significantly associated with a higher risk of death. Therefore measures to decrease mortality should include: improvement in the management of relevant comorbidities, mainly heart failure, coronary artery disease, and diabetes, together with proven global CV risk-reduction measures and healthy lifestyle changes.

Other interesting findings included:

- A significant relative risk difference in favor of the DOACs in comparison with warfarin with respect to all-cause mortality

- Significant reduction in all-cause mortality with both the HD DOAC regimens (RR: 0.91; 95% CI: 0.86 to 0.96) and LD DOAC regimens (RR: 0.89; 95% CI: 0.83 to 0.96)

There are certain limitations to study:

- There was heterogeneity across trials in absolute death rates, which are likely due to differences in baseline characteristics.

- There were methodological differences across trials in the determination of cause-specific mortality by the adjudicating committees (e.g. particularly in the subclassification of cardiac deaths or deaths due to stroke or hemorrhage).

- As with other systemic reviews and meta-analyses, the patients represent the selected populations from clinical trials, and therefore, the extrapolation to general practice should be done cautiously.

Clinical Relevance:

Oral anticoagulation therapy is standard of care in AF patients and its importance in overall treatment as well as prevention of mortality has been proved frequently. However in spite of proper treatment protocol AF patients continue to remain at high risk of death. It is vital to determine the causes of death in this population so that appropriate measures can be initiated in a timely manner.

Suggested Readings

1. Fuster V, Rydén LE, Cannom DS, et al. 2011 ACCF/AHA/HRS focused updates incorporated into the ACC/AHA/ESC 2006 guidelines for the management of patients with atrial fibrillation: a report of the American College of Cardiology Foundation/American Heart Association Task Force on Practice Guidelines. J Am Coll Cardiol 2011;57:e101-98.

2. Hohnloser SH, Oldgren J, Yang S, et al. Myocardial ischemic events in patients with atrial fibrillation treated with dabigatran or warfarin in the RE-LY (Randomized Evaluation of Long-Term Anticoagulation Therapy) trial. Circulation 2012; 125:669-76.

3. Committee for Medicinal Products for Human Use (CHMP). Pradaxa (dabigatran). Assessment report No.: EMEA/H/C/000829/X/13/G. August 23, 2011. Available at: http://www.ema.europa.eu/ docs/en_GB/ document_library/EPAR_-_Assessment_Report_-_Variation/human/000829/WC500110875. PDF.

4. Patel MR, Mahaffey KW, Garg J, et al. Rivaroxaban versus warfarin in nonvalvular atrial fibrillation. N Engl J Med 2011;365:883-91.

5. Pokorney SD, Piccini JP, Stevens SR, et al. Cause of death and predictors of all-cause mortality in anticoagulated patients with nonvalvular atrial fibrillation: data from ROCKET AF. J Am Heart Assoc 2016;4:e002197.

6. Giugliano RP, Ruff CT, Wiviott SD, et al. Mortality in patients with atrial fibrillation randomized to edoxaban or warfarin: insights from the ENGAGE AF-TIMI 48 trial. Am J Med 2016;129:850-7.

15

Dual Antiplatelet Therapy Versus Aspirin Monotherapy in Diabetics with Multivessel Disease Undergoing CABG

Ref.: Sean van Diepen, Valentin Fuster, Subodh Verma, Taye H. Hamza, F. Sandra Siami, Shaun G. Goodman, Michael E. Farkouh

Journal of the American College of Cardiology 2017, 69 (2) 119-127.

Key Points:

There is frequent use of dual antiplatelet therapy (DAPT)among patients following coronary artery bypass surgery(CABG)

However DAPT does not offer any additional benefit as compared to aspirin monotherapy

Dev Pahlajani

■ Study Objectives:

Post-operative DAPT has been recommended widely as a means of secondary prevention in patients who undergo coronary artery CABG following acute coronary syndromes (ACS). However there are no specific recommendations for diabetic patients who undergo CABG; in spite of the fact that diabetics may be a unique high-risk subgroup. The present analysis compared the long-term clinical and bleeding outcomes associated with DAPT versus aspirin monotherapy in post-bypass diabetics with multi vessel coronary artery disease from the FREEDOM (Future Revascularization Evaluation in patients with Diabetes mellitus: Optimal management of Multivessel disease) trial.

■ Protocol of the Study:

FREEDOM trial was an international multicenter study that enrolled patients ≥ 18 years of age with diabetes mellitus (DM) and with ≥ 70% stenosis of 2 or more major epicardial vessels.

- Randomization Groups in FREEDOM trial: CABG or percutaneous coronary intervention (PCI) with drug eluting stents (DES)

- Total no. of patients in this analysis: 795 patients randomized to CABG group

- DAPT: 544 patients

- Aspirin alone: 251 patients

Primary Outcome: The primary outcome was the FREEDOM trial primary endpoint of 5-year all-cause mortality, nonfatal myocardial infarction (MI), or stroke. The primary analysis here compared 5-year outcomes in patients treated with DAPT versus aspirin alone at 30-days post-CABG.

Secondary Outcomes: Included the individual components of the composite outcomes: vascular death, MI and cardiovascular hospitalization (defined as unstable angina, MI, heart failure, chest pain, arrhythmia, peripheral vascular disease, or stroke or transient ischemic attack).

Results:

- Participants who received DAPT were more frequently to be younger, non-Caucasian and had surgery performed in North America, South America, India or Israel.

- Patients who received DAPT had lower median Euro SCORE, less frequently underwent right internal mammary artery grafting, had a higher mean number of bypass grafts, and more frequently underwent endoscopic vein harvesting.

Primary Outcome:

There were no significant differences in the 5-year primary composite outcome of all-cause death, MI, or stroke (12.5% vs. 16.0%; adjusted hazard ratio [HR]: 0.83; 95% confidence interval [CI]: 0.54 to 1.27; p = 0.39). Secondary outcomes also showed not significant differences in the measured outcomes (Ref Figure).

Values are n (%) unless otherwise indicated. *All unadjusted outcomes presented as valid n (event %). Because of 0 events in 1 or more covariate categories, some covariates were excluded from specific time to event analysis as follows: † adjusted for Euro SCORE, region of enrollment, number of grafts, right internal thoracic artery graft, endarterectomy, endoscopic vein harvesting, and PPI or beta-blocker use at 1 month; ‡ adjusted for Euro SCORE, number of grafts, right internal thoracic artery graft, endarterectomy, endoscopic vein harvesting, and PPI or beta-blocker use at 1-month visit; δ adjusted for Euro SCORE, number of grafts, right internal thoracic artery graft, endarterectomy, endoscopic vein harvesting, and PPI, NSAID, or beta-blocker use at 1-month visit; k adjusted for Euro SCORE, region of enrollment, number of grafts, right internal thoracic artery graft, endarterectomy, endoscopic vein harvesting, and NSAID or beta-blocker use at 1-month visit; adjusted for Euro SCORE, region of enrollment, number of grafts, endoscopic vein harvesting, and PPI or beta-blocker use at 1 month.

Safety Outcomes:

The 5-year safety outcomes of following safety variables between DAPT- and aspirin-treated patients was also same (Fig. 1)

- Major bleeding (5.6% vs. 5.7%; HR: 1.00; 95% CI: 0.50 to 1.99; p = 0.99),

- Blood transfusions (4.8% vs. 4.5%; HR: 1.09; 95% CI: 0.51 to 2.34; p = 0.82), and

- Bleeding hospitalizations (2.6% vs. 3.3%; HR: 0.80; 95% CI: 0.31 to 2.04; p = 0.64).

Conclusions:

This post-hoc secondary analysis of the FREEDOM trial demonstrated that use of DAPT in patients with diabetes post-CABG did not show any benefits as observed with all-cause mortality, MI, or stroke. Additionally, no differences in safety outcomes were observed. The rates of bleeding, clinical indication for revascularization, complexity of coronary artery disease, completeness of revascularization, or treatment duration remained similar in both the groups. Therefore the authors suggested that routine use of DAPT in this subgroup may not be clinically warranted.

Review:

This crucial analysis in the high risk diabetic patients demonstrated no significant differences in either the primary composite outcome (all-cause death, MI, or stroke) or bleeding outcomes were observed between aspirin- and DAPT-treated patients. These findings were also applicable in subgroup analysis were patients were analyzed by pre-operative acute coronary syndrome, SYNTAX score, complete revascularization, and duration of DAPT. However approximately two-thirds of patients received DAPT for a median duration of 1 year post-CABG. This may be due to the study protocol which provided participants with up to 1 year of thienopyridine drug coverage at the discretion of their treating physician regardless of study randomization.

There are certain limitations to study:

The study outcomes were derived from prescription rates at 30 days post-CABG; thus, clinical and bleeding outcomes associated with early post-operative use cannot be inferred from this analysis. This study was not conducted with newer antiplatelet agents (ticagrelor and prasugrel); thus, results cannot be extrapolated to these agents.

Clinical Relevance:

Guidelines recommend the use of DAPT in patients who undergo a CABG for an acute coronary syndrome. However this recommendation is based only on observational studies and have not yet been supported by any randomized trials. However as mentioned with newer antiplatelet agents in the market, this results may not hold good any more. Upcoming trials with use of clopidogrel, ticagrelor and prasugrel; will be more relevant in this case and hence the results from this analysis should remain confined to the two drugs used in the study.

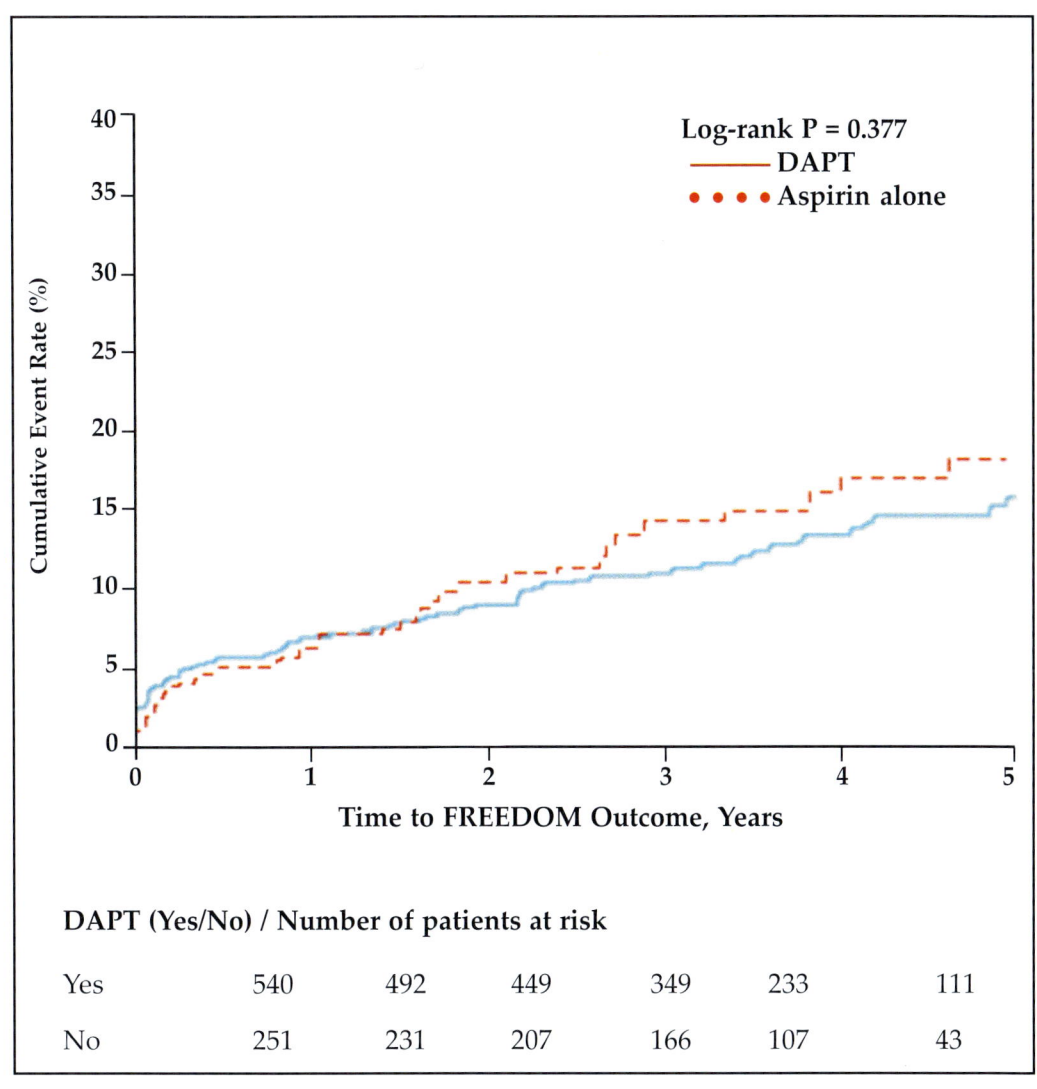

▌ Suggested Readings

1. Farkouh ME, Domanski M, Sleeper LA, et al. Strategies for multivessel revascularization in patients with diabetes. N Engl J Med 2012;367:2375-84.

2. Mohr FW, Morice MC, Kappetein AP, et al. Coronary artery bypass graft surgery versus percutaneous coronary intervention in patients with three-vessel disease and left main coronary disease: 5-year follow-up of the randomised, clinical SYNTAX trial. Lancet 2013;381:629-38.

3. Becker RC, Meade TW, Berger PB, et al. The primary and secondary prevention of coronary artery disease: American College of Chest Physicians Evidence-Based Clinical Practice Guidelines (8th edition). Chest 2008;133:776S-814S.

4. Dunning J, Versteegh M, Fabbri A, et al. Guideline on antiplatelet and anticoagulation management in cardiac surgery. Eur J Cardiothorac Surg 2008;34:73-92.

5. Farkouh ME, Dangas G, Leon MB, et al. Design of the Future Revascularization Evaluation in patients with Diabetes mellitus: optimal management of Multivessel disease (FREEDOM) Trial. Am Heart J 2008;155:215-23.

6. Kulik A, Ruel M, Jneid H, et al. Secondary prevention after coronary artery bypass graft surgery: a scientific statement from the American Heart Association. Circulation 2015;131:927-64.

7. Sun JC, Teoh KH, Lamy A, et al. Randomized trial of aspirin and clopidogrel versus aspirin alone for the prevention of coronary artery bypass graft occlusion: the Preoperative Aspirin and Postoperative Antiplatelets in Coronary Artery Bypass Grafting study. Am Heart J 2010;160:1178-84.

16

Adding Value to CAC Scoring

Improving the CAC Score by Addition of Regional Measures of Calcium Distribution. Multi-Ethnic Study of Atherosclerosis

Ref.: Michael J. Blaha, Matthew J. Budoff, Rajesh Tota-Maharaj, Zeina A. Dardari, Nathan D. Wong, Richard A. Kronmal, JohnEng, Wendy S. Post, Roger S. Blumenthal, Khurram Nasir
JACC: Cardiovascular Imaging Dec 2016, 9 (12) 1407-1416; DOI: 10.1016/j.jcmg.2016.03.001

Akshay Mehta

▮ Study Objectives:

To assess whether regional distribution of calcified plaques improves the ability of the traditional Agatston coronary artery calcium (CAC) score to predict cardiovascular events.

▮ Protocol of the Study:

Regional CAC distribution was studied in 3,262 individuals with baseline CAC > 0 from MESA (Multi-Ethnic Study of Atherosclerosis). Multivessel CAC was defined by the number of coronary vessels with CAC (scored 1 to 4, including the left main). The "diffusivity index" was calculated as: 1 - (CAC in most affected vessel/total CAC), and was used to group participants into concentrated and diffuse CAC patterns. Coronary heart disease (CHD) and cardiovascular disease (CVD) events were recorded to assess whether measures of regional CAC distribution add to the traditional Agatston CAC score.

▮ Results and Conclusions:

Addition of number of vessels with CAC significantly improved capacity to predict CHD and CVD events in survival analysis

▮ Comments:

The study shows that a simple addition of the number of vessels with CAC to the traditional Agatston score improves prediction of CHD and CVD events. This does not require re-measurement or a complicated calculation, and is available on all CAC scores that report CAC on a per-vessel basis. Also, it is more so when traditional CAC scores are in the intermediate range (1 to 300). Thus it gives increased discriminatory power in such patients for risk prediction.

This finding parallels the knowledge derived from studies which have shown that it is the total atherosclerosis burden, rather than the presence of obstructive coronary artery disease or inducible ischemia, that is the most important predictor of CVD events.

Another important information that can be derived from assessing regional distribution is the presence of higher risk plaque types. More diffuse the CAC, greater the number of with low attenuation plaques including a greater frequency of mixed plaque (higher risk) compared with fully calcified plaque.

▌ Clinical Application:

The usual CAC score does not delineate the regional distribution of calcified plaque. This measure of diffuseness of CAD adds to the traditional Agatston CAC score for the prediction of CHD and CVD events, and may be incorporated into routine reporting, particularly when CAC burden is intermediate. It may serve as one more arrow in our arsenal directed towards risk prediction.

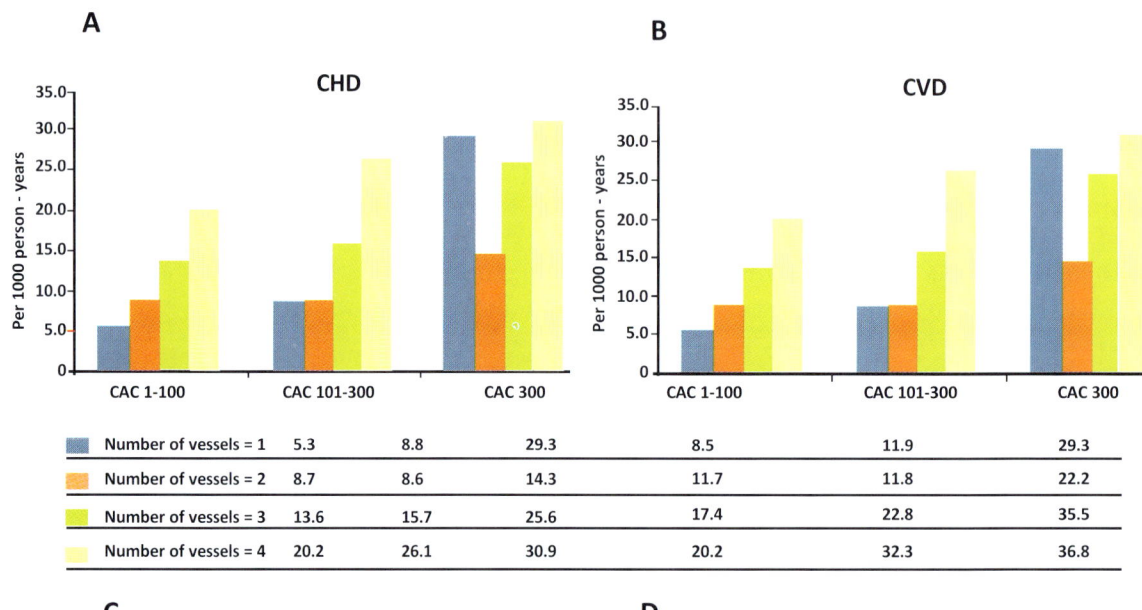

A — CHD	CAC 1-100	CAC 101-300	CAC 300	B — CVD	CAC 1-100	CAC 101-300	CAC 300
Number of vessels = 1	5.3	8.8	29.3		8.5	11.9	29.3
Number of vessels = 2	8.7	8.6	14.3		11.7	11.8	22.2
Number of vessels = 3	13.6	15.7	25.6		17.4	22.8	35.5
Number of vessels = 4	20.2	26.1	30.9		20.2	32.3	36.8

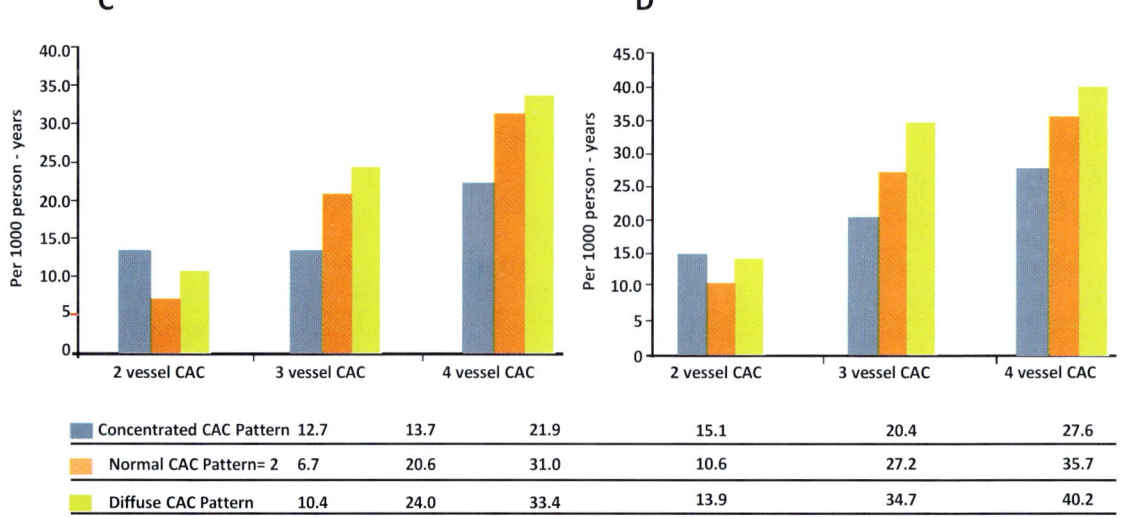

C	2 vessel CAC	3 vessel CAC	4 vessel CAC	D	2 vessel CAC	3 vessel CAC	4 vessel CAC
Concentrated CAC Pattern	12.7	13.7	21.9		15.1	20.4	27.6
Normal CAC Pattern= 2	6.7	20.6	31.0		10.6	27.2	35.7
Diffuse CAC Pattern	10.4	24.0	33.4		13.9	34.7	40.2

17

2-Year outcomes of High Bleeding Risk Patients after Polymer-Free Drug-Coated Stents

Ref.: Garot P, Morice MC, Tresukosol D, Pocock SJ, Meredith IT, Abizaid A, Carrié D, Naber C, Iñiguez A, Talwar S, Menown IB, Christiansen EH, Gregson J, Copt S, Hovasse T, Lurz P, Maillard L, Krackhardt F, Ong P, Byrne J, Redwood S, Windhövel U, Greene S, Stoll HP, Urban P; LEADERS FREE Investigators. J Am Coll Cardiol. 2017:17;69(2):162-171.

Key Points:

1. In high bleeding risk patients polymer free Biolimus A9 coated stent (DCS) maintained its superiority over bare metal stent (BMS) in primary safety end points over 2 years.
2. Lesser number of patients had cardiac events in the DCS group.
3. Bleeding risk and stent thrombosis was similar in both arms.
4. Clinically drive target vessel revascularization was .... in DC ....

Dev Pahlajani

▌ Study Objectives:

Percutaneous coronary intervention (PCI) in patients with high bleeding risk (HBR) poses several challenges which include the choice of stent and the antithrombotic management. Since it is evident that such patients receive only a short course of dual antiplatelet treatment (DAPT); a bare-metal stent (BMS) is often preferred to a drug-eluting stent (DES) for HBR patients. A prospective randomized trial compared the biofreedom biolimus A9 drug coated stent to the gazelle bare metal stent in patients with high risk of bleeding (LEADERS FREE). The trial demonstrated that during 1-year follow-up a combination of 1-month DAPT course and a polymer-free metallic drug-coated stent (DCS) was both safer and more effective than a BMS for HBR patients. The present literature evaluated the balance of the 2-year risks and the baseline and procedure correlates of the primary safety endpoint and of major bleeding events.

▌ Protocol of the Study:

Eligible patients of LEADERS FREE trial who received the BioFreedom polymer-free biolimus A9 coated stent or the control Gazelle BMS (Biosensors Europe, Morges, Switzerland; and Biosensors Interventional Technologies) were included in the analysis.

- Total no. of patients: 2,386 (98.1%) patients of 2432 were followed up to 730 days
- No. of DCS patients: 1,211
- No. of BMS patients: 1,221

Primary Safety Endpoint: Cumulative incidence of a composite of cardiac death, myocardial infarction, or definite or probable stent thrombosis.

Primary Efficacy Endpoint: The incidence of clinically driven target lesion revascularization.

Secondary Endpoints:

- All-cause and cardiac mortality, bleeding (Bleeding Academic Research Consortium [BARC] definitions)
- Myocardial infarction (third universal definition)
- Stent thrombosis (Academic Research Consortium definitions)
- Types of coronary revascularization

Results: (Fig A and B)

Primary Safety Outcome:

The primary safety outcomes (Cumulative incidence of a composite of cardiac death, myocardial infarction, or definite or probable stent thrombosis) in BMS patients = 15.3%.

The primary safety outcomes (Cumulative incidence of a composite of cardiac death, myocardial infarction, or definite or probable stent thrombosis) in DCS patients = 12.6%.

Hazard ratio [HR]: 0.80; 95% confidence interval [CI]: 0.64 to 0.99; p = 0.039.

Primary Safety Outcome:

Target lesion revascularizations - 6.8% of DCS and 12.0% of BMS patients at 2 years (HR: 0.54; 95% CI: 0.41 to 0.72; p < 0.0001)

Secondary Outcomes:

- All-cause mortality (13.1% vs. 13.8%; HR: 0.94; 95% CI: 0.75 to 1.17; p = 0.57)
- Cardiac mortality (6.6% vs. 6.9%; HR: 0.94; 95% CI: 0.69 to 1.28; p = 0.69)

Conclusions:

For HBR patients receiving a 1-month course of DAPT the risks of major bleeding and of a composite of cardiac death, myocardial infarction, or stent thrombosis were high and therefore these patients need careful evaluation of both their thrombotic and bleeding risks. The LEADERS FREE trial demonstrated, for both efficacy and safety, the sustained superiority of the Bio Freedom polymer-free biolimus A9-coated stent (DCS) compared with a similar BMS in the 2-year follow-up. There was no "catch-up" of target lesion revascularization was observed beyond 1 year in patients that had DCS.

Review:

Major bleeds in high-risk patients such as intracranial hemorrhage, gastrointestinal bleeding, and retroperitoneal bleeding, has been associated with long-term mortality. This leads to an important question of the optimal duration of DAPT in such cases. In absence of optimal antithrombotic treatment, early stent thrombosis can lead to fatal consequences. With respect to the patients at high risk of bleeding, current American College of Cardiology/American Heart Association guidelines state "In patients with ACS treated with DAPT after DES implantation who develop a high risk of bleeding (e.g., treatment with oral anticoagulant therapy), are at high risk of severe bleeding complication (e.g., major intracranial surgery), or develop significant overt bleeding, discontinuation of P2Y12 inhibitor therapy after 6 months may be reasonable". In managing these patients, rather than going back to an older stent design and using a BMS, polymer-free metallic drug-coated stents such as that studied in the LEADERS FREE trial offer an alternative strategy. The absence of any polymer on the DCS may contribute to its long-term safety despite the very short DAPT and compares favorably with stent thrombosis rates for polymercoated DES, especially in this high risk population.

These results however, cannot be applied to non-HBR patients who are likely to tolerate longer courses of DAPT. Therefore the choice of stent may also vary in these patients. The results also cannot be generalized to other DES or DCS with different drugs or slower elution kinetics.

▮ Clinical Relevance:

Intracoronary stents and anticoagulant and antiplatelet therapy have coevolved to simultaneously minimize the risk of the 2 competing and opposing evolutionary driving forces: thrombosis and bleeding. The overall clinical outcome in HBR patients undergoing PCI depends on balancing the risk of bleeding and thrombosis. The persistently high incidence of both bleeding and coronary thrombotic events in HBR patients needs wider recognition and deserves our full attention in future trials of antithrombotic therapy.

Fig. 1: *Landmark analysis at 1 year for the primary safety and primary efficacy endpoints*

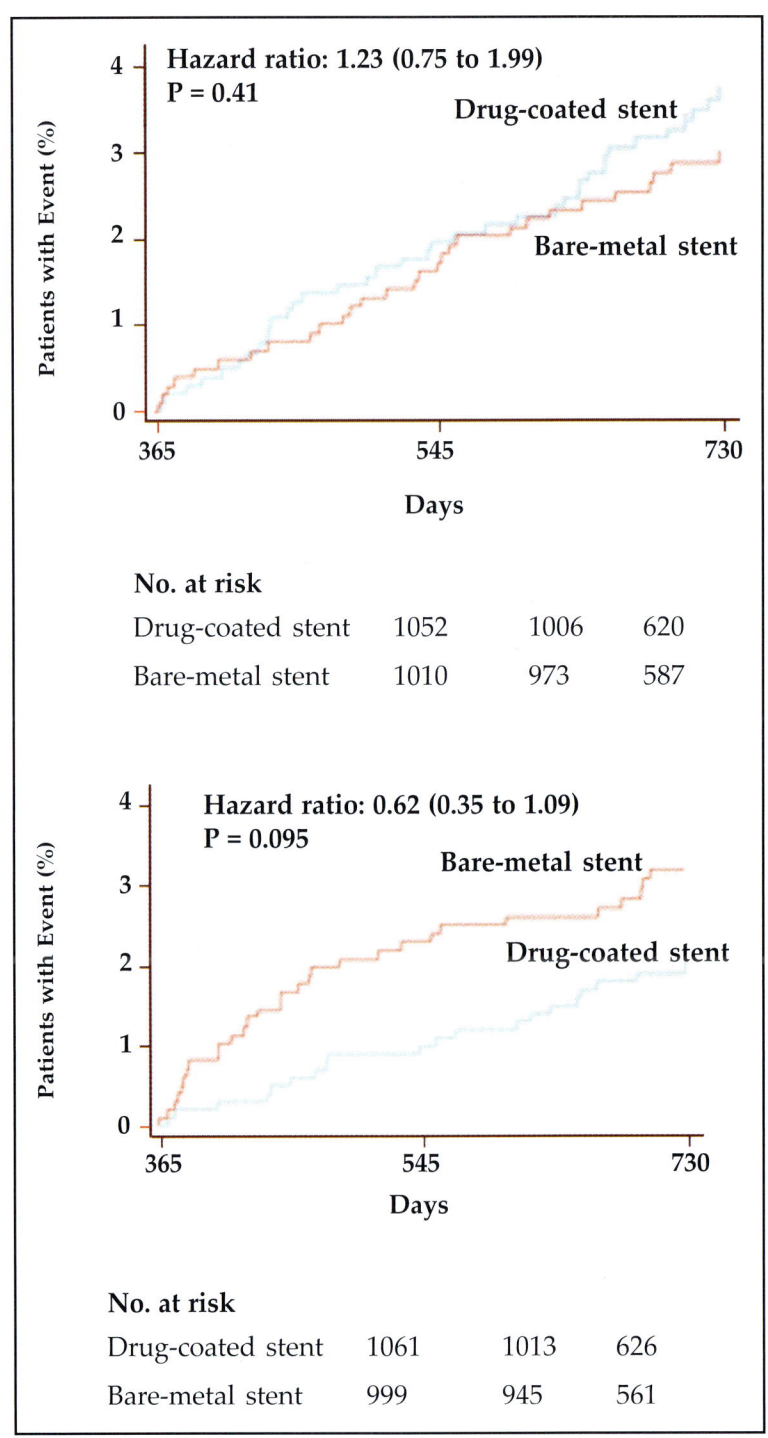

∎ Suggested Readings

1. Urban P, Meredith IT, Abizaid A, et al., for the LEADERS FREE Investigators. Polymer-free drug coated coronary stents in patients at high bleeding risk. N Engl J Med 2015;373:2038-47.

2. Ariotti S, Adamo M, Costa F, et al., for the ZEUS Investigators. Is bare-metal stent implantation still justifiable in high bleeding risk patients undergoing percutaneous coronary intervention? A pre-specified analysis from the ZEUS trial. J Am Coll Cardiol Intv 2016;9:426-36.

3. Levine GN, Bates ER, Bittl JA, et al. 2016 ACC/AHA guideline focused update on duration of dual antiplatelet therapy in patients with coronary artery disease: a report of the American College of Cardiology/American Heart Association Task Force on Clinical Practice Guidelines. J Am Coll Cardiol 2016;68:1082-115.

4. Urban P, Abizaid A, Chevalier B, et al. Rationale and design of the LEADERS FREE trial: a randomized double-blind comparison of the Bio-Freedom drug-coated stent vs the Gazelle bare metal stent in patients at high bleeding risk using a short (1 month) course of dual antiplatelet therapy. Am Heart J 2013;165:704-9.

5. Sen H, Lam MK, Löwik MM, et al. Clinical events and patient-reported chest pain in all-comers treated with Resolute integrity and Promus element stents: 2-year follow-up of the DUTCH PEERS (Durable Polymer-Based Stent Challenge of Promus ElemEnt Versus ReSolute Integrity) Randomized Trial (TWENTE II). J Am Coll Cardiol Intv 2015;8:889-99.

6. Stefanini GG, Byrne RA, Serruys PW, et al. Biodegradable polymer drug-eluting stents reduce the risk of stent thrombosis at 4 years in patients undergoing percutaneous coronary intervention: a pooled analysis of individual patient data from the ISAR-TEST 3, ISAR-TEST 4, and LEADERS randomized trials. Eur Heart J 2012;33: 1.

18

"When You Encounter Ectasia in Primary PCI"

Risk factors and outcomes in patients with Ectatic Infarct-Related Artery who underwent Primary Percutaneous Coronary Intervention after ST Elevation Myocardial Infarction

Ref.: Gokturk Ipek MD, Baris Gungor MD et al

Catheterization and Cardiovascular Interventions Volume 88, Issue 5. November 2016 Pages 748-753

Akshay Mehta

▮ Study Objectives:

Risk factors for coronary artery ectasia (CAE) as infarct-related artery (IRA) and their short-term and 1 year outcomes were retrospectively studied in 1655 patients with STEMI.

▮ Protocol of the Study:

Patients were divided into two groups according to their coronary anatomy as ectasia (99) and control groups (1556). Demographic features, angiographic results, and clinical events were compared. Multivariate analysis was performed to assess the association of the features with CAE in STEMI.

▮ Results and Conclusions:

The study showed an incidence of ectatic IRA of about 5% and that hypertension and smoking were independently associated with CAE as IRA among patients with STEMI. Also, despite there being higher no-reflow rates, short-term and 1 year survival in the CAE group were similar with the control group. Revascularization rates at 1 year also did not differ between the groups.

▮ Comments:

This is probably the first large study comparing interventional and clinical outcomes between ectatic IRA and a control group in a large cohort of STEMI patients. Prior studies have been either small or without a comparator arm. Guidelines too do not mention special recommendations about thrombus aspiration, deferred stenting and pharmacotherapy in patients with ectatic IRA-all of which may find a special place in such patients.

Indeed, in his editorial comments, Samuel M. Butman (1) advocates use of aspiration thrombectomy, venous access for bradycardia treatment if required, delivery of a vasodilator distally and avoiding post-dilatation, if possible.

It may be intriguing to know what the results of deferred stenting or plain balloon angioplasty could be in such IRA's. Unfortunately, use of this strategy in only 8 patients, though successful, in the study precludes any meaningful conclusions being drawn.

The study suffers from some limitations such as its retrospective design, lack of data about medication after discharge and during follow-up, the insufficient number of ectatic patients to determine accurate statistical associations between risk factors and ectatic IRA and under-representation of female gender in the study.

Yet, the study is reassuring about the short and long term outcomes in such patients despite higher rates of no -reflow.

▌ Suggested Readings

1. Samuel M. Butman. The newly occluded ectatic vessel: Not an ecstatic time: Comment. Catheterization and Cardiovascular Interventions Volume 88, Issue 5. November 2016 (pages 753-754).

19

Culprit Vessel Versus Multi vessel Versus In-Hospital Staged Intervention for Patients with ST-Segment Elevation Myocardial Infarction and Multi vessel Disease. Stratified Analyses in High-Risk Patient Groups and Anatomic Subsets of Non Culprit Disease

Ref.: M. Bilal Iqbal, Imad J. Nadra, Lillian Ding, Anthony Fung, Eve Aymong, Albert W. Chan, Steven Hodge, Anthony Della Siega, Simon D. Robinson, British Columbia Cardiac Registry Investigators

JACC: Cardiovascular Interventions 2017:10 (1) 11-23.

Key Points:
In patients with ST Elevation Myocardial Infarction (STEMI) strategy of culprit vessel only or staged percutaneous coronary intervention (PCI) is associated with lower death rate and repeat revascularization as compared to multi vessel primary PCI.

Dev Pahlajani

▌ Study Objectives:

Approximately 60% patients with ST Elevation Myocardial Infarction (STEMI) have multi vessel coronary artery disease and is associated with poor prognosis. While there is unanimity that primary percutaneous coronary intervention (PCI) is the prefered form of treatment for STEMI there are continuing debates regarding performing culprit only or staged PCI. Several observational studies, registries and randomized control trials have provided conflicting results.

The current study includes 6503 STEMI patients with multi vessel disease who underwent primary PCI. The investigators compared the outcomes with 3 different PCI strategies during primary PCI.

1. Multi vessel intervention.

2. Culprit vessel intervention only.

3. Culprit vessel intervention with staged revascularization. The end points were all cause mortality and repeat revascularization at 2 years.

▌ Results:

Multivessel PCI was associated with higher adverse outcomes as compared to culprit only intervention (HR 0.78 p=0.023) as well as with culprit vessel intervention with staged PCI (HR 0.55 p=0.004).

The lowest mortality was in the patients with culprit vessel intervention at the time of primary PCI and staged PCI of the non-culprit vessel.

There was increased risk of repeat revascularization with culprit vessel only intervention as compared to culprit vessel intervention with staged PCI.

Culprit vessel intervention was associated with lower mortality in the presence of non-culprit left circumflex and right coronary artery disease.

However, when the non-culprit vessel was LAD the culprit vessel intervention and multi vessel intervention had similar results (Fig. & Table 1).

Conclusion:

The results of this study indicate that STEMI patients with multi vessel involvement have lower mortlity with culprit only and staged PCI as compared to multi vessel PCI during primary PCI. However in selected patients with LAD involvement as a non culprit vessel performing multi vessel PCI carry similar outcomes.

Reviewers Comments:

Current ACC/AHA guidelines recommend PCI of the culprit vessel only during STEMI, except in patients with cardiogenic shock. However, some of the recent trials like PRAMI or CvLPRIT have indicated that performing multi-vessel PCI during primary angioplasty could actually be associated with better outcomes. There are concerns that non culprit vessels may actually could be "culprit but non occlusive or non ruptured" that is waiting to rupture. This could lead to acute coronary syndrome while waiting for staged PCI. In the light of the current study it seems that larger randomized control trials will offer clear cut directions and guidelines.

Clinical Relevance:

Since results of the study confirm the recommendations of current guidelines it seems reasonable that patients with STEMI should undergo primary PCI of culprit vessel only and PCI of circumflex and or right coronary artery should be performed before discharge during index hospitalization. However multi vessel PCI in patients with non culprit LAD lesion could be an exception for performing multi vessel PCI.

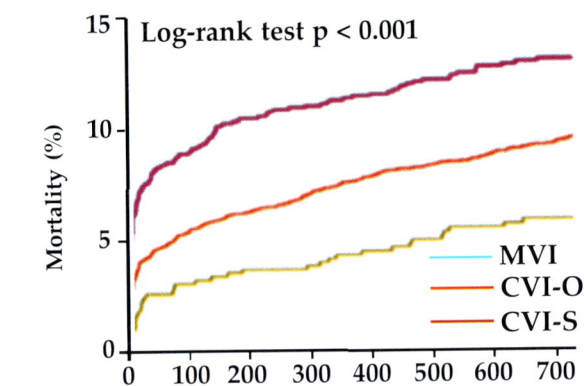

Number at risk

MVI	1325	1207	1187	1096	1011	946	869	819
CVI-O	4520	4274	4238	4018	3802	3600	3408	3201
CVI-S	658	635	634	608	576	552	518	490

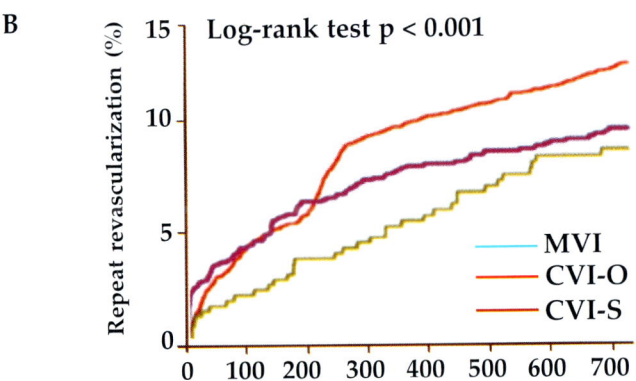

Number at risk

MVI	1325	1267	1240	1137	1044	971	802	833
CVI-O	4520	4323	4255	4022	3795	3594	3392	3160
CVI-S	658	428	421	403	379	362	333	314

Table 1: Unadjusted outcomes

	CVI-O	CVI-S	MVI	p Value		
				MVI vs. CVI-O	MVI vs. CVI-S	MVI vs. CVI-S
Mortality						
30 days	4.2	2.6	7.5	< 0.001	< 0.001	< 0.048
1-year	7.5	4.3	11.2	< 0.001	< 0.001	< 0.002
2-year	9.1	5.6	12.6	< 0.001	< 0.001	< 0.003
Repeat revascularization						
30-days	2.3	1.1	2.9	0.152	0.009	0.046
1-year	9.8	3.6	7.8	0.030	< 0.001	< 0.001
2-year	12.1	5.5	9.1	0.002	0.005	< 0.001

Values are %. All outcomes are compared the Z-test (2-tailed).
Abbreviation as in Table 1.

▊ Suggested Readings

1. Bagai A, Thavendiranathan P, Sharieff W, Al Lawati HA, Cheema AN. Non-infarct-related artery revascularization during primary percutaneous coronary intervention for ST-segment elevation myocardial infarction: a systematic review and meta-analysis. Am Heart J 2013;166:684-93.e681.

2. Bainey KR, Mehta SR, Lai T, Welsh RC. Complete vs culprit-only revascularization for patients with multivessel disease undergoing primary percutaneous coronary intervention for ST-segment elevation myocardial infarction: a systematic review and meta-analysis. Am Heart J 2014;167:1-14 e12.

3. Gershlick AH, Khan JN, Kelly DJ, et al. Randomized trial of complete versus lesion-only revascularization in patients undergoing primary percutaneous coronary intervention for STEMI and multivessel disease: the CVLPRIT trial. J Am Coll Cardiol 2015;65:963-72.

4. Wald DS, Morris JK, Wald NJ, et al. Randomized trial of preventive angioplasty in myocardial infarction. N Engl J Med 013;369:1115-23.

5. Engstrom T, Kelbaek H, Helqvist S, et al. Complete revascularisation versus treatment of the culprit lesion only in patients with st-segment elevation myocardial infarction and multivessel disease (danami-3-primulti): an open-label, randomised controlled trial. Lancet 2015;386:665-71.

6. Hanratty CG, Koyama Y, Rasmussen HH, Nelson GI, Hansen PS, Ward MR. Exaggeration of nonculprit stenosis severity during acute myocardial infarction: Implications for immediate multivessel revascularization. J Am Coll Cardiol 2002; 40:911-6.

7. Song YJ, Shin HC, Yang JI, et al. Preventive versus culprit-only percutaneous coronary intervention in ST-elevation myocardial infarction patients with multivessel disease: a meta-analysis. J Interv Cardiol 2015;28:1-13.

8. Iqbal MB, Ilsley C, Kabir T, et al. Culprit vessel versus multivessel intervention at the time of primary percutaneous coronary intervention in patients with ST-Segment-Elevation Myocardial Infarction and multivessel disease: Real-world analysis of 3984 patients in London. Circ Cardiovasc Qual Outcomes 2014;7:936-43.

20

Is the Stroke Risk same with All Patterns of Atrial Fibrillation? Stroke and Mortality Risk in Patients with Various Patterns of Atrial Fibrillation

Results From the ENGAGE AF-TIMI 48 Trial (Effective Anticoagulation with Factor Xa Next Generation in Atrial Fibrillation-Thrombolysis in Myocardial Infarction 48)

Ref.: Mark S. Link, Robert P. Giugliano, Christian T. Ruff, Benjamin M. Scirica, Heikke Huikuri, Ali Oto, Andrea E. Crompton, Sabina A. Murphy, Hans Lanz, Michele F. Mercuri, Elliott M. Antman, Eugene Braunwald and on behalf of the ENGAGE AF-TIMI 48 Investigators

https://doi.org/10.1161/CIRCEP.116.004267

Circulation: Arrhythmia and Electrophysiology. 2017;10:e004267. Originally published January 11, 2017

Akshay Mehta

A detailed analysis of risk/benefit of anticoagulation by AF pattern was done in ENGAGE AF-TIMI 48 trial (Effective Anticoagulation with Factor Xa Next Generation in Atrial Fibrillation-Thrombolysis in Myocardial Infarction 48).

▋ Protocol of the Study:

Efficacy and safety outcomes were evaluated during the 2.8 years median follow-up in 21,105 patients categorized as having paroxysmal (< 7 days duration), persistent (≥ 7 days but < 1 year), or permanent (≥ 1 year or failed cardioversion) AF patterns at randomization.

▋ Results:

In subjects who were all undergoing oral anticoagulation therapy, paroxysmal AF was associated with a lower stroke risk of 1.49% per year compared with persistent AF (1.83% per year; P=0.015) and permanent AF (1.95% per year; P=0.004). Also, all-cause mortality was lower in paroxysmal than in persistent or permanent AF, probably because patients with permanent AF may have more advanced heart disease and more comorbidities.

AF pattern did not modify the efficacy and the safety of edoxaban compared to Vitamin K antagonist.

▋ Comments:

The strength of this analysis is in the numbers comprising 21,105 patients, with a long follow-up period, providing data on > 650 primary outcome events of stroke and systemic embolism. Although the patients analysed were on OAC, the pattern of influence of type of AF on stroke risk mirrors that in patients who were not on OAC's in trials such as ACTIVE A and in the AVERROES (Apixaban Versus Acetylsalicylic Acid to Prevent Stroke in Atrial Fibrillation Patients Who Have Failed or Are Unsuitable for Vitamin K Antagonist Treatment) trials.

▮ Clinical Application:

The message from the study is that though all patients of AF benefit from OAC, there is a difference in risk of thromboembolism among patients with paroxysmal versus persistent and permanent AF. The latter are PARTICULARLY at higher risk and deserve utmost care.

▮ Suggested Readings

1. McManus DD, Rienstra M, Benjamin EJ. An update on the prognosis of patients with atrial fibrillation. Circulation. 2012;126:e143-e146. doi: 10.1161/CIRCULATIONAHA.112.129759.

2. Healey JS, Connolly SJ, Gold MR, Israel CW, Van Gelder IC, Capucci A, Lau CP, Fain E, Yang S, Bailleul C, Morillo CA, Carlson M, Themeles E, Kaufman ES, Hohnloser SH; ASSERT Investigators. Subclinical atrial fibrillation and the risk of stroke. N Engl J Med. 2012;366:120-129. doi: 10.1056/NEJMoa1105575.

3. Kannel WB, Abbott RD, Savage DD, McNamara PM. Coronary heart disease and atrial fibrillation: the Framingham Study. Am Heart J. 1983;106:389-396.

4. Petersen P, Godtfredsen J. Embolic complications in paroxysmal atrial fibrillation. Stroke. 1986; 17:622-626.

5. Shimomura K, Ohe T, Uehara S, Matsuhisa M, Kamakura S, Sato I. Significance of atrial fibrillation as a precursor of embolism. Am J Cardiol. 1989;63:1405-1407.

21

Crushed Prasugrel Tablets in Patients with STEMI Undergoing Primary Percutaneous Coronary Intervention

Ref.: Fabiana Rollini, Francesco Franchi, Jenny Hu, Megha Kureti, Niti Aggarwal, Ashwin Durairaj, Yongwhi Park, Michael Seawell, Pedro Cox-Alomar, Martin M. Zenni, Luis A. Guzman, Siva Suryadevara, Patrick Antoun, Theodore A. Bass, Dominick J. Angiolillo

http://www.onlinejacc.org/content/67/17 1994 ? ijkey =623886e 2f494d0a 554f6d8ce 1db2e 113e 97be 2d7 & keytype2=tf_ipsecsha.

JACC, 2016, 67, 17, 1994-2004.

Key Points:

In patients undergoing primary percutaneous coronary intervention, better therapeutic effect is achieved with crushed prasugrel tablets as compared to whole tablets.

Dev Pahlajani

STUDY OBJECTIVES:

Prasugrel is an orally administered third-generation thienopyridine that irreversibly inhibits the platelet P2Y12 receptor resulting in more prompt, potent, and predictable antiplatelet effects than other medicines in the category. This potential effect of prasugrel is of great importance in managing atherothrombotic events in patients with acute coronary syndrome (ACS) undergoing percutaneous coronary intervention (PCI). However reduction of the time of onset of action of all antiplatelet agents, including prasugrel, is the next domain of study since in STEMI patients undergoing primary PCI, a delay of therapeutic action is often observed. Therefore, the aim of this study was to investigate whether crushing prasugrel is associated with more favorable drug bioavailability and platelet inhibitory effects compared with whole tablets in STEMI patients undergoing primary PCI.

▮ Protocol of the Study:

Study design: prospective, randomized, open-label, parallel-design study

- Study Period: October 15, 2014, and August 12, 2015

- Total no. of patients randomized: 52 (whole tablets, n = 26; crushed tablets, n = 26)

- Study treatment: 60-mg loading dose (LD) of prasugrel administered as whole (Group A) or crushed tablets (Group B) in STEMI patients undergoing primary PCI

- Other treatment: standard of care, which included 325 mg aspirin and 4,000 IU

Primary Endpoint: Comparison of platelet reactivity units (PRU) determined by VN-P2Y12 between whole and crushed prasugrel at 2 hr post-LD administration (time point at which optimal platelet inhibition should be achieved in non-ST-segment elevation ACS patients following a 60mg LD administration).

Secondary Outcomes:

1. Platelet reactivity, at each time point as well as over time.

2. Rates of high on treatment platelet reactivity.

3. Pharmacokinetic parameters.

Results:

Fig. 1: *The effect of crushing prasugrel on pharmacokinetic and pharmacodynamic profiles. STEMI = ST-segment elevation myocardial infarction.*

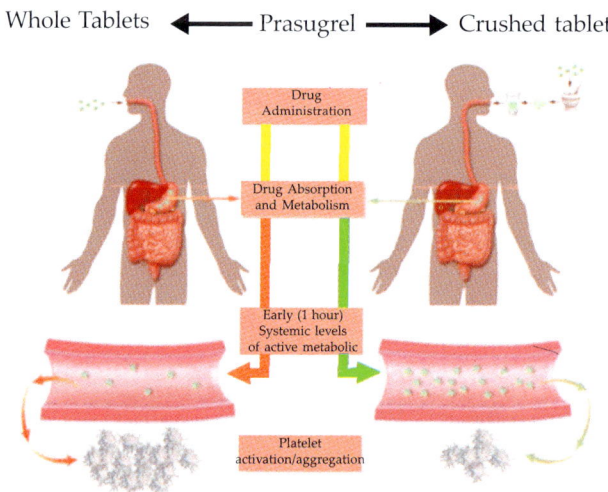

Primary Outcome:

1. PRU levels significantly decreased over time in both groups (p < 0.001 for both), however since platelet reactivity had reduced by 30 min in patients treated with crushed prasugrel; the PRU levels declined more rapidly in this group.

2. PRU at 2 hrs after LD administration: Group B (164) vs. Group A (95); least-square means difference = 68; 95% CI: 10 to 126; p = 0.022.

3. 24 hours difference: p = 0.008.

Secondary Outcomes:

Rates of HPR: significantly reduced rates at 30 min, 1 hr, and 2 hrs after drug administration.

▮ Conclusions:

The above study demonstrated that crushed prasugrel administration is associated with faster drug absorption and more prompt and potent antiplatelet effects compared with whole tablet ingestion in the study population described. However larger randomized trials are warranted to generalize the findings of this study.

▮ Review:

The journey of intracoronary stents and antiplatelet agents has been a remarkable one and both of these have often met the milestones together. However there is lot of investigation and revolution happening and the goal remains the same prevention of mortality and morbidity in ACS patients. One of the key aspects to the pharmacological development is to enhance the PK of any drug and thereby improve its pharmacodynamics (PD) and overall efficacy. To this effect this was the first trial that assessed the PK and PD profiles associated with crushing prasugrel tablets (60-mg LD). The results demonstrated that crushed prasugrel was associated with an over 3-fold faster drug absorption and nearly 2-fold higher maximal plasma concentration of its active metabolite compared with whole tablet administration. Although patients had similar exposure to P-AM during the overall study time course, this was approximately 3.5-fold higher with crushed prasugrel during the first 2 h post-LD.

▮ Clinical Relevance:

Though the study showed remarkable changes in PK/PD parameters; there was no clinical evaluation. In other words the study did not show whether these changes can translate into clinical efficacy. Many other aspects such as comparison with other P2Y12 receptor antagonist such as cangrelor and the effect of drug-drug interaction should be accounted for when considering the results of the study. Nevertheless this study gives a new direction of thinking and the ever evolving therapies may benefit in long run.

▌ Suggested Readings

1. Franchi F., Angiolillo D.J. (2015) Novel antiplatelet agents in acute coronary syndrome. Nat Rev Cardiol 12:30-47.

2. Montalescot G., Wiviott S.D., Braunwald E., et al. (2009) Prasugrel compared with clopidogrel in patients undergoing percutaneous coronary intervention for ST-elevation myocardial infarction (TRITON-TIMI 38): double-blind, randomised controlled trial. Lancet 373:723-731.

3. Heestermans A.A., van Werkum J.W., Taubert D., et al. (2008) Impaired bioavailability of clopidogrel in patients with a ST-segment elevation myocardial infarction. Thromb Res 122:776-781.

4. Alexopoulos D., Makris G., Xanthopoulou I., et al. (2014) Onset of antiplatelet action with high (100 mg) versus standard (60 mg) loading dose of prasugrel in patients with ST-segment-elevation myocardial infarction undergoing primary percutaneous coronary intervention: pharmacodynamic study. Circ Cardiovasc Interv 7:233-239.

5. Alexopoulos D., Barampoutis N., Gkizas V., et al. (2016) Crushed versus integral tablets of ticagrelor in ST-segment elevation myocardial infarction patients: a randomized pharmacokinetic/pharmaco dynamic study. Clin Pharmacokinet 55:359-367.

6. Diodati J.G., Saucedo J.F., French J.K., et al. (2013) Effect on platelet reactivity from a prasugrel loading dose after a clopidogrel loading dose compared with a prasugrel loading dose alone: Transferring From Clopidogrel Loading Dose to Prasugrel Loading Dose in Acute Coronary Syndrome Patients (TRIPLET): a randomized controlled trial. Circ Cardiovasc Interv 6:567-574.

22

Women are from Venus - for early PCI following NSTE ACS

Outcomes of Women and Men with Acute Coronary Syndrome Treated with and without Percutaneous Coronary Revascularization

Ref.: Jacob A. Udell, Maria Koh, Feng Qiu, Peter C. Austin, Harindra C. Wijeysundera, Akshay Bagai, Andrew T. Yan, Shaun G. Goodman, Jack V. Tu, Dennis T. Ko Journal of the American Heart Association. 2017;6:e0043 19 January 2017 - Volume 6, Issue 1.

Akshay Mehta

Study Objectives:

To assess whether clinical outcomes differ between women and men presenting with ACS treated with an early invasive strategy.

Protocol of the Study:

In a population-based cohort of 23 473 hospitalized ACS patients who received early cardiac catheterization from 2008 to 2011 in Ontario, Canada, and followed for up to 2 years, clinical outcomes were compared stratified by the use of coronary revascularization.

The primary outcome of the study was defined as a composite of all-cause mortality or recurrent hospitalization for ACS (myocardial infarction or unstable angina) within 1 year. Secondary outcomes were the incidence of the individual components of the composite outcome events. Events were captured at the time of ACS hospitalization to the end of 2 years of follow-up.

Results:

Out of all ACS patients who received cardiac catheterization during an index hospitalization, 66.1% of men and 51.8% of women received coronary revascularization. In the propensity-weighted cohort of patients who received coronary revascularization, the 1-year rate of death or recurrent ACS was 10.6% for men compared with 13.1% for women (hazard ratio 1.24; 95% CI 1.16-1.33). In contrast, outcomes for patients who did not receive coronary revascularization were higher in both and did not differ significantly between women and men at 1 year (17.8% versus 16.9%; hazard ratio 1.06; 95% CI 0.99-1.14) or at longer follow-up.

Conclusion:

Among revascularized patients, women had consistently higher risk for major adverse cardiovascular events compared with men, predominantly driven by recurrent ACS and not mortality. In contrast, men and women managed with medical therapy after early invasive evaluation had overall higher, but relatively similar, outcomes after ACS at longer term.

▮ Review:

Older age at presentation, a higher burden of comorbidities, late presentation, more atypical symptoms compared with men, and lesser use of an early invasive strategy are usually regarded as the factors responsible for higher risk of women having ACS.

What if the last factor is equally applied to both sexes? Whether greater use of early coronary revascularization can mitigate sex-based risk differences in outcomes following ACS, adjustments being made for other factors?

Well, the present study suggests that sex differences in outcomes remain among patients who undergo early revascularization. One reason was higher rates of bleeding and blood transfusion in women than men in the coronary revascularization group, both known to be associated with negative consequences.

Other reasons could be that women with ACS are more likely to have nonobstructive epicardial coronary disease, smaller epicardial coronary arteries, less traditional focal plaque rupture on angiography, and have more microvascular dysfunction, diffuse disease, or plaque erosion as some studies have suggested in the past.

Sex-based disparities in outcomes following cardiac catheterization for ACS persisted despite the use of early revascularization in women. Whether inherent differences in underlying comorbidities or response to invasive therapy and adjunct treatment are responsible in impacting the outcomes remains to be studied.

The chief limitation of the study is its observational design which is subject to the potential influence of confounding even though a propensity matching method was utilized.

▮ Clinical Application:

Although the study suggests women had worse outcomes than men after early revascularization, this should not be construed as a reason to withhold revascularization in appropriately selected women presenting with ACS, because data from randomized trials have shown that an early invasive strategy reduces adverse cardiovascular events to a similar extent in higher risk ACS men and women, particularly when presenting with positive biomarkers. The study suggests that careful monitoring of weight and renal function be factored when selecting antithrombotic dosing to reduce bleeding, as well as use of other bleeding avoidance strategies.

23

First-in-Human Evaluation of a Novel Polymer-Free Drug-Filled Stent: Angiographic, IVUS, OCT and Clinical Outcomes From the RevElution Study.

Ref.: Worthley SG, Abizaid A, Kirtane AJ, Simon DI, Windecker S, Brar S, Meredith IT, Shetty S, Sinhal A, Almonacid AP, Chamié D, Maehara A, Stone GW; RevElution Investigators.
JACC: Cardiovascular Interventions 2017, 10 (2) 147-156.

Key Points:
Drug filled polymer free stent is associated with significantly less late lumen loss, 0% binary angiographic restenosis, and more or less complete stent strut coverage.

Dev Pahlajani

■ Study Objectives:

To study the safety and efficacy of the drug filled stent (DFS) in the treatment of patients with coronary artery disease.

■ Protocol:

RevElution trial enrolled 100 patients with de novo 1 or 2 coronary lesions. The patients underwent angiographic intravascular ultrasound and clinical evaluation at 9 and 24 months. The vessel diameter was 2.25 - 3.5 mm with length equal to or less than 27 mm. There were 2 cohorts of 50 patients each. Fifty patients in 1 cohort were followed for 9 months while the other cohort of 50 patients was followed for 24 months. In each group 30 patients underwent OCT. The primary end point was angiographic in-stent late lumen loss at 9 months which was compared with Resolute Zotarolimus eluting stent by historical control data.

■ Results:

The in-stent late lumen loss was 0.26 ± 0.28 mm in DFS treated patients and 0.36 ± 0.52 mm in Resolute treated patients ($p = < 0.001$ for non inferiority). Binary restenosis was 0%. The median stent coverage by OCT was 91%, 95.6% and 99.1% at 1, 3 and 9 months respectively. While there was no stent thrombosis, one patient developed non Q-wave myocardial infarction (Ref. Fig) .

■ Conclusion:

In this first in man trial data shows that the safety and efficacy of DFS is non inferior to zotarolimus eluting resolute stent.

Reviewers Comments:

DES has become a standard of care for patients with obstructive coronary artery disease undergoing percutaneous coronary revascularization. The drug coated on the stent is delivered through a polymer which could be either biocompatible or bioabsorbable. However, it has been noted that polymer can be inflammatory and could crack with high deployment pressure. This cracked polymer could be a nidus for the development of stent thrombosis or accelerated neo atherosclerosis. Histopathological studies have demonstrated late inflammatory reaction to polymer that could lead to late and very late stent thrombosis. This has created need for pronged dual antiplatet therapy (DAPT). Lately several polymer free stents have been used to treat obstructive coronary artery disease with the aim of reducing inflammation produced by polymer. Though the current stents are coated with bioabsorbable or biocompatible polymer the risk of late or very late stent thrombosis though considerably reduced still remains. Polymer free stents are used with the expectation that the duration of the DAPT will be reduced. In the LEADERS FREE trial, Biolimus A9 stent was associated with similar efficacy and stent thrombosis as bare metal stent with 1 month duration of DAPT. DFS is a polymer free stent consisting of trilayered continuous wire while the inner core of material is removed to create a continuous lumen. The inner layer of the lumen is coated with sirolimus while the middle layer is tantalum which provides better radio-opacity while the outer layer is made up of cobalt chromium which provides stent strength and the strut thickness of 81 microns. The holes are on the abluminal surface which elutes the drug directly to the arterial wall without the polymer. The initial results are encouraging. The safety and efficacy has been proved that is comparable to zotarolimus resolute stent in the current Revolution study. However lesions treated are simple and only upto two de novo lesions were permitted to be treated. Follow up is also for 9 and 24 months in 2 cohorts. Will the stent reduce the duration of DAPT needs to be established by larger number of patients with multi vessel and multi lesion complex disease since these are the patients who need prolonged duration of DAPT with conventional DES.

▌ Clinical Relevance:

If proved to be efficacious and safe in complex lesions duration of DAPT could be reduced to avoid risk of bleeding assocaited with DAPT particularly in patients with high bleeding risk or needing urgent non cardiac surgery.

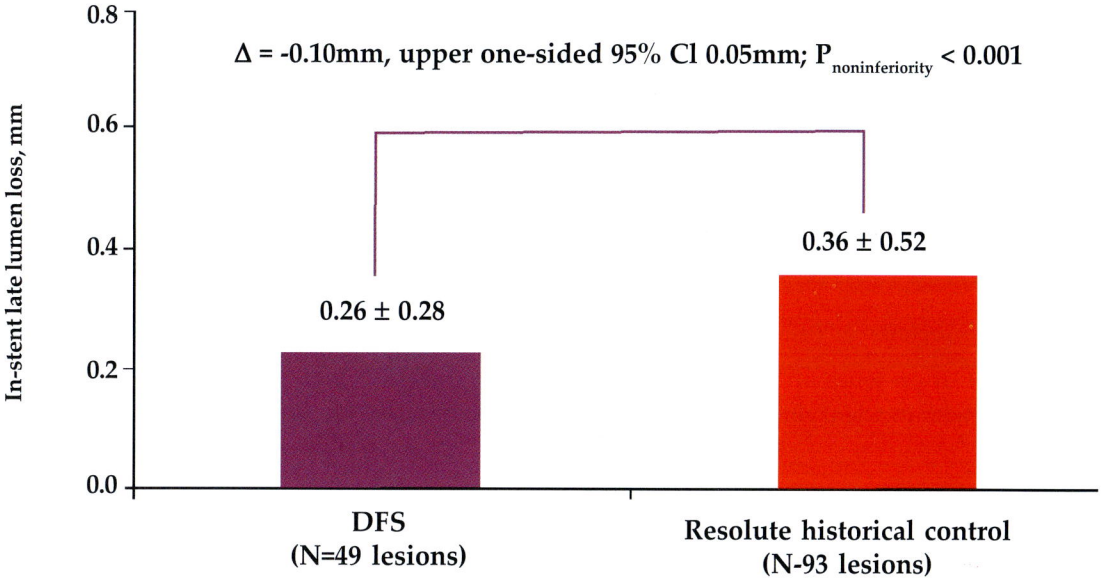

Fig. 1: *The powered primary endpoint, 9-month late Lumen Loss with the DFS compared with 8-months late Lumen Loss from the historical Control Resolute Zotarolimus-Eluting stent*

■ Suggested Readings

1. Stone GW, Kirtane AJ, Abizaid A, et al. Preclinical results with a novel internally loaded drug-filled coronary stent. Presented at: American College of Cardiology; March 14-16, 2015; San Diego, CA.

2. Kim S.J., Lee H., Cho J.M., et al. (2013) Comparison of zotarolimus-eluting stent and everolimus-eluting stent for vascular healing response: serial 3-month and 12-month optical coherence tomography study. Coron Artery Dis 24:431-439.

3. Kim J.S., Jang I.K., Fan C., et al. (2009) Evaluation in 3 months duration of neointimal coverage after zotarolimus-eluting stent implantation by optical coherence tomography: the ENDEAVOR OCT trial. J Am Coll Cardiol Intv 2:1240-1247.

24

Catching Them Young-Important for South Asians !

Association of Coronary Artery Calcium in adults 32 to 46 years with Incident Coronary Heart Disease and Death.

Ref.: Carr JJ, Jacobs DR, Terry JG, et al.
JAMA Cardiol 2017; DOI:10.1001/jamacardio.2016.5493

Akshay Mehta

▌ Study Objectives:

To find out if presence of Coronary Artery Calcium in young adults (aged 32 to 46 years) is associated with incident clinical CHD, CVD, and all-cause mortality during 12.5 years of follow-up.

▌ Protocol of the Study:

The Coronary Artery Risk Development in Young Adults (CARDIA) Study is a prospective community-based study that involved studying 5115 black and white participants aged 18 to 30 years from March 25, 1985, to June 7, 1986 for 30 years, with CAC measured 15, 20 and 25 years after recruitment. The mean follow-up period for incident events was 12.5 years, i.e. from the year 15 of computed tomographic scan through 2014.

There were two outcomes measured:

1. Incident CHD which included fatal or nonfatal myocardial infarction, acute coronary syndrome without myocardial infarction, coronary revascularization, or CHD death, incident CVD, which included CHD, stroke, heart failure, and peripheral arterial disease, and death which included all causes.

2. The probability of developing CAC by age 32 to 56 years was estimated using clinical risk factors measured 7 years apart between ages 18 and 38 years. This was based on participant age, race/ethnicity, sex, educational level, field center, smoking status, LDL cholesterol, body-mass index, systolic BP, presence of diabetes, and use of medication(s) for BP and lipid control.

▌ Results and Conclusions:

1. Overall, the prevalence of CAC was 10.2% at year 15, 20.1% at year 20, and 28.4% at year 25.

2. After adjusting for demographics, risk factors, and treatments, those with any CAC experienced a 5-fold increase in CHD events and 3-fold increase in CVD events.

3. Within CAC score strata of 1-19, 20-99, and 100 or more, the HRs for CHD were 2.6, 5.8 and 9.8 respectively. A CAC score of 100 or more had an incidence of 22.4 deaths per 100 participants.

4. Risk factors for CVD in early adult life identified those above the median risk for developing CAC. If so applied, a selective CAC screening strategy could reduce the number of people to be screened for CAC by 50% and the number imaged needed to find 1 person with CAC from 3.5 to 2.2.

▌ Comments:

The study shows that presence of any CAC among the young (between age 32 and 46 years) was associated with increased risk of fatal and nonfatal CHD during 12.5 years of follow-up. CAC score of 100 or more was associated with early death.

Most current guidelines exclude people below 40 years age (due to absence of relevant data) for risk stratification and recommend screening for CAC as an option with threshold CAC scores of 100, 300, and 400 only for people in whom risk is uncertain.

This keeps the young outside the ambit of risk stratification and CAC scoring, which is especially relevant for India where CHD is so prevalent in the young.

What this paper suggests is that coronary calcium is a very specific biomarker of identifying young people who are anywhere from a 10% to 25% risk of having a clinical event over next 10 to 15 years which can be prevented with life style advice and statins.

▌ Clinical Application:

Of course, the study doesn't mean that all young adults should get a CT scan. As the study shows, if CACS is restricted to only people at high risk (measured by usual criteria), the number of people needed to image to find 1 person with CAC will be just 2.

Also many people get CT scans for other causes, and those scans could be checked for CAC levels.

Thus, selective use of screening for CAC might be considered in individuals with risk factors in early adulthood to inform discussions about primary prevention.

25

Anticoagulation Versus Antiplatelet or No Therapy in Patients Undergoing Bioprosthetic Valve Implantation: A Systematic Review and Meta-Analysis.

Ref.: Ahmad Masri, A Marc Gillinov, Douglas M Johnston, Joseph F Sabik, Lars G Svensson, L Leonardo Rodriguez, Samir R Kapadia, William J Stewart, Richard A Grimm, Brian P Griffin, Milind Y Desai Heart 2017;103:40-48.

Dev Pahlajani

Background:

Patients who have irreparable structural degeneration of native valves can only depend on valve replacement as the definitive therapy. Current guidelines recommend bioprosthetic valve implantation in aortic and mitral position as a reasonable option for patients who are older than 65 years and for a certain select patients who are younger than 65 years, keeping patient preference in mind too.

Current guidelines don't recommend prolonged anticoagulation for patients with bioprosthetic valves, however guidelines recommend using a Vit. K antagonist (VKA) in the three months after surgery but this remains controversial. VKA is recommended on the belief that there may be early thrombus formation, on the valve sewing ring before the completion of endotheliasation.

Several bioprosthetic valve implants are done yearly, but there are no large randomized clinical trials which evaluate the benefit of VKA in the first three months after their implantation.

Study Objectives:

There has always been a controversy about the usage of VKA versus antiplatelet (AP)/no therapy post bioprosthetic valve implantation.

This study aims to:

- Develop a systematic review from the published literature comparing the use of VKA versus AP/no treatment
- Meta-analysis to study the risks and benefits of using VKA as compared with AP/no therapy

Methods:

Five databases were examined:

- PubMed
- Medline

- Embase
- Ovid
- Cochrane

From these databases randomised clinical trials and observational studies were picked which compared VKA (group I) versus AP/no therapy (group II).

14 studies were included: two randomised trials, 12 observational studies and one conference abstract

No. of patients: 31,740

Outcome was after surgical intervention.

Mantel-Haenszel odds ratio (OR) was calculated - random-effects meta-analysis was used for the outcome.

Heterogeneity was assessed by I2 statistics.

▌ Results:

There are two groups: group I (VKA) and group II (AP/no therapy). No differences in thromboembolic events were observed (145 (1%) vs. 262 (1.5%), OR 0.96 (95% CI 0.60 to 1.52)), all-cause mortality (351 (3.5%) vs. 415 (2.9%), OR 1.48 (95% CI 0.87 to 2.50)) or need for redo surgery (47 (3.3%) vs. 55 (3.2%); OR 0.81 (95% CI 0.42 to 1.58)). However, there were more bleeding events in group I versus group II (292 (2.6%) vs. 189 (1.1%); OR 2.26 (95% CI 1.67 to 3.05)).

▌ Reviewers Comments:

In this meta-analysis, it was proven that there was no benefit of adding VKA in the treatment regimen of patients who had undergone bioprosthetic valve implantation regarding thromboembolism or mortality. However, use of a VKA was associated with increased risk of major bleeding, with an absolute increased risk of 1.5%.

▌ Clinical Relevance:

There is a need for a large and well-done randomised clinical trial to understand the imapct of adding or not adding VKA in the treatment regimen. There is a pressing need for an individually customized assessment and an open discussion with patients regarding impact on thromboembolism or mortality, with a potential increased risk of bleeding.

▌ Suggested Readings

1. Nishimura RA, Otto CM, Bonow RO, et al. 2014 AHA/ACC Guideline for the Management of Patients With Valvular Heart Disease: Executive Summary: a Report of the American College of Cardiology/ American Heart Association Task Force on Practice Guidelines. J Am Coll Cardiol 2014;63:2438-88.

2. Colli A, Verhoye JP, Heijmen R, et al. Antithrombotic therapy after bioprosthetic aortic valve replacement: ACTION Registry survey results. Eur J Cardiothorac Surg 2008;33:531-6.

3. Stein B, Fuster V, Halperin JL, et al. Antithrombotic therapy in cardiac disease. An emerging approach based on pathogenesis and risk. Circulation 1989;80:1501-13.

Cardiac Symptoms Before Sudden Cardiac Death Caused by Hypertrophic Cardiomyopathy

A Nationwide Study Among the Young in Denmark

Ref.: Thomas Hadberg Lynge; Bjarke Risgaard; Reza Jabbari; Charlotte Glinge; Henning Bundgaard; Barry Maron; Stig Haunsø; Bo GregersWinkel; Jacob Tfelt-Hansen
Europace. 2016;18(12):1801-1808

Akshay Mehta

1. Hypertrophic cardiomyopathy (HCM) is a frequent cause of sudden cardiac death (SCD) among the young (SCDY).

2. To assess symptoms before SCDY due to HCM, all SCDs in Danes aged 1-35 years in 2000-2009 were identified. In the 10-year study period, out of 431 autopsied SCDY cases 38 cases (9%) were included for the study.

3. For comparison, a control group consisting of traffic accident victims (n = 74) was included.

4. Antecedent cardiac symptoms (those occurring within a year to 1 h before death) were present in 21 (55%) of the cases, and 13 (34%) had prodromal symptoms (possible cardiac symptoms occurring < 1 hr before death), while 7 (18%) cases had both antecedent and prodromal symptoms prior to death.

5. A total of 28 (74%) cases had at least 1 cardiac symptom prior to death; 1 cardiac symptom was documented in 11 (29%) cases, 9 (24%) had two cardiac symptoms, and 8 (21%) had 3 or more cardiac symptoms before death. The most common cardiac symptoms were chest pain (n = 13, 34%), dyspnoea (n = 11, 29%), syncope/presyncope, and seizures (n = 13, 34%).

6. The majority (n = 33, 87%) of deaths occurred during sleep or while the individuals were awake and relaxed (e.g. lying, sitting, standing, gardening, or walking).

7. In 5 (13%) cases, death occurred during high-intensity activity.

8. In this nationwide study, it was found that nearly 74% of the young SCD cases who died of HCM had possible cardiac symptoms prior to death. The majority of patients had symptoms more than 24 hrs prior to death, which gives enough time for evaluation for the need for ICD implantation.

9. Indeed, the majority of patients with witnessed cardiac arrests had a shockable rhythm upon initial evaluation and there were at least 9 cases with a risk factor for sudden death (i.e. the 9 cases with reported syncope), which would have justified consideration for an implantable cardioverter defibrillator (ICD).

Influenza Vaccine as a Coronary Intervention for Prevention of Myocardial Infarction

Ref.: C Raina MacIntyre, Abela Mahimbo, Aye M Moa, Michelle Barnes
Heart 2016;102:1953-1956.

Dev Pahlajani

▮ Background:

In the recent times, cardiovascular disease (CVD) has taken over other diseases to become the leading cause of mortality in the world, beating even communicable diseases, which incidentally were leading for many years. CVD now approximately causes 13% of deaths globally. Such a huge global burden makes it imperative that risk factors need to be identified for necessary prevention and management of coronary heart disease.

To reduce the burden of coronary heart disease (CHD), certain strategies are adopted worldwide:

● Smoking cessation

● Lifestyle changes

● Improved nutrition

● Statins usage

● Correct antihypertensive regimen

Next in line is the influenza vaccine - can this vaccine be useful as an additional strategy to decrease the burden of CHD?

▮ Influenza as a Trigger for Acute Myocardial Infarction:

Evidence shows that there is an association between influenza infection and acute myocardial infarction (AMI). There is an increase in both - influenza and AMI deaths in winter.

In atherosclerosis there is an inflammatory response which results in the formation of a plaque comprising of a core rich in lipids, inflammatory cells and cytokines and also a fibrous cap. It is believed that there are several mechanisms by which influenza acts: inflammatory release of cytokines resulting in a pro-thrombotic state, disruption of plaques, certain effects such as hypoxia and tachycardia - all leading to obstruction of coronary arteries that may be sub-critically stenosed.

Influenza infection may precipitate AMI by several mechanisms as shown in the following Fig. 1.

Fig. 1: *Mechanisms by which influenza infection may precipitate acute myocardial infarction.*

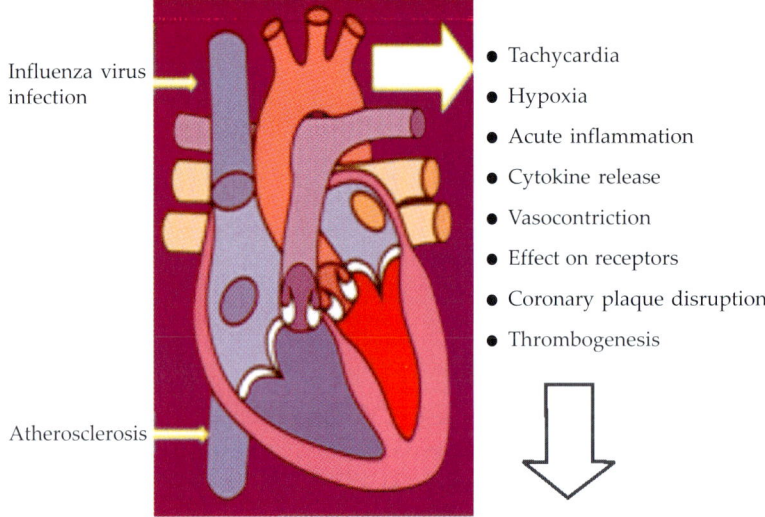

Acute Myocardial Infarction

▌ Influenza Vaccine for Secondary Coronary Prevenetion:

Several studies showcase the fact that influenza vaccine has effective protection against AMI. A meta analysis of certain studies indicates that influenza vaccine has a summary effectiveness to the tune of 29% against AMI. Certain major findings of several studies are as follows:

- Influenza vaccine is protective against AMI but the pooled estimate is not statistically significant

- Influenza vaccine is effective against composite coronary morbidity and mortality outcomes

- Influenza vaccine decreased major cardiovascular events by 10% in patients with acute coronary syndromes during a 12-month follow-up period.

The mechanism by which influenza vaccine protects the heart against AMI is by prevention of influenza infection triggered by the various mechanisms listed above. Also, it is postulated that the interaction between vaccine-induced antibody and the human bradykinin receptor could lead to an increased production of nitrous oxide which in turn increases the cardiac blood flow.

▌ Smoking Cessation for Secondary Prevention:

There is a huge and significant body of evidence which clearly shows that smoking cessation is extremely imperative and effective in the secondary prevention of AMI and also in reduction of AMI mortality rates.

Statins for Secondary Prevention

Studies show that statin efficacy in prevention of AMI ranges from 19% to 30%.

Antihypertensive Medication for Secondary Prevention:

Several randomized clinical trials have proven that antihypertensive treatment regimen has an established efficacy of 20-25% in secondary prevention of AMI.

Does Influenza Vaccine have a place in routine Coronary Prevention?

In spite of increasing body of evidence, vaccination for coronary prevention is unfortunately not a priority amongst physicians. In fact, influenza vaccination is a cheap, safe and effective strategy in prevention of both influenza and AMI. This is true especially for high risk people.

Clinical Relevance:

Several well-powered clinical trials of influenza vaccine in the prevention of AMI are definitely the need of the hour, it would tremendously add to the evidence. This will definitely help in bringing about the paradigm shift that vaccination in the risk groups is for prevention of CHD more importantly rather than prevention of the influenza infection. This will encourage the physicians to view influenza vaccine as an important, cheap and effective part of their armamentarium in the fight to prevent CHD.

Suggested Readings

1. World Health Organization (WHO). Cardiovascular diseases (CVDs). http://www. who.int/mediacentre/factsheets/fs317/en.

2. Chow CK, Jolly S, Rao-Melacini P, et al. Association of diet, exercise, and smoking modification with risk of early cardiovascular events after acute coronary syndromes. Circulation 2010;121:750-8.

3. Corrales-Medina VF, Suh KN, Rose G, et al. Cardiac complications in patients with community-acquired pneumonia: a systematic review and meta-analysis of observational studies. PLoS Med 2011;8:e1001048.

4. MacIntyre RC, Heywood AE, Kovoor P. Influenza virus vaccine reduces risk of ischemic events: time for a large-scale randomized trial? Future Cardiol 2014;10:35-7.

5. Phrommintikul A, Kuanprasert S, Wongcharoen W, et al. Influenza vaccination reduces cardiovascular events in patients with acute coronary syndrome. Eur Heart J 2011;32:1730-5.

6. Veljkovic V, Glisic S, Veljkovic N, et al. Influenza vaccine as prevention for cardiovascular diseases: possible molecular mechanism. Vaccine 2014;32:6569-75.

28

Association between early Q Waves and Reperfusion Success in Patients with ST-Segment-Elevation Myocardial Infarction Treated with Primary Percutaneous Coronary Intervention

A Cardiac Magnetic Resonance Imaging Study

Ref.: Divan Gabriel Topal, Jacob Lønborg, Kiril Aleksov Ahtarovski, Lars Nepper-Christensen, Steffen Helqvist, Lene Holmvang, Frants Pedersen, Peter Clemmensen, Kari Saünamaki, Erik Jørgensen, Kasper Kyhl, Ali Ghotbi, Mikkel Malby Schoos, Christoffer Göransson, Litten Bertelsen, Dan Høfsten, Lars Køber, Henning Kelbæk, Niels Vejlstrup, Thomas Engstrøm

Circulation: Cardiovascular Interventions. 2017;10:e004467

Akshay Mehta

▌ Key Points:

1. To ascertain the benefit of primary PCI in STEMI patients presenting with early onset Q waves, their myocardial salvage index and microvascular obstruction (MVO) was studied.

2. The presence of early QW in patients presenting with a first time STEMI was associated with a large area at risk, larger MVO and smaller myocardial salvage index as assessed by CMR. However, final myocardial salvage at 3 months was still substantial in patients with early QW.

3. Patients presenting with significant ST-segment-elevations within 12 hours after onset of clinical relevant symptoms with early QW should therefore not be excluded from treatment with primary PCI.

▌ Summary:

This is the first study to evaluate the association between early QW and myocardial salvage index and MVO in STEMI patients treated with primary PCI. Five hundred fifteen patients (from DANAMI 3 trial) with their first STEMI treated with primary PCI constituted the study population and were studied prospectively by ECG and cardiac magnetic resonance imaging scan (CMR). They underwent a CMR at day 1 and again at day 92. Early QW was observed in 108 (21%) patients and was associated with larger area at risk, infarct size, greater extent of MVO and lower LV ejection fraction with lesser degree of myocardial salvage. However, final myocardial salvage was still substantial in these patients. In addition, LV ejection fraction increased substantially between the acute phase and follow-up at 3 months later in this early QW group.

The presence of QW remained associated with outcome whether symptom onset to wire was more or less than 3 hours. Thus, QW presence is better estimate of the success from primary PCI than time from symptom onset to wire. This is in accordance with the previous findings that the benefit from reperfusion by primary PCI compared with thrombolysis seems to be more pronounced among patients with non-QW. Yet, as shown by this study, a considerable myocardial salvage after primary PCI is possible in patients with early QW, and these patients should not be rejected from immediate angioplasty.

Some limitations of the study were 1. Study population was already selected (from DANAMI 3 trials population) for primary PCI based on ECG and clinical presentation which may cause some risk of selection bias. Also 2. Although patients with known previous myocardial infarction were excluded from this study, inclusion of patients with unknown previous myocardial infarct cannot be ruled out.

▮ Clinical Application:

About 1 in 5 patients with STEMI present with a pathological Q wave (QW) before primary percutaneous coronary intervention (PCI). Early QW is known to be associated with larger infarct size and adverse prognosis and doubts remain about the benefit of primary PCI in such patients.

This study shows for the first time that STEMI patients with early QW treated with primary PCI have large area at risk, smaller myocardial salvage and larger microvascular obstruction as assessed by cardiac magnetic resonance imaging, but the myocardial salvage was still > 50%, at 3 months suggesting that this patient group benefits from primary PCI and should undergo immediate angioplasty.

Thus whether Q waves are present or not, in STEMI patients presenting within 12 hours of symptom onset, the goal should be to open the artery as best as one can and expect substantial long term benefits.

29

Outcomes of Intensive Blood Pressure Lowering in Older Hypertensive Patients

Ref.: Chirag Bavishi, Sripal Bangalore, Franz H. Messerli
JACC. 2017 69, 5, DOI: 10.1016/j.jacc.2016.10.077.

Key Points:

In older patients lowering of blood pressure < 140 mm Hg decreases major adverse cardiac complications and cardiovascular mortality.

Dev Pahlajani

◾ Study Objectives:

Earlier the Joint National Committee (JNC) recommendation was that the systolic blood pressure (BP) should be < 140 mm Hg in patients ≥ 60 years of age. The 2014 8th JNC report changed this recommendation to < 150 mm Hg in patients ≥ 60 years of age. This study aims to evaluate the efficacy and safety of such intensive BP-lowering strategies in older hypertensive patients (age ≥ 65 years).

◾ Protocol:

All relevant randomized controlled trials were examined ranging from a period of 1965 through July 1, 2016.

Adverse events evaluated were:

- Cardiovascular (major adverse cardiovascular events [MACE]
- Cardiovascular mortality
- Stroke
- Myocardial infarction
- Heart failure
- Safety (serious adverse events and renal failure)

Pooled relative risks (RRs) and 95% confidence intervals (CIs) were calculated using random and fixed effects analysis.

Results:

4 high-quality trials were analysed:

- Number of patients: 10,857 older hypertensive patients with a mean follow-up of 3.1 years
- When compared with standard BP lowering, intensive BP lowering was associated with:
  - 29% reduction in MACE (RR: 0.71; 95% CI: 0.60 to 0.84)
  - 33% in cardiovascular mortality (RR: 0.67; 95% CI: 0.45 to 0.98)
  - 37% in heart failure (RR: 0.63; 95% CI: 0.43 to 0.99)
- Between the two groups, no differences seen in:
  - Incidence of serious adverse events (RR: 1.02; 95% CI: 0.94 to 1.09)
  - Renal failure (RR: 1.81; 95% CI: 0.86 to 3.80)
- Rates of myocardial infarction and stroke

The fixed effects model did yield almost similar results, but an increase was seen in the risk of renal failure (RR: 2.03; 95% CI: 1.30 to 3.18) with intensive BP-lowering therapy.

Fig. 1: *Effects of Intensive BP-lowering in Older (≥ 65 Years) Hypertensive Patients*

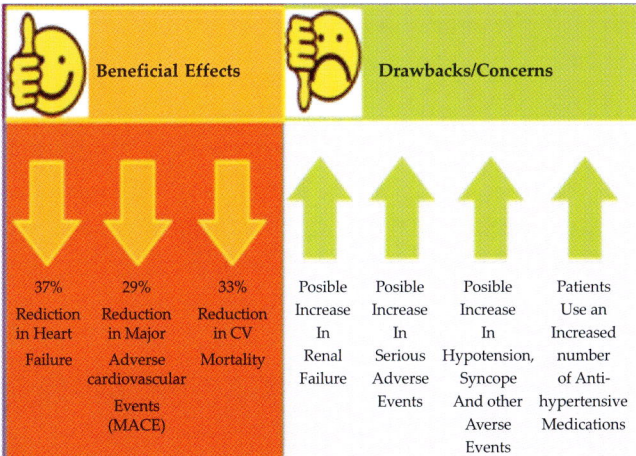

Conclusion:

When intensive BP control was initiated in elder hypertensive patients, the following were decreased:

- MACE
- Cardiovascular mortality
- Heart failure

There seemed an increased risk of renal failure and limited data was available on adverse events.

■ Reviewer's Comments:

One of the hottest topics of debate in the recent years has been optimal target BP. Recent JNC 8 report recommends quite a liberal systolic BP target of < 150 mm Hg in patients age ≥ 60 years. This however, has been received with a lot flak and criticism. The reason this liberal goal was set because it was observed that in this elderly group of patients a goal of systolic BP lower than 140 mm Hg provides no incremental benefit when compared with a higher goal SBP of 140 to 160 mmHg or 140 to 149 mmHg.

■ Clinical Relevance:

When setting strict or intensive BP control targets, all clinicians should carefully analyze and evaluate the benefits versus the potentila risks of treatment. In elderly hypertensive patients, there's a reduction in MACE, heart failure, cardiovascular mortality with intensive BP control (systolic BP < 140 mmHg) but may increase the renal failure risk. Hence all future randomized trials should aim at investigation of safety intensive BP control in elderly patients.

■ Suggested Readings

1. James P.A., Oparil S., Carter B.L., et al. (2014) 2014 evidence-based guideline for the management of high blood pressure in adults: report from the panel members appointed to the Eighth Joint National Committee (JNC 8). JAMA 311:507-520.

2. Ogihara T., Saruta T., Rakugi H., et al. (2010) Target blood pressure for treatment of isolated systolic hypertension in the elderly: valsartan in elderly isolated systolic hypertension study. Hypertension 56:196-202.

3. Wei Y., Jin Z., Shen G., Zhao X., Yang W., Zhong Y., Wang J. (2013) Effects of intensive antihypertensive treatment on Chinese hypertensive patients older than 70 years. J Clin Hypertens 15:420-427.

4. Williamson J.D., Supiano M.A., Applegate W.B., et al. (2016) Intensive vs standard blood pressure control and cardiovascular disease outcomes in adults aged ?75 years: a randomized clinical trial. JAMA 315: 2673-2682.

30

Patient and Lesion-Specific Characteristics Predict Risk of Major Adverse Cardiovascular Events Among Patients with Previous Percutaneous Coronary Intervention Undergoing Noncardiac Surgery

Ref.: Ehrin J. Armstrong MD, MSc, Laura Graham MPH, Stephen W. Waldo MD, Javier A. Valle MD, MSc, Thomas M. Maddox MD, MSc, Mary T. Hawn MD
Catheterization and Cardiovascular Interventions Volume 89, Issue 4, March 1, 2017, Pages 617-627

Akshay Mehta

▮ Key Points:

1. The objective of the study was to identify predictors of postoperative MACE among 12,621 patients with a history of prior PCI who underwent subsequent noncardiac surgery and were linked to VA and non-VA surgical records.

2. The strongest predictors of postoperative MACE were urgency of the operation, revised cardiac risk index, the indication for the prior PCI, and timing of the surgery after the PCI.

3. Lesion characteristics that were independently associated with postoperative MACE included PCI to a distal or ostial lesion and lesion calcification but stent length and target vessel (particularly left main or left anterior descending locations) as well as chronic total occlusion were not independently associated with outcomes.

▮ Summary:

Usual factors thought to contribute to an increased risk of postoperative adverse outcomes post PCI are patient comorbidities, the type and urgency of surgery, and perioperative antiplatelet management.

Hitherto, few studies have addressed the association between procedural characteristics of the initial PCI and risk of major adverse cardiac events (MACE) after subsequent noncardiac surgery.

In this study records of the initial PCI procedures within the Veterans' Administration, were linked to outcomes after subsequent noncardiac surgery within the next 2 years.

Expectedly, the following were strong predictors of events after non cardiac surgery

1. Urgency of the operation

2. Revised cardiac risk index

3. The indication for the prior PCI, and

4. Timing of the surgery after the PCI.

Interestingly, there were independent procedural characteristics of the initial PCI that predicted postoperative MACE. These included:

1. Lesion calcification

2. PCI to an ostial or distal lesion

3. And placement of a bare metal stent.

Surprisingly, lesion length, number of lesions treated at the time of PCI, location at left main or chronic total occlusion PCI did not predict post operative events as was shown in smaller studies earlier.

These could reflect the effectiveness of PCI with drug-eluting stent implantation in left main, left anterior descending, and chronically occluded lesions whereas distal or ostial lesions, or lesion with severe calcification are more likely to face a suboptimal PCI due to the possibility of following technical pitfalls.

About 52% increased odds of MACE in ostial PCI could be increased risk of stent thrombosis due to the presence of uncovered stent struts in the ostium. A 43% increased odds of MACE after PCI to a distal lesion could be due to greater possibility of restenosis and demand supply imbalance in the post-op period. The 29% increased risk of MACE after PCI on calcific lesions could be due to increased chances of inadequate stent expansion, stent deformation or stent fracture and/or increased platelet activation.

Some limitations of the study were : a possible bias in that patients with high-risk lesion characteristics may have had their surgeries delayed beyond 2 years due to concern for potential adverse postoperative outcomes, chiefly a male cohort from the VA system, a likely inherent selection bias in the placement of BMS vs. DES among patients who subsequently required surgery, lack of information on residual coronary artery stenosis and/or ischemia after the initial PCI (e.g., residual SYNTAX score), which could be a determinant of outcomes after subsequent non-cardiac surgery, entry of data by the treating physician at the time of the procedure and not by a core laboratory, lack of information on what percentage of events was related to stent thrombosis, possibility that the relative contribution of PCI lesion characteristics to outcomes could vary based on surgery type and non availability of details of perioperative antiplatelet use or bridging.

Despite the limitations, the large sample size of the cohort allowed multivariable adjustment for numerous risk factors and the ability to test for lesion-specific predictors of adverse outcomes.

❚ Clinical Application:

The findings from the study convey an important message that following the treatment of ostial, distal, or calcified lesions, it is advisable to delay surgery as much as possible. Possibly the use of intravascular imaging may be useful whenever treating these complex lesions to avoid under-expansion and guarantee adequate lesion coverage.It also suggests that besides patient and surgical characteristics, some procedural characteristics of the initial PCI could be useful in predicting the risk of adverse events among patients requiring subsequent noncardiac surgery.

31

Outcomes Associated with Resuming Warfarin Treatment after Hemorrhagic Stroke or Traumatic Intracranial Hemorrhage in Patients with Atrial Fibrillation

Ref.: Peter Brønnum Nielsen, PhD; Torben Bjerregaard Larsen, PhD; Flemming Skjøth, PhD; et al. JAMA Intern Med. Published online February 20, 2017. doi:10.1001/jamainternmed.2016.9369

Dev Pahlajani

▪ Study Objectives:

A very common dilemma in atrial fibrillation (AF) patients is the resumption of warfarin therapy. There is an increase in the risk of bleeding with antithrombotic therapy. In the absence of randomized clinical trials, certain observational studies act as a guide and help in proper decision making. This analysis is an investigation of the prognosis which goes with the resumption of warfarin treatment in AF patients who have suffered either hemorrhagic stroke or traumatic intracranial hemorrhage.

Design, Setting and Participants:

- Nationwide study: AF patients with incident ICH event (during warfarin treatment)

- Period: 1st Jan, 1998 - 28th Feb, 2016

- Evaluation: resumption of warfarin treatment post discharge from hospital.

▪ Exposures:

- Nither oral anticoagulation therapy nor warfarin therapy was a part of the time-dependent exposure.

▪ Main Outcomes and Measures:

- One-year observed event rates per 100 person-years were measured and calculated. All treatment strategies were compared. Time-dependent Cox proportional hazards regression models were used; adjustments were made for concomitant medication use, existing comorbidities, age, sex and length of stay.

▪ Results:

No. of AF patients with ICH event: 2415

No. of male patients: 1481 (61.3%)

No. of female patients: 934 (38.7%)

Mean (SD) age: 77.1 years (9.1 years)

No. of events attributed to hemorrhagic stroke: 1325

No. of events attributed to trauma: 1090

Lower rate of ischemic stroke or systemic embolism was associated with resumption of warfarin therapy (adjusted hazard ratio [AHR], 0.49; 95% CI, 0.24-1.02). An increment was observed in the rate of recurrent ICH when warfarin was not resumed (AHR, 1.31; 95% CI, 0.68-2.50), however these difference do not have statistical significance. In patients who have sustained hemorrhagic stroke, resumption of warfarin resulted in lower rate of recurrent ICH (AHR, 0.45; 95% CI, 0.26-0.76). In patienst with traumatic ICH, resumption of warfarin treatment resulted in lower rate of ischemic stroke or systemic embolism (AHR, 0.40; 95% CI, 0.15-1.11). A reduction in mortality was seen with resuming warfarin treatment among patients with hemorrhagic stroke (AHR, 0.51; 95% CI, 0.37-0.71) and those with traumatic ICH (AHR, 0.35; 95% CI, 0.23-0.52).

▌ Conclusions:

Post spontaneous hemorrhagic stroke in AF patients was associated with a lesser rate of ischemic events and an icreased rate of recurrent ICH when warfarin treatment was resumed. However, in patients with traumatic ICH, a relatively lesser risk of recurrent ICH (and a similar increased risk of ischemic events) was seen after resuming warfarin treatment.

▌ Reviewer's Comments:

What is the difference in prognosis of both patient subgroups? The additional risk of resuming oral anticoagulant therapy in traumatic intracranial hemorrhage or hemorrhagic stroke patients suggests a decrease in thromboembolism in both subgroups. The difference in both subgroups was that patients who suffered a hemorrhagic stroke tend to have a higher rate of intracranial hemorrhage after the resumption of treatment. On the other hand, patients who had sustained a traumatic intracranial hemorrhage did not experience this.

▌ Clinical Application:

This study reveals that all atrial fibrillation patients who have survived a traumatic intracranial hemorrhage or a hemorrhagic stroke will have different prognoses. Hence different recommendations have to be made in order to resume oral anticoagulant treatment.

32

Clinical Outcomes After PCI Treatment of Very Long Lesions with the XIENCE V Everolimus Eluting Stent; Pooled Analysis from the SPIRIT and XIENCE V USA Prospective Multicenter Trials.

Ref.: Georgios Bouras MD, MSC, PhD, Sunny Jhamnani MD et al
Catheterization Cardiovascular Interventions Volume 89, issue 6, May 2017, Pages 984-991

Akshay Mehta

▮ Study Objectives:

To assess the safety and efficacy of second-generation drug eluting stents in very long coronary lesions (≥ 35 mm).

▮ Study Protocol:

A patient level pooled analysis of 13,266 patients undergoing planned overlapping stent treatment of very long coronary lesions with the XIENCE V everolimus eluting coronary stent system from 6 trials evaluating the XIENCE V stent (Spirit II, III, IV, V, Spirit Small Vessel and XIENCE V USA) was done.

Patients were divided into two cohorts, a very long lesion (VLL) group (lesions ≥ 35 mm) and a control group (lesions > 24 to < 35 mm). The primary outcome measures were Target Lesion Failure (TLF), Major Adverse Cardiac Events (MACE), and Academic Research Consortium (ARC) defined definite and probable stent thrombosis at 1 year.

▮ Results and Conclusions:

A comparison of 323 patients with 328 total lesions with a mean lesion length of 47.1 ± 13.7 mm (the VLL group) with controls comprising of 482 patients with 500 total lesions with mean lesion length of 28.1 ± 2.4 mm, out of a total of 13,266 patients, revealed no significant difference in the rates of TLF between the VVL and control groups (8.9 vs. 10%, P = 0.63), MACE (9.2 vs. 10%, P = 0.74) or stent thrombosis (1.6 vs. 1.5%, P = 0.92) at 1 year.

Thus, the XIENCE V stent appears as safe and effective in the treatment of very long coronary lesions as PCI for long lesions.

▮ Comments:

Diffuse coronary disease, present in about 20% of patients presenting for PCI creates a therapeutic dilemma due to the unsuitability of target vessel for grafting as well as hitherto variable results with first and second generation DES.

This is the largest analysis evaluating patients undergoing multiple, overlapping EES stent implantation in very long coronary lesions. The results show acceptable clinical outcomes with EES used.

It reaffirms the safety and efficacy of the cobalt-chromium EES with thin struts, a biocompatible and thrombo-resistant fluoropolymer and an optimal dose of everolimus.

Although the strength of the study is in its numbers, a short follow up of only 1 year is a limitation. It would be interesting to know the rates of late and very late stent thrombosis and TLR.

❚ Clinical Application:

Based on this study, percutaneous coronary treatment of very long lesions with the XIENCE V stent appears as safe and effective as PCI for long lesions. Also, the study highlights one more situation where benefit from more potent and prolonged dual antiplatelet therapy may be derived.

33

Atherothrombotic Risk Stratification and Ezetimibe for Secondary Prevention

Ref.: Erin A. Bohula, David A. Morrow, Robert P. Giugliano, Michael A. Blazing, Ping He, Jeong-Gun Park, Sabina A. Murphy, Jennifer A. White, Y. Antero Kesaniemi, Terje R. Pedersen, Adrian J. Brady, Yale Mitchel, Christopher P. Cannon, Eugene Braunwald.
Journal of the American College of Cardiology 2017, 69 (8) 911-921.

Key Points:
1. In patients with high risk of atherothrombosis addition of ezetimibe to statin therapy provides greater benefit of prevention of acute coronary syndrome.
2. Patients with high risk derive the maximum benefit of combination therapy.
3. Patients should be risk stratified.

Dev Pahlajani

∎ Study Objectives:

Patients who have been stabilized after acute coronary syndrome (ACS) show an improvement in cardiovascular outcomes (CV) when ezetimibe is added to their existing statin therapy. This study analyses the hypothesis that atherothrombotic risk stratification may prove beneficial in identification of post-ACS patients who stand to benefit greatly from the addition of ezetimibe to ongoing statin therapy.

∎ Protocol:

This study used the TIMI risk stratification tool. TIMI (Thrombolysis In Myocardial Infarction) Risk Score for Secondary Prevention (TRS 2°P) is a simple 9-point risk stratification tool. The TIMI Score tool has been previously developed in a large population with atherothrombosis. This tool is used in prediction of myocardial infarction (MI), cardiovascular (CV) death, and ischemic stroke (CV death/MI/ischemic cerebrovascular accident (iCVA).

No. of patients where TIMI was used: 17,717 (post-ACS patients)

These post-ACS patients were randomized to either 1. ezetimibe and simvastatin or 2. placebo and simvastatin (in IMPROVE-IT trial).

Treatment efficacy was assessed by the following:

- Baseline risk for CV death/MI/iCVA
- The IMPROVE-IT composite endpoints (CE)
- Individual component endpoints at 7 years

Results: (Ref Fig)

- All 9 clinical variables in the TRS 2°P were independent risk indicators for CV death/MI/ iCVA ($p < 0.001$).

- The integer-based scheme showed a strong graded relationship with the rate of CV death/MI/ iCVA, the trial CE, and the individual components (p trend <0.0001 for each).

- High-risk patients (n = 4,393; 25%), defined by ≥3 risk indicators, had a 6.3% (95% confidence interval: 2.9% to 9.7%) absolute risk reduction in CV death/MI/iCVA at 7 years with ezetimibe/ simvastatin, thus translating to a number-needed-to-treat of 16.

- Intermediate-risk patients (2 risk indicators; n = 5,292; 30%) had a 2.2% (95% confidence interval: -0.3% to 4.6%) absolute risk reduction. Low-risk patients (0 to 1 risk indicators; n = 8,032; 45%) did not appear to derive benefit from the addition of ezetimibe (p interaction = 0.010).

- Similar findings were observed for the IMPROVE-IT primary CE.

Conclusions:

Atherothrombotic risk stratification utilizing the TRS 2°P helps in identification of high-risk patients who benefit from addition of ezetimibe to ongoing statin therapy.

Clinical Application:

Ezetimibe improves CV outcomes when it is given as an add-on therapy to statin therapy in patients who have been stabilized after ACS. This study aimed to analyse whether higher-risk populations of patients could be identified who have the greatest potential for benefit from such an addition by using the TRS 2°P (a simple 9-point risk stratification tool). In this secondary analysis, it was found that in patients who conditions were stabilized after ACS in IMPROVE-IT, the TRS 2°P the following was identified: 1) a strong gradient of risk for recurrent CV events; and, importantly; 2) an increasingly favorable relative and absolute benefit from the addition of ezetimibe to simvastatin therapy with increasing risk profile.

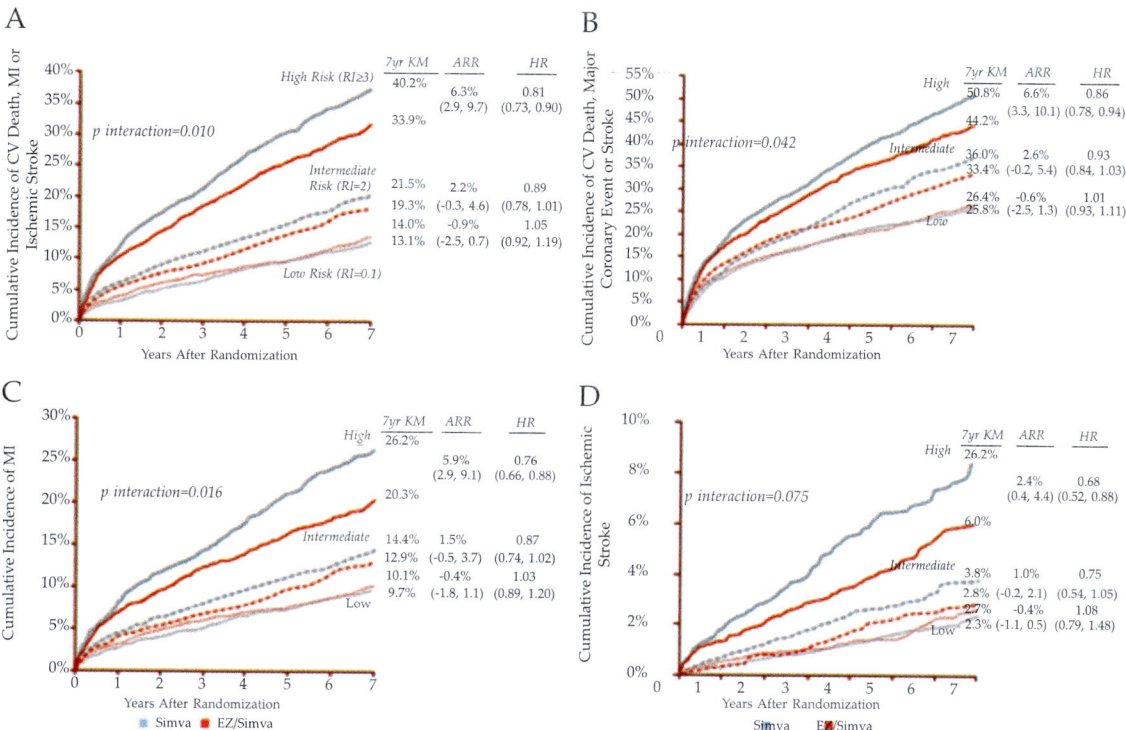

Fig. 1: Outcomes by category and randomized treatment

Simva   EZ/Simva

Suggested Readings

1. Cannon C.P., Blazing M.A., Giugliano R.P., et al. (2015) Ezetimibe added to statin therapy after acute coronary syndromes. N Engl J Med 372:2387-2397.

2. Bohula E.A., Bonaca M.P., Braunwald E., et al. (2016) Atherothrombotic risk stratification and the efficacy and safety of vorapaxar in patients with stable ischemic heart disease and previous myocardial infarction. Circulation 134:304-313.

3. Morrow D.A., Braunwald E., Bonaca M.P., et al. (2012) Vorapaxar in the secondary prevention of atherothrombotic events. N Engl J Med 366:1404-1413.

4. Scirica B.M., Bonaca M.P., Braunwald E., et al. (2012) Vorapaxar for secondary prevention of thrombotic events for patients with previous myocardial infarction: a prespecified subgroup analysis of the TRA 2 degrees P-TIMI 50 trial. Lancet 380:1317-1324.

34

Tips thru Tables

Back to LDLC (and other) Targets

> **Ref.:** 2017 American Association of Clinical Endocrinologists and American College of Endocrinology Guidelines for Management of Dysimpidemia and Prevention of Cardiovascular Disease

Akshay Mehta

Atherosclerotic Cardiovascular Disease Risk Categories and Treatment Targets

Risk category	Risk factorsa/ 10-year riskb (mg/dL)	Treatment goals		
		LDL-C (mg/dL)	Non-HDL-C (mg/dL)	Apo B
Extreme risk	- Progressive ASCVD including unstable angina in patients after achieving an LDL-C < 70 mg/dL - Established clinical cardiovascular disease in patients with DM, CKD 3/4, or HeFH - History of premature ASCVD (< 55 male, < 65 female)	< 55	< 80	< 70
Very high risk	- Established or recent hospitalization for ACS, coronary, carotid or peripheral vascular disease, 10-year risk > 20% - Diabetes or CKD 3/4 with 1 or more risk factor(s) - HeFH	< 70	< 100	< 80
High risk	- ≥ 2 risk factors and 10-year risk 10-20% - Diabetes or CKD 3/4 with no other risk factors	< 100	< 130	< 90
Moderate risk	≤ 2 risk factors and 10-year risk < 10%	< 100	< 130	< 90
Low risk	0 risk factors	< 130	< 160	NR

Abbreviations: ACS = acute coronary syndrome; ASCVD = atherosclerotic cardiovascular disease; CKD = chronic kidney disease; DM = diabetes mellitus; HDL-C = high-density lipoprotein cholesterol; HeFH = heterozygous familial hypercholesterolemia; LDL-C = low-density lipoprotein cholesterol; MESA = Multi-Ethnic Study of Atherosclerosis; NR = not recommended; UKPDS = United Kingdom Prospective Diabetes Study.

a. Major independent risk factors are high LDL-C, polycystic ovary syndrome, cigarette smoking, hypertension (blood pressure ≥ 140/90 mmHg or on hypertensive medication), low HDL-C (< 40 mg/dL), family history of coronary artery disease (in male, first-degree relative younger than 55 years; in female, first-degree relative younger than 65 years), chronic renal disease (CKD) stage 3/4, evidence of coronary artery calcification and age (men ≥ 45; women ≥ 55 years). Subtract 1 risk factor if the person has high HDL-C.

b. Framingham risk scoring is applied to determine 10-year risk.

▌ Suggested Readings

1. Reproduced with permission from Garber et al. Endocr Pract. 2017;23:207-238.

35

Valvular Heart Disease Patients on Edoxaban or Warfarin in the ENGAGE AF-TIMI 48 Trial

Ref.: Raffaele De Caterina, MD, PHD,a Giulia Renda, MD, PHD,a Anthony P. Carnicelli, MD,b Francesco Nordio, PHD,b Marco Trevisan, MSC, b Michele F. Mercuri, MD,c Christian T. Ruff, MD, MPH,b Elliott M. Antman, MD,b Eugene Braunwald, MD,b Robert P. Giugliano, MD, SMb ABSTRACT BACKGROUND The use of non-vitamin K antagonist oral anticoagulants (NOACs) instead of vitamin K antagonists.

JACC; Vol 69,11,2017,1372-82

Key Points:

1. Patients with atrial fibrillation and concomitant valvular heart disease have higher risk of death, major adverse cardiovascular events and bleeding as compared to those with no valvular heart disease

2. Similar efficacy to warfarin was observed with high dose edoxaban and far less major bleeding as compared to warfarin

Dev Pahlajani

■ Objectives:

Non Vitamin-K antagonists oral coagulation (NOACs) are being increasingly used for stroke prevention in non valvular atrial fibrillation. However, the efficacy and safety in atrial fibrillation with valvular heart disease has not been established so far. Recently conducted trials have excluded patients with significant valvular heart disease particularly cases with severe mitral stenosis with atrial fibrillation and prosthetic heart valves from their studies.

Investigators of ENGAGE AF-TIMI trial studied the safety and efficacy outcomes in 18222 patients with no valvular heart disease and 2824 patients valvular heart disease with atrial fibrillation. The study included moderate aortic or mitral regurgitation, aortic stenosis, prior valve surgery, bioprosthesis replacement, valve repair and valvuloplasty. However, patients with severe mitral stenosis and mechanical heart valves were excluded. Outcomes of stroke, systemic embolic events, major bleeding were compared in patients with valvular heart disease versus non valvular heart disease and further efficacy and safety with net clinical outcomes were studied in patients with or without valvular heart disease comparing Edoxaban versus Warfarin.

■ Results:

Rate of stroke or systemic embolization were similar in patients with valvular heart disease versus non valvular heart disease with atrial fibrillation. However, those with valvular heart disease had higher risk of death major adverse cardiac events (MACE) and major bleeding. Higher dose of

Edoxaban with 60 mg daily and further adjusted to 30 mg for patients with low creatinine clearance, weight less than 60 kg were compared with Warfarin. The efficacy of reduction in systemic embolism was similar to Warfarin in patients with valvular heart disease when compared to non valvular heart disease. The risk of bleeding with Edoxaban was also lower as compared to Warfarin (Fig. 1 & 2).

▌ Conclusion:

Atrial Fibrillation in patients with valvular heart disease have high risk of death, MI and MACE and major bleeding as compared to those without valvular heart disease. When treated with higher dose of Edoxaban the clinical efficacy was similar to Warfarin and was associated with decreased major bleeding.

Fig. 1 : *Forest plot for efficacy outcomes in patients treated with higher-Dose edoxaban versus those treated with warfarin, with or without VHD*

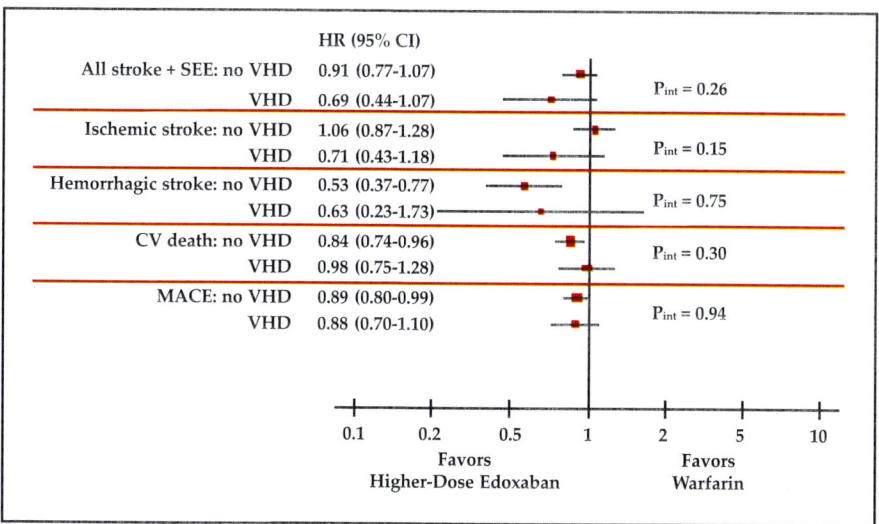

Fig. 2 : *Forest plot for safety outcmes in patients treated with higher-Dose edoxaban versus those treated with warfarin, with or without VHD*

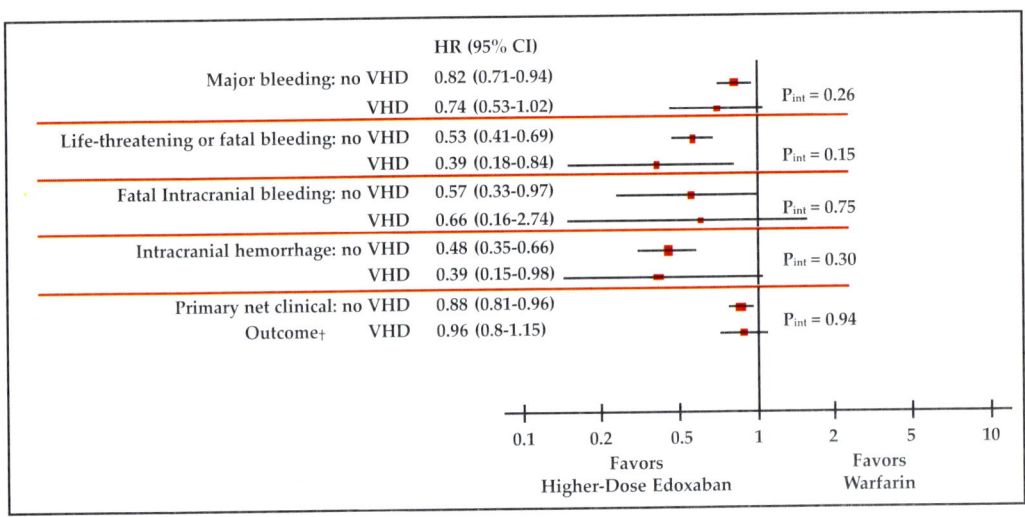

Suggested Readings

1. Gupta DK, Shah AM, Giugliano RP, et al. Left atrial structure and function in atrial fibrillation: ENGAGE AF-TIMI 48. Eur Heart J 2014;35:1457-65.

2. Breithardt G, Baumgartner H, Berkowitz SD, et al. Clinical characteristics and outcomes with rivaroxaban vs. warfarin in patients with non-valvular atrial fibrillation but underlying native mitral and aortic valve disease participating in the ROCKET AF trial. Eur Heart J 2014;35:3377-85.

3. Giugliano RP, Ruff CT, Braunwald E, et al. Edoxaban versus warfarin in patients with atrial fibrillation. N Engl J Med 2013;369:2093-104.

4. Ruff CT, Giugliano RP, Antman EM, et al. Evaluation of the novel factor Xainhibitor edoxaban compared with warfarin in patients with atrial fibrillation: design and rationale for the Effective anticoagulation with factor x A next Generation in Atrial Fibrillation-Thrombolysis In Myocardial Infarction study 48 (ENGAGE AF-TIMI 48). Am Heart J 2010;160:635-41.

5. Avezum A, Lopes RD, Schulte PJ, et al. Apixaban in comparison with warfarin in patients with atrial fibrillation and valvular heart disease: findings from the Apixaban for Reduction in Stroke and Other Thromboembolic Events in Atrial Fibrillation (ARISTOTLE) trial. Circulation 2015; 132:624-32.

36

Anticoagulation for Pregnant Women with Mechanical Heart Valves: A Systematic Review and Meta-analysis

Ref.: Rohan D'Souza Jackie Ostro Prakesh S. Shah Candice K. Silversides Ann Malinowski Kellie E. Murphy Mathew Sermer Nadine Shehata
Eur Heart J (2017) 38 (19): 1509-1516.

Akshay Mehta

▌ Study Objectives:

To compare maternal and foetal outcomes in women with mechanical heart valves (MHVs) treated with vitamin-K antagonists (VKAs), first-trimester heparin followed by VKAs (sequential treatment), low molecular weight heparin (LMWH) and unfractionated heparin (UFH) during pregnancy.

▌ Study Protocol:

Pooled incidence was calculated for maternal and foetal outcomes from a meta-analysis that included 46 publications, all of which were non-randomized prospective and retrospective studies, totalling 2468 pregnancies in women with a mechanical heart valve because of rheumatic or congenital heart disease, mostly single-tilting discs or bi-leaflet valves.

▌ Results and Conclusions:

Maternal mortality and thromboembolic complications (TECs) were lower with VKAs (with the recommended INR targets of 2.5-3.5 throughout pregnancy) (0.9% & 2.7%) when compared to sequential treatment (2% & 5.8%)and LMWH. (2.9% & 8.7%)However, VKAs were associated with more miscarriages and more embryo- and foetopathy (2%). Anticoagulation with heparin followed by VKAs eliminated VKA-related embryopathy, but not the risks of foetopathy, with an estimated risk of (1.4%) of foetal and neonatal anomalies. This regimen also carried a higher risk of thrombotic events compared with VKAs throughout pregnancy. In women with LMWH throughout pregnancy, there was no embryopathy or foetopathy related to the anticoagulant therapy, but thrombotic complications were highest.

▌ Comments :

VKAs are still the only oral anticoagulants for the long-term prevention of valve thrombosis in patients with mechanical heart valve prostheses.

Among the many limitations of VKAs, the risk of embryopathyis and foetopathy are important concerns. These defects occur when there is exposure to VKAs between the sixth and 12th week of pregnancy and in the 2nd and 3rd trimester respectively.

Both the ESC and AHA/ACC guidelines currently recommend the use of VKA throughout pregnancy in patients with a low daily dosing of a VKA and include the sequential anticoagulation of heparin during the first trimester to eliminate embryopathy, followed by a VKA during the second and third trimester of the pregnancy.

However, VKAs also carry a risk of neurological anomalies in the second and third trimester (foetopathy), and expose the neonate to a risk of bleeding, particularly intracranial haemorrhage during labour.

At the end of the pregnancy, to lessen the bleeding risk for both foetus and mother, oral anticoagulation with VKAs is switched to i.v. heparin or s.c. low molecular weight heparin (LMWH) before labour is expected. In the case of urgent delivery while on VKAs, the administration of vitamin K together with vitamin K-dependent coagulation factors will promptly revert the anticoagulation of the mother, but not of the foetus, and hence a caesarian section is advisable to reduce the risk of neonatal intracranial haemorrhage.

The present analysis found that VKAs were associated with fewest maternal complications but also with fewest livebirths, and significant number of embryopathies and foetopathies. Sequential treatment was associated with higher maternal complications when compared with VKAs and did not eliminate anticoagulant-related foetopathy. Finally LMWH was associated with the most livebirths and lowest incidence of fetal complications, albeit with a higher rate of TEC.

The latter may partly be explained by inappropriate low dosing. Twice-daily dosing with frequent measurement of peak and trough anti-Xa levels and adjusting dose to target anti-Xa levels may mitigate the risk of valve thrombosis.

Also the use of aspirin in addition, which was not analyzed may help reduce TEC.

Finally, the use of concurrent low dose VKA: When VKA was used throughout pregnancy, with a first-trimester warfarin daily dose of ≤ 5mg, the reported rate of live births was 84% vs. 44% with a warfarin daily dose of > 5 mg. Also there were fewer foetal anomalies (2.3% vs. 12%) with lower doses compared with higher doses of warfarin.

Hence, for best maternal and fetal outcomes, options that need to be studied are a combination of carefully dose monitored twice daily LMWH throughout pregnancy with low dose aspirin or low dose VKA. Also, fondaparinux, although not studied or proven except in isolated case reports, may offer the advantage of more convenient once daily dosing.

Till new studies throw more light, the dilemma for pregnant women with prosthetic heart valves still remains.

37

Complete or Culprit only Revascularization for Patients with Multivessel Coronary Artery Disease Undergoing PCI.

A Pairwise and Network Meta-analysis of Randomized Trials.

Ref.: Islam Y. Elgendy, Ahmed N. Mahmoud, Dharam J. Kumbhani, Deepak L. Bhatt, Anthony A. Bavry
JACC Cardiovascular Interventions 2017 Vol 10, no 4,315-24.

Key Points:
Complete revascularization during primary percutaneous coronary intervention is associated with similar outcomes of all cause death, spontaneous reinfarction as compared to staged or culprit only strategy.

Dev Pahlajani

■ Introduction:

Current guidelines recommend culprit only percutaneous coronary intervention (PCI) for patients undergoing primary PCI for acute myocardial infarction except those with hemodynamic compromise

Current study is a network meta-analysis of 10 trials that included 2285 patients.

Investigators analyzed the outcomes of four different revascularization strategies.

a. Complete revascularization at the index procedure

b. Staged procedure during index hospitalization

c. Staged procedure after discharge

d. Culprit only revascularization

Complete revascularization at the index procedure or staged procedure during hospitalization was associated with lower risk of urgent revascularization.

However, the risk of all cause mortality and spontaneous reinfarction was similar in all four strategies.

Irrespective of the timing of non culprit artery revascularization reduction of major adverse cardiac events (MACE) was similar with all four strategies.

The reduction in the MACE was significantly attributed to the reduction in the urgent revascularization (Ref. Fig).

Clinical Relevance:

The study points to the safety and benefit of complete revascularization either during index procedure or index hospitalization or staged procedure after discharge. The results are in agreement with the results of PRAMI and CvLPRIT trials.

Table 1 : Summary estimates for the outcomes in the pairwise meta-analysis

Outcome	Incidence complete/ Culpit-only, %/%	Risk Ratio	95% Confidence Interval	p Value	I^2, %
Major adverse cardiac events	14.6/24.4	0.57	0.42-0.77	< 0.0001	57
All-cause mortality	4.6/5.8	0.76	0.52-1.12	0.17	2
Spontaneous reinfarction	3.1/5.5	0.54	0.23-1.27	0.16	47
Urgent revascularization	9.0/18.6	0.44	0.30-0.66	< 0.0001	56

Suggested Readings

1. Gershlick AH, Khan JN, Kelly DJ, et al. Randomized trial of complete versus lesion-only revascularization in patients undergoing primary percutaneous coronary intervention for STEMI and multivessel disease: the CvLPRIT Trial. J Am Coll Cardiol 2015;65:963-72.

2. Engstrøm T, Kelbæk H, Helqvist S, et al. Complete revascularization versus treatment of the culprit lesion only in patients with ST-segment elevation myocardial infarction and multivessel disease (DANAMI-3-PRIMULTI): an open-label, randomized controlled trial. Lancet 2015;386:665-71.

3. Bhatt DL. Do we really know the CvLPRIT in myocardial infarction? Or just stent all lesions? J Am Coll Cardiol 2015;65:973-5.

38

Comparison of Coronary Artery Calcification, Carotid intima-media thickness and Ankle-brachial index for Predicting 10-year incident Cardiovascular Events in the General Population

Ref.: Marie Henrike Geisel Marcus Bauer Frauke Hennig Barbara Hoffmann Nils Lehmann Stefan Möhlenkamp Knut Kröger Kaffer Kara Tobias Müller Susanne Moebus
Eur Heart J (2017) 38 (23): 1815-1822

Akshay Mehta

▌ Study Objectives:

To determine which of the three markers : coronary artery calcification (CAC), carotid intima-media thickness (CIMT) and ankle-brachial index (ABI) in a primary prevention cohort improves cardiovascular (CV) risk discrimination best in 3 different risk groups.

▌ Study Protocol :

CAC, CIMT, and ABI were studied and quantified in 3108 subjects without prevalent CV diseases from the population-based Heinz Nixdorf Recall study. Associations with incident major CV events were assessed during a follow-up period of 10.3 ± 2.8 years with Cox proportional regressions in the total cohort and stratified by Framingham risk score (FRS) groups. Discrimination ability was evaluated with Harrell's C.

▌ Results & Conclusions:

All three markers were associated with raised hazard for CV events. However, CAC lead to highest reclassification in the total cohort, while also for CIMT and ABI significant improvement in net-reclassification was observed.

Stratifying by risk group, only CAC led to a significant improvement in risk prediction for subjects in the low and intermediate risk group. Comparing the other two measures, CIMT had a higher discriminative value for subjects with low risk, while ABI provided better discrimination for subjects with high risk according to traditional risk factors. The results confirmed that CAC-scoring outperforms CIMT and ABI in its overall predictive ability.

▌ Comments:

Prediction of cardiovascular risk based on risk factor profiles has limitations. Presence of subclinical atherosclerosis is a strong predictor clinical events and hence can be added to classical methods of risk prediction.

In this study on 3108 randomly selected apparently healthy population, coronary artery calcification (CAC), carotid intima-media thickness (CIMT) and ankle-brachial index (ABI) were studied and correlated with events over a 10 year period and compared with risk prediction by classical Framingham Risk Scores.

Significant differences of three measures of subclinical atherosclerosis (CAC-scoring, CIMT and ABI) regarding risk prediction were found.

CAC-score is best to improve risk prediction in the low and intermediate risk group. In contrast, ABI <0.9 improves prediction only in subjects with very high risk, but is a rare finding in subjects within the low or intermediate risk group.

Although a negative CIMT is reassuring in the low risk group, its assessment is prone to measurement errors which may limit its value in clinical practice, especially when performed by less experienced hands.

According to current ACC/AHA guidelines, assessment of CIMT is no longer recommended for risk estimation in the primary prevention. The results of this study confirm that in the intermediate and high risk cohort, CIMT is inferior to CAC and ABI.

Analysing the components of the primary endpoint, (coronary event, stroke, CV death), it was found that CAC was associated with all three components, CIMT with stroke and CV death and ABI with stroke.

Some limitations of the study were that

1. Predominant European population used; hence, generalization of the results to other ethnic groups is undetermined.

2. Carotid plaque measurements were not available for this analysis.

3. Finally, increased CIMT can also be altered by media layer increase as seen in hypertension.

❚ Clinical Application:

The value of these markers of atherosclerosis is mainly for the low and intermediate risk groups for their better reclassification which can help decision making for lipid lowering therapy.

However, it should be noted that absence of these markers in high risk patients according to FRS does not rule out elevated risk and such people deserve intensive preventive efforts independent of these markers of subclinical atherosclerosis.

39

Long-Term Outcomes of Stenting the Proximal Left Anterior Descending Artery in the PROTECT Trial

Ref.: Ariel Roguin, MD, PHD, Edoardo Camenzind, MD, Arthur Kerner, MD, Rafael Beyar, MD, DSC, Eric Boersma, MD, Laura Mauri, MD, Ph. Gabriel Steg, MD, William Wijns, MD
JACC: Cardiovascular Interventions 2017:Vol. 10, No. 6, 548-556

Key Points:

1. Stenting of proximal LAD is associated with higher rates of myocardial infarction as compared to non LAD lesions ...... long following period

2. However death, target vessel failure (TVF) and overall major adverse cardiac event rates are similar in LAD and non LAD locations

Dev Pahlajani

Disease of proximal left anterior descending artery (LAD) could lead to larger size myocardial infarction and severe LV dysfunction with higher mortality rates as compared to the lesions in the circumflex or right coronary artery. Proximal LAD supplies 40-45% of the LV myocardium. Additionally through the septal perforators it supplies the conduction system. Thus the resultant signicant loss of myocardium complete heart block is associated with high mortality and morbidity. Considering its importance, the guidelines recommend coronary artery bypass graft (CABG) in patients with multivessel disease where the LAD obstruction is a common denominator. However, the outcomes of percutaneous coronary interventricular (PCI) of LAD when compared to the RCA and/or circumflex lesions are not known.

▌ Methods:

In the PROTECT study 8709 patients were enrolled. The study was a multicenter PCI trial, the aims of which were to compare outcomes of zotarolimus stent versus sirolimus coated Cypher stent. Amongst the patients enrolled in the trial there were 2534 patients who had stents implanted in the proximal LAD and 6172 patients received stents in non LAD coronary arteries. The follow up was 4 years.

▌ Results:

At the end of 4 years the death rates were identical in both the groups (5.8% versus 5.8%). However, the patients who underwent PCI in proximalLAD had greater incidence of myocardial infarction

(6.2% versus 4.9% p = 0.015). The risk of clinically driven target vessel failure (TVF) or major adverse cardiac events (MACE) and stent thrombosis were similar .

Conclusion:

PCI of proximal LAD is not associated with any more increased risk of death as compared to non-LAD PCI except there is a higher incidence of myocardial infarction. MACE that included all cause death, myocardial infarction, emergency CABG surgery and clinically indicated TLR whereas TVF which included death, Target vessel MI, clinically driven TLR was also similar in both groups. Safety of LAD PCI has also been reported in earlier 2 meta-analysis which indicated that there was no difference in mortality, MI or stroke between PCI and CABG in patients who underwent revascularization for LAD lesions. With the currently available 2nd and 3rd generation drug eluting stents the results of PCI for LAD seem to be comparable to those achieved with CABG.

Suggested Readings

1. Aziz O, Rao C, Panesar SS, et al. Meta-analysis of minimally invasive internal thoracic artery bypass versus percutaneous revascularization for isolated lesions of the left anterior descending artery. BMJ 2007;334:617-21.

2. Kapoor JR, Gienger AL, Ardehali R, et al. Isolated disease of the proximal left anterior descending artery comparing the effectiveness of percutaneous coronary interventions and coronary artery bypass surgery. J Am CollCardiolIntv 2008;1:483-91.

3. Camenzind E, Wijns W, Mauri L, et al. Stent thrombosis and major clinical events at 3 years after zotarolimus-eluting or sirolimus-eluting coronary stent implantation: a randomised, multicentre, open-label, controlled trial. Lancet 2012; 380:1396-405.

4. Hannan EL, Zhong Y, Walford G, et al. Coronary artery bypass graft surgery versus drug-eluting stents for patients with isolated proximal left anterior descending disease. J Am CollCardiol 2014;64:2717-26.

40

Early use of N-Acetylcysteine (NAC) with Nitrate Therapy in Patients Undergoing Primary Percutaneous Coronary Intervention for ST-Segment Elevation Myocardial Infarction Reduces Myocardial Infarct Size (The NACIAM Trial)

Ref.: SivabaskariPasupathy, Rosanna Tavella, Suchi Grover, Betty Raman, Nathan E.K. Procter, Yang T. Du, Gnanadevan Mahadavan, Irene Stafford, Tamila Heresztyn, Andrew Holmes, Christopher Zeitz, Margaret Arstall, Joseph B. Selvanayagam, John D. Horowitz, John F. Beltrame
Circulation 2017; CIRCULATION AHA. 117.027575 Originally published June 20, 2017.

Key Points

1. Effects of intravenous high dose N-acetylcysteine (NAC, 29 g over 2 days) with background low-dose nitroglycerin (NTG, 7.2 mg over 2 days) on early cardiac magnetic resonance (CMR) imaging-assessed infarct size, and CMR-determined myocardial salvage and creatine kinase (CK) kinetics as secondary endpoints were assessed.

2. This small study on 75 patients showed that high dose intravenous NAC administered with low dose intravenous NTG is associated with reduced infarct size in STEMI patients undergoing PCI.

Akshay Mehta

■ Introduction:

Micro embolization following PTCA and ischemia-reperfusion injury, due to increased release of reactive oxygen species, are the Achilles heals of reperfusion therapy in STEMI and are responsible for substantial loss of myocardium despite an open epicardial artery.

NTG is a pro-drug that releases nitric oxide and N-acetylcysteine (NAC), a sulfhydryl-containing antioxidant, potentiates the vasodilator and anti-aggregatory effects of NTG. Also, NAC is an antioxidant with reactive oxygen species scavenging properties which thus may be a potentially beneficial therapy in primary PCI.

■ Methods:

All patients underwent emergency coronary angiography, with angioplasty/stenting, antiplatelet therapy (including aspirin, a P2Y12 receptor antagonist ± intravenous glycoprotein IIb/IIIa inhibitors) at the discretion of the interventional cardiologist.

Of 112 randomized STEMI patients, 75 (37 in NAC & 38 in Placebo) underwent early CMR imaging and were the subjects of analysis. Patients received either placebo or intravenous NAC infusion at 20mg/min in the first hour of admission followed by 10mg/min for the remaining 47 hours, accounting for at least a total of 29 grams over 48 hours. Both NAC and placebo were delivered in a 5% dextrose solution. In addition, both placebo- and NAC-treated patients received an NTG infusion through nonadsorbent tubing, with infusion rate held at 2.5 µg/min for 48 hours.

The pre-specified primary study endpoint was myocardial infarct size as measured by CMR imaging within 7 days (early) from the acute presentation. Secondary efficacy endpoints included both pre-specified (pre-PCI infarct-related artery patency and creatine kinase (CK) release kinetics) and post-hoc endpoints (CMR imaging assessed myocardial salvage and chest pain resolution).

Results:

Those randomized to NAC showed an absolute 5.5% reduction in CMR-assessed infarct size relative to placebo (median 11.0% vs 16.5%; p = 0.02). Myocardial salvage was approximately doubled in the NAC group (60% [37, 79%]) compared to placebo (27% [14, 42%], p < 0.01) and median CK areas under the curve were 22,000 IU hours and 38,000 IU hours in the NAC and placebo groups, respectively (p = 0.08).

NAC treatment was associated with more rapid resolution of chest pain. Late CMR imaging performed on 55 patients showed a significantly reduced infarct size in the NAC group.

Conclusions:

High dose intravenous NAC administered with low dose intravenous NTG on admission is associated with reduced infarct size in STEMI patients undergoing PCI with improved myocardial salvage, more rapid resolution of chest pain, a favorable in-hospital safety profile, and sustained evidence of infarct size reduction at 3 months post-STEMI.

Comments:

The strength of the study is that it is a randomized, double-blind, placebo-controlled, multicenter study done with these agents for the first time for STEMI patients, showing substantial benefits. Limitations are in the numbers and a lack of mechanism of action being delineated. Hence it requires a larger study to substantiate the claims made by this study.

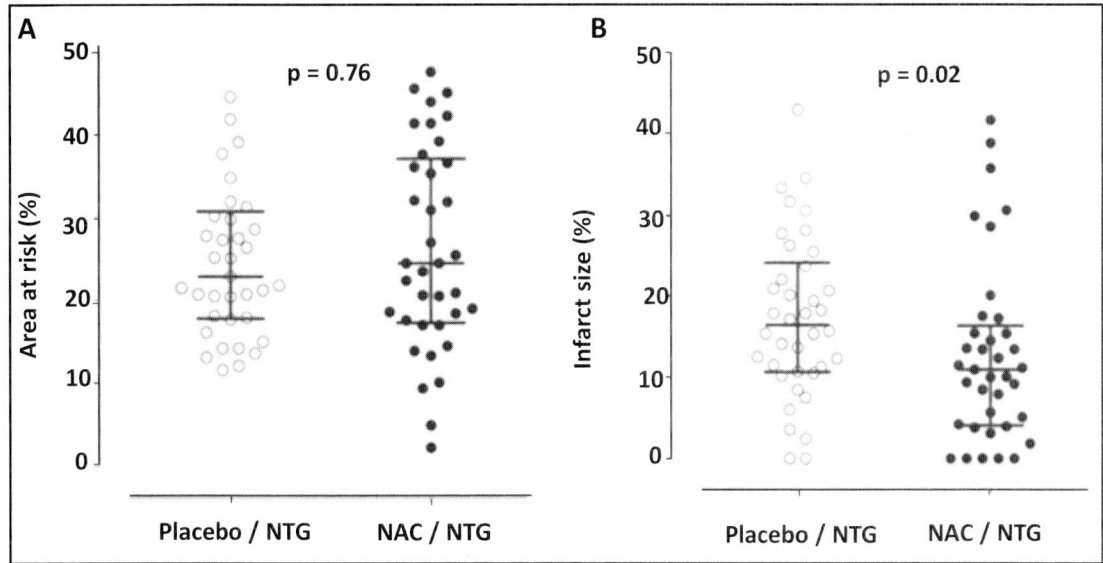

Individual patient data showing area at risk (A) and infarct size (B) for both placebo/nitroglycerin (NTG) and N-acetylcysteine (NAC)/NTG groups.

41

Safety and Efficacy of Bioabsorbable Polymer Coated Everolimus Eluting Coronary Stent in Patients with Diabetes, The Evolve II Diabetes Sub Study

Ref.: Dean J. Kereiakes, MD; Ian T. Meredith, AM, MBBS, PhD; Monica Masotti, MD; Didier Carrié, MD, PhD; Raul Moreno, MD; Andrejs Erglis, MD; Shamir R. Mehta, MD, MSc; Simon Elhadad, MD; Jacques Berland, MD; Bernardo Stein, MD; Juhani Airaksinen, MD; R. Lee Jobe, MD; Arthur Reitman, MD; Luc Janssens, MD; Thomas Christen, MD, PhD; Keith D. Dawkins, MD; Stephan Windecker, MD

LINK: Eurointervention 2017;12:1987-1994

Key Points:

1. Bioabsorbable polymer coated everolimus eluting coronary stent demonstrates safety in patients with diabetes.

2. Pre specified event rates of target lesion failure (TVF) were low.

3. 2 year target lesion failure (TLF) of cardiac death, target vessel myocardial infarction, ischemia driven target lesion revascularization (TLR) and stent thrombosis events are low number of patients.

Dev Pahlajani

■ **Methods:**

The current study is an analysis of outcomes from a pre-specified sub study of EVOLVE II trial. The aim was to evaluate the safety and effectiveness of the SYNERGY stent in patients with diabetes.

Diabetes is a single most important determinant of restenosis, stent thrombosis, myocardial infarction (MI) following stent implantation. The inflammatory reaction to polymer is of great concern which itself could add to increased burden of stent related complications. SYNERGY stent from Boston Scientific is coated as bioabsorbable polymer with everolimus drug. The earlier data had demonstrated similar 2 years TLF when compared to permanent polymer DES. The rates of stent thrombosis from 24 hours to two years were also extremely low. However, the outcomes in diabetics are ill-defined.

In this current study pre-specified data was collected from EVOLVE II study in diabetic patients. The primary end point was the rate of 12 month TLF which included composite of TVF, all deaths, all MI and TVR and stent thrombosis.

EVOLVE II diabetics included 466 patients and 2 year clinical follow up was available in 488 patients. The primary end point occurred in 7.5% patients with diabetes in the SYNERGY treated patients which was significantly lower than the performance goal of 14.5% (p = < 0.0001). The

2-year TLF was 11.2% which included cardiac death, 1.5% target vessel (TV) MI, 6.4% ischemia driven TLR and stent thrombosis in 1.1%. Thus the EVOLVE II sub study indicates that the bioabsorbable polymer coated everolimus eluting stent is associated with one sided 97.5% upper confidence limit which is significantly below the pre specified performance goal. The outcomes are comparable to those observed in overall patients in SYNERGY stent treated patients (6.7% and 9.4% respectively) which were enrolled in EVOVLE II trial.

The angiographic characteristics indicated the prevalence of a very small TV reference diameter in 27% and significant number of them had long length lesions. The trial also included significant number of complex target lesion morphology. There was a high prevalence of insulin treatment in whom the incidence of MI and stent thrombosis was low.

▌ Study Limitations:

It is a single arm evaluation. It is not a randomized trial.

Clinical application: The data is encouraging for using bioresorbable polymer coated drug eluting stent.

▌ Suggested Readings

1. Kereiakes DJ, Meredith IT, Windecker S, Lee Jobe R, Mehta SR, Sarembock IJ, Feldman RL, Stein B, Dubois C, Grady T, Saito S, Kimura T, Christen T, Allocco DJ, Dawkins KD. Efficacy and safety of a novel bioabsorbable polymer-coated, everolimuseluting coronary stent: the EVOLVE II Randomized Trial. Circ Cardiovasc Interv. 2015;8(4).

2. Wilson GJ, Marks A, Berg KJ, Eppihimer M, Sushkova N, Hawley SP, Robertson KA, Knapp D, Pennington DE, Chen YL, Foss A, Huibregtse B, Dawkins KD. The SYNERGY biodegradable polymer everolimus eluting coronary stent: Porcine vascular compatibility and polymer safety study. Catheter Cardiovasc Interv. 2015;86:E247-57 trial. Interv. 2008;1:699-709.

3. Kandzari DE, Amjadi N, Caputo C, Rowe SK, Williams J, Tamboli HP, Christen T, Allocco DJ, Dawkins KD. One-Year Outcomes in "Real-World" Patients Treated With a Thin-Strut, Platinum-Chromium, Everolimus-Eluting Stent (from the PROMUS Element Plus US Post-Approval Study [PE-Plus PAS]). Am J Cardiol. 2016;117:539-45.

4. Silber S, Serruys PW, Leon MB, Meredith IT, Windecker S, Neumann FJ, Belardi J, Widimsky P, Massaro J, Novack V, Yeung AC, Saito S, Mauri L. Clinical outcome of patients with and without diabetes mellitus after percutaneous coronary intervention with the resolute zotarolimus-eluting stent: 2-year results from the prospectively pooled analysis of the international global RESOLUTE program. JACC Cardiovasc Interv. 2013;6:357-68. -eluting stents. JAMA. 2005;293:2126-30.

5. de la Torre Hernández JM, Tejedor P, Camarero TG, Duran JM, Lee DH, Monedero J, Laso FS, Calderón MA, Veiga G, Zueco J. Early healing assessment with optical coherence tomography of everolimus-eluting stents with bioabsorbable polymer (synergy™) at 3 and 6 months after implantation.Catheter Cardiovasc Interv. 2016;88:E67-73.

6. Xu B, Gao R, Yang Y, Cao X, Qin L, Li Y, Li Z, Li X, Lin H, Guo Y, Ma Y, Wang J, Nie S, Xu L, Cao E, Guan C, Stone GW; PANDA III Investigators. Biodegradable Polymer-Based SirolimusEluting Stents With Differing Elution and Absorption Kinetics: The PANDA III Trial. J Am Coll Cardiol. 2016;67:2249-58. 32. Nakano M.

42

Time-to-Furosemide Treatment and Mortality in Patients Hospitalized with Acute Heart Failure

Ref.: Yuya Matsue, Kevin Damman, Adriaan A. Voors, Nobuyuki Kagiyama, Tetsuo Yamaguchi, Shunsuke Kuroda, Takahiro Okumura, Keisuke Kida, Atsushi Mizuno, Shogo Oishi, Yasutaka Inuzuka, Eiichi Akiyama, Ryuichi Matsukawa, Kota Kato, Satoshi Suzuki, Takashi Naruke, Kenji Yoshioka, Tatsuya Miyoshi, Yuichi Baba, Masayoshi Yamamoto, Koji Murai, Kazuo Mizutani, Kazuki Yoshida, Takeshi Kitai

Journal of the American College of Cardiology

Volume 69, Issue 25, June 2017DOI: 10.1016/j.jacc.2017.04.042

Key Points

1. REALITY-AHF (Registry Focused on Very Early Presentation and Treatment in Emergency Department of Acute Heart Failure) was a prospective, multicenter, observational cohort study that primarily aimed to assess the association between time to loop diuretic treatment and clinical outcome in patients with AHF admitted through the emergency department (ED).
2. Early treatment with intravenous loop diuretics was associated with lower in-hospital mortality.

Akshay Mehta

▮ Introduction:

Based on studies that have highlighted the time dependency of efficacy of any intervention/treatment in acute HF, recent HF guidelines and recommendations have emphasized the importance of immediate diagnosis and treatment of patients presenting with AHF.

However, this concept has only been evaluated using retrospective data, whereasthe REALITY-AHF study was a prospective multicenter study to evaluate the association between time to treatment with furosemide and clinical outcome in patients with AHF presenting at the ED.

▮ Methods:

For all patients admitted with AHF to the emergency department (ED), and given intravenous furosemide within 24 hours, door-to-furosemide (D2F) time was defined as the time from patient arrival at the ED to the first intravenous furosemide injection. Patients with a D2F time <60 min were pre-defined as the early treatment group. Primary outcome was all-cause in-hospital mortality.

▮ Results and Conclusions:

Out of 1,291 AHF patients treated with intravenous furosemide within 24 hrs of ED arrival, 481 patients (37.3%) were categorized as the early treatment group. In-hospital mortality was significantly lower in the early treatment group (2.3% vs. 6.0% in the nonearly treatment group; p = 0.002). In multivariate analysis, earlier treatment remained significantly associated with lower in-hospital mortality (odds ratio: 0.39; 95% confidence interval: 0.20 to 0.76; p = 0.006).

Thus this prospective multicenter, observational cohort study shows that early treatment with intravenous loop diuretics was associated with lower in-hospital mortality.

▌ Comments:

The benefits of early opening of the infarct related artery in acute STEMI is well established.

This REALITY-AHF study, with the help of prospective data now shows that time may be an important factor determining the success of decongestive therapy in acute HF also.

Interestingly, although the early treatment group had more moribund patients with more signs of congestion compared with the non-early treatment group, their in-hospital mortality was significantly lower. Thus this treatment strategy might be even more effective in high-risk patients with AHF.

Another interesting facet of the results was that delaying D2F time steeply increased the mortality risk till the first approximately 100 min, but after this effect leveled off, thus emphasizing that the first 1 hour is crucial for treatment.

With regards to the mechanism of benefit with early treatment, a recent sub-study of RELAX-AHF showed that some organ damage markers (including high-sensitivity troponin) increased over time in the first 2 days in placebo groups which was associated with mortality. Early treatment with serelaxin significantly attenuated the increase in high-sensitivity troponin within 2 days and decreased mortality. Thus, myocardial damage is a progressive phenomenon in the acute phase among patients with AHF, and that early decongestive treatment, by mitigating this organ damage might consequently improve outcomes.

Although the study is an observational one (it would be impossible ethically to randomize patients into early and late treatment groups), and the event numbers are small, it should have an impact on clinical practice, since, with aging population and decreasing mortality of patients with coronary artery disease, patients with HF are on the rise.

▌ Suggested Readings

1. Ponikowski P., Voors A.A., Anker S.D., et al. (2016) 2016 ESC Guidelines for the diagnosis and treatment of acute and chronic heart failure. Eur J Heart Fail 18:891-975.

2. Mebazaa A., Yilmaz M.B., Levy P., et al. (2015) Recommendations on pre-hospital and early hospital management of acute heart failure: a consensus paper from the Heart Failure Association of the European Society of Cardiology, the European Society of Emergency Medicine and the Society of Academic Emergency Medicine. Eur J Heart Fail 17:544-558.

43

Quality of Life After Surgery or DES in Patients With 3-Vessel or Left Main Disease

Ref.: Mouin S. Abdallah, Kaijun Wang, Elizabeth A. Magnuson, Ruben L. Osnabrugge, A. Pieter Kappetein, Marie-ClaudeMorice, Friedrich A. Mohr, Patrick W. Serruys, David J. Cohen
Journal of the American College of Cardiology 2017; 69, 16, 2039-2050.

Key Points:

1. Revascularization in 3 vessel or left main disease with CABG or percutaneous coronary intervention provides substantial improvement in quality of life over 5 years

2. Greater relief in angina is achieved with CABG

Dev Pahlajani

❚ Introduction:

Coronary artery bypass graft surgery (CABG) and percutaneous coronary intervention(PCI) with drug eluting stents (DES) are two useful modalities of revascularization that have improved the outcomes in patients with triple vessel and left main coronary artery disease. Several randomized control trials and registries have reported similar rates of mortality during short and medium term follow up with both strategies. However symptom relief and need for repeat revascularization has been reported to be in favor of CABG. Several earlier reports have indicated that the quality of life and symptom relief is better with CABG. The current study was undertaken to compare the quality of life improvement with CABG versus PCI in 1800 patients enrolled in the SYNTAX trial. In SYNTAX trial 897 were randomized to CABG and 903 to PCI. The trial compared outcome of death, MI and repeat revascularization up to 5 years follow up with both revascularization strategies.

In the current study the authors compared the quality of life and assessed the health status by Seattle Angina Questionnaire and a 36 item questionnaire to assess the generic health status.

❚ Results:

At the end of 5 years follow up patients who underwent CABG had better relief of angina frequency and better physical function including physical and emotional scales of questionnaire as compared to patients treated with PCI. The authors further analyzed the quality of life improvement and its correlation with SYNTAX score. Those patients who had low and intermediate SYNTAX score had similar relief in angina and similar quality of life improvement with both strategies. However, the maximum benefit was observed with CABG in patients with high SYNTAX score. At one year follow up 76.8% patients with CABG were angina free as compared to 71.5% treated with PCI (p = 0.01). At 5 years follow up

78.8% patients in CABG group were angina free versus 71.4% in the PCI group (p = 0.03). Among patients with high SYNTAX score 82.2% in CABG group were angina free as against 73.3% in the PCI group. However, there was no significant difference in the low and intermediate score patients.

▌ Discussion:

Some of the earlier trials like RITA, ARTS II and FREEDOM have reported similar conclusions. While the mortality and MI has been similar, relief of angina and repeat revascularization is better with CABG as compared to PCI.

▌ Conclusions:

The results of the data confirms the conclusions of some of the earlier trials that for patients with triple vessel and left main disease with complex coronary anatomy, CABG should be considered as a preferred mode of revascularization.

▌ Suggested Readings

1. Cohen DJ, Van Hout B, Serruys PW, et al. Quality of life after PCI with drug-eluting stents or coronary-artery bypass surgery. N Engl J Med 2011;364:1016-26.

2. Mohr FW, Morice MC, Kappetein AP, et al. Coronary artery bypass graft surgery versus percutaneous coronary intervention in patients with three-vessel disease and left main coronary disease: 5-year follow-up of the randomised, clinical SYNTAX trial. Lancet 2013;381:629-38.

3. Van Domburg RT, Daemen J, Morice MC, et al. Short- and long-term health related quality-of-life and anginal status of the Arterial Revascularisation Therapies Study part II, ARTS-II: sirolimus-eluting stents for the treatment of patients with multivessel coronary artery disease. Euro Intervention J 2010;5:962-7.

4. Abdallah MS, Wang K, Magnuson EA, et al. Quality of life after PCI vs CABG among patients with diabetes and multivessel coronary artery disease: a randomized clinical trial. JAMA 2013; 310:1581-90.

44

How Much is the Lay Public Aware About Risk Factors, Early Symptoms and Treatment of Heart Attack and Cardiac Arrest?

Public Knowledge of Cardiovascular Disease and Response to Acute Cardiac Events in Three Cities in China and India

Ref.: Herbert C Duber1,2, Claire R McNellan1, Alexandra Wollum1, Bryan Phillips1, Kate Allen1, Jonathan C Brown1, Miranda Bryant1, R B Guptam3, Yichong Li4, Piyusha Majumdar3, Gregory A Roth1,5, Blake Thomson1, Shelley Wilson1, Alexander Woldeab1, Maigeng Zhou4, Marie Ng1

Heart Published Online First: 29 June 2017. doi: 10.1136/heartjnl-2017-311388

Key Points

1. To get a baseline assessment of public awareness and practices about cardiovascular disease (CVD) risk factors, acute myocardial infarction (AMI) symptoms, cardiopulmonary resuscitation (CPR) and automated external defibrillators (AEDs), a household survey, supplemented by focus group and individual interviews, was used in 2 cities in China and one in India.

2. Knowledge of CVD risk factors and AMI symptoms were low to modest, CPR training was infrequentand there was little understanding of AEDs.

Akshay Mehta

■ Study Protocol:

This was a cross-sectional descriptive study in which data about knowledge, attitudes and practices (KAP) pertaining to

1. CVD risk factors,

2. AMI and SCA symptoms,

3. CPR and AED awareness, and

4. Emergency service utilization were collected from the general public, ages 18 and older, in Shanghai, Beijing and Bangalore through two complementary mechanisms:

   - A structured household survey, and

   - Key informant interviews and focus groups, between April and June 2015 (Shanghai, Beijing)and between September and November 2015 (Bangalore)

■ Results:

Knowledge of risk factors : Sixty eight percent of respondents in Beijing identified hypertension as a risk factor, and just under half identified high cholesterol, high blood glucose and obesity. In Shanghai these numbers were almost same. In Bangalore, only 20% of respondents identified high blood glucose as a risk factor, while even fewer named physical inactivity. Hypertension was mentioned by just under half of respondents, while hypercholesterolaemia was noted by 55% of the respondents. Over 90% of individuals surveyed in Bangalore named smoking as a CVD risk factor, the highest percentage of any risk factor identified in all three cities.

University or college education was associated with a statistically higher probability of naming a larger number of CVD risk factors.

■ AMI Symptoms:

Almost60% of respondents in each city named chest pain/discomfort as asymptom of AMI and pain/numbness or radiation to back/jaw/neck/arm/hand was listed by 57% of respondents in Bangalore. Symptoms such as diaphoresis, dizziness and nausea were mentioned less frequently.About 15%, 18% and 21% of respondents in Beijing, Shanghai and Bangalore were unable to name any AMI symptoms respectively.

Surprisingly, although higher education was found to be correlated with the ability to name AMI symptoms in Beijing and Shanghai, in Bangalore, those who had received a higher education actually named fewer AMI symptoms.

Focus group and patient interviews in Bangalore suggested that there was little public education covering this topic of AMI symptoms.

■ CPR and AED Awareness and Training:

About 92% of respondents in Bangalore had never heard of CPR, and very few (3%) were CPR-trained. The proportions of CPR-aware and CPR-trained individuals were greatest in Beijing. Even so, less than one-third of respondents reported any prior CPR training in that city. Higher education was found to be highly correlated with CPR knowledge.

Although respondents in all cities expressed interest in training, they were apprehensive about administering it due to fear of inadvertently injuring someone, incorrectly administering the procedure and/or potential legal implications.

Only 22% in Beijing, 15% in Shanghai and only 6% in Bangalore recognised the AED device on showing its picture.Athough recognition was lowest in Bangalore, respondents were substantially more likely to report willingness to use an AED (80%), whereas out of the respondents in Beijing and Shanghai, only 13% in each city reported willingness to use an AED. Majority of all who reported having received CPR training in the past in all three cities said that AED use was not explained during trainings.

■ Emergency Service Utilisation:

This was low in all cities, where reporting or first calling or visiting their doctor was more common. Logistics of transport and traffic were cited as reasons for low use of EMS.

■ Comments:

Besides being the first study to comprehensively examine public awareness around CVD risk factors, AMI symptoms and SCA response in China or India, it is an important study because knowing the level of existing awareness is the basis or the first step towards planning or disseminating heart related education to the public.

As the study shows, public awareness about risk factors and early warning signals of heart attack are rather low, indicating a wider need for educational activities among the public.

The new and simplified "hands only" CPR protocol will make bystander CPR more acceptable and successful and needs to be publicized. Also the spectacular improvement in the CPR results of out of hospital cardiac arrests in Seattle and other cities prods us to spread this awareness and utilization of these modalities to cover wider population than ever before.

If prevention and early interventions have to succeed in improving outcomes for patients with acute cardiac events we will need to improve general public knowledge, bystander responses, access to care and EMS capabilities. Gauging the present level of awareness is the first step in that direction which the present study importantly defines.

Bleeding Related Deaths in Relation to the Duration of Dual Antiplatelet Therapy After Coronary Stenting

Ref.: Tullio Palmerini, Letizia BacchiReggiani, Diego Della Riva, Mattia Romanello, Fausto Feres, Alexandre Abizaid,Martine Gilard, Marie-Claude Morice, Marco Valgimigli, Myeong-Ki Hong, Byeong-Keuk Kim, Yangsoo Jang, Hyo-Soo Kim, Kyung Woo Park, Antonio Colombo, Alaide Chieffo, Jung-Min Ahn, Seung-Jung Park, Stefanie Schüpke,Adnan Kastrati, Gilles Montalescot, Philippe Gabriel Steg, Abdourahmane Diallo, Eric Vicaut, Gerard Helft,Giuseppe Biondi-Zoccai, Bo Xu, Yaling Han, Philippe Genereux, Deepak L. Bhatt, Gregg W. Stone.
LINK: J Am Coll Cardiol 2017;69,16:2011-2022

Key Points:
1) Bleeding after percutaneous coronary intervention is an independent risk factor mortality within 1 year.
2) Shorter duration of dual antiplatelet therapy as compared to longer duration is associated with lower risk of bleeding.

Dev Pahlajani

Dual antiplatelet therapy (DAPT) is recommended as standard of care for patients who undergo percutaneous coronary intrervention (PCI) particularly with drug eluting stents (DES). However there is significant risk of bleeding among patients who receive DAPT for longer duration particularly those with comorbidities that predisposes them to risk of bleeding. Several trials in the past have shown bleeding to be an important risk factor for mortality and myocardial infarction. Recommended duration for dual antiplatelet therapy varies between 6 and 12 months and for some complicated cases DAPT has been continued for longer duration of up to two years. Not enough data is available that compares the risk of bleeding and death related to the duration of DAPT.

In the current meta-analysis individual patient data was obtained from randomized and aggregate data from 12 randomized control trials. The individual patient data meta-analysis included 11473 randomized patients. Out of these 5730 received shorter duration DAPT and 5743 were treated with longer duration DAPT. Shorter duration was defined as < 6 months and longer was defined as ≥ one year.

Conclusions:

Incidence of bleeding was significantly lower in the shorter duration treated patients as compared to the patients who received DAPT for longer duration (HR 0.66 p = 0.004). The mortality attributed to bleeding was defined as the one that occurred up to one year. Mortality was directly related to bleeding. There were 189 patients who developed bleeding and out of these 36 died (19%). In 13.4% death occurred within 30 days while 18.84% died at one year. Time adjustment multivariate analysis indicated bleeding to be an independent predictor of all-cause mortality within 30 days (p = < 0.001) and between one month and one year (p = 0.005).

Other co-morbidity conditions that were associated with all-cause death were age, diabetes, acute coronary syndrome.

Thus in the present study the investigators found that there was time-related association between bleeding and mortality and the bleeding was related to the duration of DAPT.

Discussion:

Since bleeding is an important risk factor contributing to higher mortality, efforts have been on to reduce the risk of bleeding by deploying stents which do not warrant longer duration DAPT. Recently stents with bioabsorbable polymers or polymer free stents have been used with reduced duration of DAPT. In the LEADERS FREE trial polymer free drug coated stent showed promising results which were better than the results of BMS with one month DAPT. Not only polymer free but second generation DES also have shown low adverse event rates with shorter duration DAPT. In the ZEUS trial zotarolimus eluting second generation stent has reported superior results as compared to BMS with one months' DAPT. The current meta-analysis does not provide information on the use of different types of P2Y12 inhibitors and their relation to bleeding and mortality. All the same the message is clear for interventional cardiologist to trim down the duration of DAPT particularly in the older population patients with cancer, gastro-intestinal pathology, diabetics and those at high risk of bleeding.

▌ Suggested Readings

1. Levine G.N., Bates E.R., Bittl J.A., et al. (2016) 2016 ACC/AHA guideline focused update on duration of dual antiplatelet therapy in patients with coronary artery disease: a report of the American College of Cardiology/American Heart Association Task Force on Clinical Practice Guidelines. J Am Coll Cardiol 68:1082-1115.

2. Palmerini T., Stone G.W. (2016) Optimal duration of dual antiplatelet therapy after drug-eluting stent implantation: conceptual evolution based on emerging evidence. Eur Heart J 37:353-364.

3. Colombo A., Chieffo A., Frasheri A., et al. (2014) Second-generation drug-eluting stent implantation followed by 6- versus 12-month dual antiplatelet therapy: the SECURITY randomized clinical trial. J Am Coll Cardiol 64:2086-2097.

4. Park S.J., Park D.W., Kim Y.H., et al. (2010) Duration of dual antiplatelet therapy after implantation of drug-eluting stents. N Engl J Med 362:1374-1382.

5. Yeh R.W., Secemsky E.A., Kereiakes D.J., et al. (2016) Development and validation of a prediction rule for benefit and harm of dual antiplatelet therapy beyond 1 year after percutaneous coronary intervention. JAMA 315:1735-1749.

6. Urban P, Abizaid A, Chevalier B, et al. Rationale and design of the LEADERS FREE trial: a randomized double-blind comparison of the Bio Freedom drug-coated stent vs the Gazelle bare metal stent in patients at high bleeding risk using a short (1 month) course of dual antiplatelet therapy. Am Heart J 2013;165:704-9.

7. Windecker S, Serruys PW, Wandel S, et al. Biolimus-eluting stent with biodegradable polymer versus sirolimuseluting stent with durable polymer for coronary revascularisation (LEADERS): a randomised non-inferiority trial. Lancet 2008;372:1163-73.

8. Martine Gilard, Paul Barragan, Arif A.L. Noryani, Hussam A. Noor, Talib Majwal, et al. 6-Versus 24-Month Dual Antiplatelet Therapy After Implantation of Drug-Eluting Stents in Patients Non resistant to Aspirin The Randomized, Multicenter ITALIC Trial. JACC 2015;65(8):805-815.

46

Outcome in Middle-Aged Individuals with Anomalous Origin of the Coronary Artery from the Opposite Sinus: A Matched Cohort Study

Ref.: Christoph Gräni, Dominik C. Benz Dominik A. Steffen Olivier F. Clerc Christian Schmied Mathias Possner Jan Vontobel Fran Mikulicic Cathérine Gebhard Aju P. Pazhenkottil
Eur Heart J (2017) 38 (25): 2009-2016.

Key Points

1) Whether anomalous origin of a coronary artery from the opposite sinus (ACAOS) is as much associated with adverse cardiac events in the middle-aged as in the young is not firmly established.
2) The outcome in middle-aged patients with newly diagnosed ACAOS by coronary computed tomography angiography (CCTA) was compared with that in a matched cohort over an observation period averaging 4 years
3) In the medium term, overall outcome of middle-aged patients with ACAOS was favourable and not statistically different from the matched control cohort without coronary artery anomalies regardless of intra- arterial course (IAC).

Akshay Mehta

■ Introduction:

Although the prevalence of anomalous origin of the coronary artery from the opposite sinus (ACAOS) is low (around 1% in the general population), it has been known to be associated with increased risk of sudden death in the young, whether the anomaly is right coronary artery origin from the left coronary sinus (right-ACAOS) or left coronary artery origin from the right coronary sinus (left-ACAOS). The following features are especially associated with high risk : ACAOS with an inter-arterial course (IAC, i.e. a vessel course between the aorta and the pulmonary artery), slit-like ostium, acute-angle take-off and intramural aortic course.

The increasing use of coronary computed tomography angiography (CCTA) for evaluation of suspected coronary artery disease (CAD)in middle-aged patients with a low-to-intermediate cardiovascular risk, has the propensity to incidentally pick up more and more cases of ACAOS. This poses a challenge in decision making for treatment which mostly is surgical.

■ Study Protocol:

After retrospectively identifying 66 patients (mean age 56 years) with newly diagnosed ACAOS by CCTA at a single center in Switzerland between March 2003 and May 2015 from among patients referred for evaluation of suspected or known CAD, they were matched to 132 controls without

ACAOS and followed up for an average for 4 years. End points looked at were major adverse cardiac events (i.e. myocardial infarction, revascularization and cardiac death). Forty (65%) patients were classified as having ACAOS with IAC.

Results and Conclusions:

The annual event rate of ACAOS vs. controls was 4.9 and 4.8%, the hazard ratio (HR) 0.94 (0.39-2.28, P=0.89). The annual event rate of ACAOS with IAC compared with their matched controls was 5.2 and 4.3%, and the HR 1.01 (95% CI 0.39-2.58, P=0.99). No cardiovascular death occurred in the cohort of ACAOS and no difference in outcome was found in patients with ACAOS and IAC vs. ACAOS without IAC or in right-ACAOS vs. left-ACAOS compared with their controls. The study also found no evidence for a higher incidence of obstructive or non-obstructive CAD among anomalous vs. non-anomalous coronary arteries.

Thus the mid- term outlook of newly diagnosed ACAOS and possible concomitant CAD in middle aged patients is favorable and comparable to a matched control cohort without coronary artery anomaly, regardless of whether ACAOS with or without IAC variants are present.

Comments and Clinical Application:

This is hitherto the largest study attempting to answer the question whether newly diagnosed ACAOS in middle-aged adults predisposes them to adverse cardiac events. The results clearly show that the answer is negative. Although the sample size was rather small and patients were identified retrospectively posing a selection bias, ACAOS is rare and selection bias would equally affect both the ACAOS as well as the control cohort.

The reason why ACAOS in older patients might be less relevant compared with younger patients could be that with increasing age stiffening of the anomalous vessels and the aortic wall occurs which may be protective against dynamic compression of the anomalous vessel which can occur with anatomic features such as IAC, slit-like ostium, acute angle take-off, intramural course, elliptical vessel course, and proximal vessel narrowing of the anomalous vessel. These characteristics may pose risk as a direct consequence of scissor-like shearing, kinking or lateral dynamic compression of the anomalous vessel due to increased pressure in both the aorta and the pulmonary artery during strenuous physical exercise.

Other reasons could be natural selection of inherently low-risk patients who survived through young age,or that with ageing, the risk for cardiovascular morbidity and mortality due to ACAOS is overshadowed by the increasing risk due to CAD.

Whatever the cause, the study shows that the risk of ACAOS in middle-aged patients is low and supports conservative approach in these patients.

47

Vasomotor Response to Nitroglycerine Over 5 Years Follow-Up After Everolimus-Eluting Bioresorbable Scaffold Implantation

Ref.: Dariusz Dudek, MD, PHD, ukasz Rzeszutko, MD, PHD, Yoshinobu Onuma, MD, PHD, Yohei Sotomi, MD, Rafa Depukat, Susan Veldhof, RN, Divine Ediebah, MS,Peter Staehr, MD, Wojciech Zasada, MD, PHD, Krzysztof P. Malinowski, MS, Grzegorz L. Kaluza, MD, PHD, Patrick W. Serruys, MD, PHD.
LINK: JACC: Cardiovascular Iinterventions 2017; 10(8): 786 -795.

Key Points:

1) There is no statistically significant increase of vasomotor response to intracoronary nitroglycerine (NTG) after implantation of ABSORB stent.

2) Maximum lumen diameter increased over period extending from 2 to 5 years.

3) Only modest improvement in the vasomotor tone over 5 years period consistent with degradation of bioresorption of the polymer stent.

Dev Pahlajani

Introduction:

Everolimus eluting polymer stent - ABSORB is expected to result in the progressive increase in the vasomotor tone over a period of 1-5 years -period that it takes for the polymer struts to completely absorb. However, the demonstration of such an increase has not been studied in great detail.

In the current study, the authors performed the quantitative coronary angiography of the segment stented by ABSORB scaffold along with vasomor response of the proximal and distal adjacent segments by infusing 200 µg of NTG diminished intra coronary. The study was conducted at two, three and five years follow up after PCI . The maximal and mean luminal diameter response of these segments was calculated. Patients were enrolled from ABSORB Cohort B trial which was a multicenter single arm unblinded trial that evaluated safety and feasibility of 3 x 18 mm ABSORB stent. The trial enrolled 101 patients and scaffold was imaged with intracoronary ultrasound imaging. The mean lumen diameter after NTG in the scaffold segment increased from 0.03 ± 0.09 at two years to 0.05 ± 0.12 mm at 3 years and up to 0.07 ± 0.08 mm at 5 years. The change was statistically insignificant. As opposed to this, the maximal lumen diameter change increased significantly from two years to 3 years to 5 years (p=0.04). Nonetheless the increments were small (0.03 ± 0.14 mm at 2 years, 0.06 ± 0.16 mm at 3 years and 0.11 ± 0.1 mm at 5 years). There was no change at the distal and adjacent segment for response to NTG from two years versus 5 years.

Discussion:

Advantage and one of the most important selling point of ABSORB - a bioresorbable Everolimus coated stent has been the hypothesis, that the vascular healing is better as compared to metallic stents and thus the vasomotor response and endothelial function would be preserved while the polymer of the stent undergoes absorption. We should therefore expect a progressive increase in vasomotor tone over 1-5 years. In the current study though there was a statistically significant increase in maximum lumen diameter the response was not dramatically great. Also, the mean lumen diameter did not show significant change. Recently published data of ABSORB 2 study also did not show significant superiority of vasomotor tone preservation as compared to the Xience V stent after 3 years. This could be due to the change in the design of the scaffold in the ABSORB II trial. Since numerically the change in numbers is small at 5 years following deployment of the scaffold could this mean that one has to wait for still longer post scaffold period to observe greater changes to have significant impact on the vasomotor tone and patient outcomes? Since there was unexpected improvement in the vasomotor tone in the Xience V stent arm in ABSORB II, similar large scale trials would be required to study vasomotor regain with scaffold and "metallic cages" with OCT and IV US.

▌ Suggested Readings

1. Brugaletta S, Heo JH, Garcia-Garcia HM, et al. Endothelial-dependent vasomotion in a coronary segment treated by ABSORB everolimus-eluting bioresorbable vascular scaffold system is related to plaque composition at the time of bioresorption of the polymer: indirect finding of vascular reparative therapy? Eur Heart J 2012; 33:1325-33.

2. Sarno G, Bruining N, Onuma Y, et al. Morphological and functional evaluation of the bioresorption of the bioresorbable everolimus-eluting vascular scaffold using IVUS, echogenicity and vasomotion testing at two year follow-up: a patient level insight into the ABSORB A clinical trial. Int J Cardiovasc Imaging 2012;28:51-8.

3. Serruys PW, Chevalier B, Sotomi Y, et al. Comparison of an everolimus-eluting bioresorbable scaffold with an everolimus-eluting metallic stent for the treatment of coronary artery stenosis (ABSORB II): a
    3 year, randomised, controlled, single-blind, multicentre clinical trial. Lancet 2016;388:2479-91.

4. Ormiston JA, Serruys PW, Onuma Y, et al. First serial assessment at 6 months and 2 years of the second generation of absorb everolimus-eluting bioresorbable vascular scaffold: a multi-imaging modality study. Circ Cardiovasc Interv 2012;5:620-32.

5. Shin DI, Kim PJ, Seung KB, et al. Drug-eluting stent implantation could be associated with longterm coronary endothelial dysfunction. Int Heart J 2007;48:553-67.

6. Hofma SH, van der Giessen WJ, van Dalen BM, et al. Indication of long-term endothelial dysfunction after sirolimus-eluting stent implantation. Eur Heart J 2006;27:166-70.

7. Sabate M, Kay P, van der Giessen WJ, et al. Functional assessment of coronary arteries previously treated with angioplasty and intracoronary radiation. Circulation 1999;100:1623-9.

8. Serruys PW, Ormiston JA, Onuma Y, et al. A bioabsorbable everolimus-eluting coronary stent system (ABSORB): 2-year outcomes and results from multiple imaging methods. Lancet 2009;373:897-

9. Serruys PW, Onuma Y, Dudek D, et al. Evaluation of the second generation of a bioresorbable everolimus-eluting vascular scaffold for the treatment of de novo coronary artery stenosis 12-month clinical and imaging outcomes. J Am Coll Cardiol 2011;58:1578-88.

10. Onuma Y, Serruys PW, Perkins L, et al. Intracoronary Optical coherence tomography and histology at 1 month and 2, 3, and 4 years after implantation of everolimus-eluting bioresorbable vascular scaffolds in a porcine coronary artery model: an attempt to decipher the human optical coherence tomography images in the ABSORB trial. Circulation 2010;122:2288-300.

11. Otsuka F, Pacheco E, Perkins LE, et al. Long-term safety of an everolimus-eluting bioresorbable vascular scaffold and the cobaltchromium XIENCE V stent in a porcine coronary artery model. Circ Cardiovasc Interv 2014;7: 330.

48

The Effects of Public Access Defibrillation on Survival After Out-of-Hospital Cardiac Arrest: A Systematic Review of Observational Studies

Ref.: JosefineBækgaard, SørenViereck, Thea Møller, Annette Ersbøll, Freddy Lippert and Fredrik Folke Circulation. 2017; Circulation AHA. 117.029067, originally published 2017

Key Points

1) To evaluate the effect of public access defibrillation (PAD) and different PAD strategies on survival after out-of-hospital cardiac arrest (OHCA), the authors searched Pubmed, Embase, and the Cochrane Library for observational studies reporting survival to hospital discharge in OHCA patients in whom an AED was used by non-emergency medical services.

2) PAD was divided into three groups according to who applied the defibrillator: 1. Non-dispatched lay first responders (available on site), 2. Professional first responders (firefighters/police) dispatched by the Emergency Medical Dispatch Center (EMDC) or 3. Lay first responders dispatched by the EMDC.

3) Whereas a median overall survival of 40% for OHCA patients treated by PAD was found, defibrillation by non-dispatched lay first responders was found to correlate with the highest impact on survival (53%) compared to EMDC-dispatched professional first responders (28.6%).No studies describing long-termsurvival after defibrillation performed by EMDC-dispatched lay first responders were identified.

Akshay Mehta

▌ Introduction:

At present the average survival after out-of-hospital cardiac arrest (OHCA) treated by EMS aloneremains below 10%. In fact the chance of survival decreases by 7-10% for every minute that passes without defibrillation.When bystander CPR is provided, the decline in survival is more gradual and averages 3-4% per minute delay to defibrillation. Besides, the proportion of victims in VF can be as high as 76% when the rhythm is recorded soon after collapse, but may deteriorate to asystole later.

Hence both the 2015 American Heart Association Guidelines as well as the 2015 European Resuscitation Council Guidelines recommend PAD based onstudies demonstrating increased survival after OHCA following defibrillation with an AEDprior to the arrival of EMS.

The present review not only shows a median survival to hospital discharge after OHCA of 40% when patients were defibrillated before EMS arrival by PAD, but also distinguishes between the different types of PAD strategies.

Methods:

From a systematic search of Pubmed, Embase, and the Cochrane Library for observational studies reporting survival to hospital discharge in OHCA patients where an AED had been used by non-emergency medical services, 18 reported PAD by non-dispatched lay first responders, 20 reported PAD by EMDC-dispatched professional first responders (firefighters/police) and three reported both. No qualified studies reporting survival after PAD by EMDC-dispatched lay first responders were found.

Results and Conclusions:

The results showed a median survival to hospital discharge after OHCA of 40% when patients were defibrillated before EMS arrival by PAD. In fact, the survival after OHCA seemed to be higher when the patient was defibrillated by non-dispatched lay first responders (53% median survival to hospital discharge) compared to EMDC-dispatched professional first responders (firefighters/police) (28.6% median survival to hospital discharge). The study does not throw light on how effective the 3rd method of PAD namely EMDC-dispatched lay first responders, would be, from the literature search they did.

Clinical Implications:

Early defibrillation, especially by on site lay first responders increases the chances of survival maximally, followed by EMDC-dispatched professional first responders (fire fighters/police) - both much above the 10% chances when only EMS is deployed. Although the study could not evaluate the effectiveness of EMDC-dispatched lay first responders, there is a great need of this mode of PAD because they can reach OHCA patients in residential areas where most (about 70%) of cardiac arrests occur. Already, recent studies from Sweden and Netherlands have shown benefits of activating lay persons via a mobile-phone positioning system and sending them to OHCAs within 500 to 1000 meters.

Thus, now there is a great need to deploy laypersons not only to use an on-site AED, but also dispatch them via the dispatch center to the OHCA victim.

The hitherto dismal scenario of OHCA is poised to change for the better with wider dissemination of CPR knowledge and greater availability of AED's in the community.

Suggested Readings

1. Perkins GD, Handley AJ, Koster RW, Castrén M, Smyth MA, Olasveengen T, Monsieurs KG, Raffay V, Gräsner J-T, Wenzel V, Ristagno G, Soar J. European Resuscitation Council Guidelines for Resuscitation 2015: Section 2. Adult basic life support and automated external defibrillation. Resuscitation. 2015;95:81-99.

2. Ringh M, Rosenqvist M, Hollenberg J, Jonsson M, Fredman D, Nordberg P, Järnbert-Pettersson H, Hasselqvist-Ax I, Riva G, Svensson L. Mobile-Phone Dispatch of Laypersons for CPR in Out-of-Hospital Cardiac Arrest. N Engl J Med. 2015;372:2316-2325.

49

Contemporary Incidence, Management and Long Term outcomes of PCI for Chronic Coronary Artery Total Occlusions

Ref.: Insights From The VA CART PROGRAM

LINK: JACC: Cardiovascular InterventionsVolume 2017;10,9:879 - 888

Key Points:

Chronic total occlusion is encountered in about 30% of patients with obstructive coronary artery disease. Over years there is progressive improvement in success rate to 80%. Successful PCI of CTO is associated with improved survival. Patients with unsuccessful CTO-PCI have higher comorbidities.

Dev Pahlajani

■ Introduction:

Chronic total occlusion of a coronary artery (CTO) is observed in about 20-30% patients with obstructive coronary artery disease who undergo coronary angiography. Over last 15 years there has been a progressive increase in the success rate of CTO PCI. There have been several single center and observational studies that have reported on the incidence, treatment and outcomes of patients who undergo CTO - PCI. However, the large scale detailed analysis of CTO success, incidence and outcomes is scanty. Current study was undertaken by the investigators to ascertain the incidence of CTO, success rate with PCI and complications with long term outcomes.

■ Methods:

The study enrolled 111273 patients who had obstructive coronary artery disease from 79 hospitals of USA. Out of these 29,399 (26.4%) had at least one CTO. The maximum distribution was in the right coronary artery (64.6%). Out of these 2393 (8.1%) underwent elective CTO PCI with success rate of 79.9%.

■ Results:

Patients with CTO were older, had higher co-morbidities like hypertension, hyperlipidemia, diabetes, history of smoking, dialysis, congestive heart failure, CVA, COPD, PVD, chronic depression, sleep apnea, prior dialysis, prior PCI, prior MI and prior CABG.

Those patients not on dialysis and non right coronary artery lesions had greater chance of success. Also patients with calcified CTO lesions had lesser success rate.

Patients with LAD CTOs had greater chance of success as compared to right coronary artery CTO.

Patients with successful PCI had lesser incidence of complications as compared to unsuccessful PCI (3.5% versus 7.5%). There was a progressive increase in the success rate over successive years.

Cumulative 2 years survival was higher among patients with successful versus failed PCI. Successful CTO-PCI was an independent predictor of 2 year survival (p=0.02).

However, the freedom from MI did not differ significantly while patients with unsuccessful CTO PCI had greater risk of undergoing CABG at 2 years (Ref. Fig).

■ **Comments:**

The data from the current study is in agreement with earlier studies that have reported incidence of 18-35% CTOs in patients with obstructive coronary artery disease. The number of patients subjected to CTO PCI in most of the studies has been low. CTO PCI is challenging coronary intervention due to procedural complexity, prolonged time and questionable long term benefits. In centers not familiar with different strategies of performing CTO-PCI are likely to encounter higher complication and lower success rates and patients are invariably referred for CABG. Familiarity with the procedure and improved devices and hardware and higher success rates of CTO PCI have been reported in the earlier trials as well. However, part of the decreased survival could be related to greater atherosclerotic burden and associated co-morbidities associated with unsuccessful PCI.

Fig. 1: *Kaplan-Meier Estimate for Coronary Artery Bypass Graft Surgery*

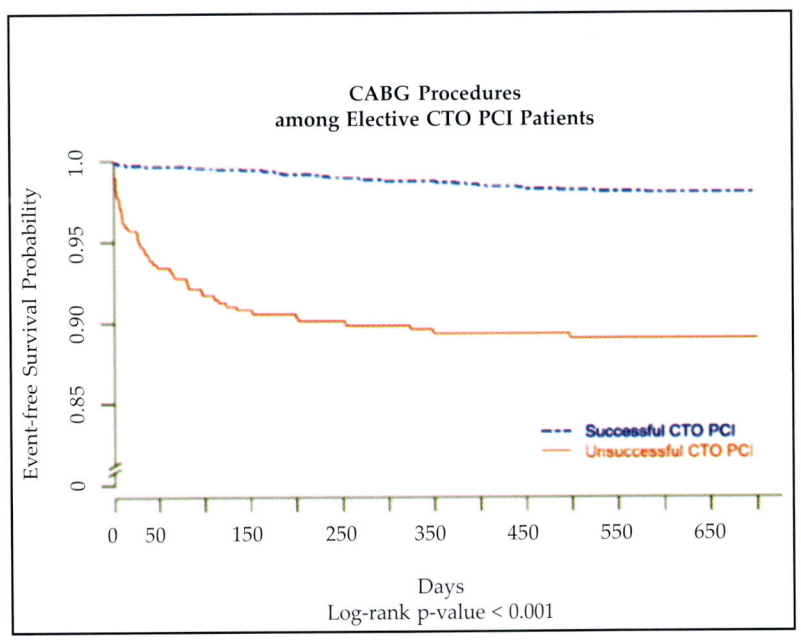

Suggested Readings

1. Fontenla A, Martínez-Ferrer JB, Alzueta J, et al. Incidence of arrhythmias in a large cohort of patients with current implantable cardioverter defibrillators in Spain: results from the UMBRELLA registry. Europace 2015;18:1726-34.

2. Sirnes PA, Myreng Y, Mølstad P, Bonarjee V, Golf S. Improvement in left ventricular ejection fraction and wall motion after successful recanalization of chronic coronary occlusions. Eur Heart J 1998;19:273-81.

3. Baks T, van Geuns RJ, Duncker DJ, et al. Prediction of left ventricular function after drug-eluting stent implantation for chronic total coronary occlusions. J Am CollCardiol 2006;47:721-5.

4. Werner GS. The role of coronary collaterals in chronic total occlusions. Curr Cardiol Rev 2014;10: 57-64.

5. Généreux P, Palmerini T, Caixeta A, et al. Quantification and impact of untreated coronary artery disease after percutaneous coronary intervention: the residual SYNTAX (Synergy Between PCI with Taxus and Cardiac Surgery) score. J Am Coll Cardiol 2012;59:2165-74.

6. Nombela-Franco L, Urena M, Jerez-Valero M, et al. Validation of the J-chronic total occlusion score for chronic total occlusion percutaneous coronary intervention in an independent contemporary cohort. Circ Cardiovasc Interv 2013;6: 635-43.

7. Cardona M, Martín V, Prat-Gonzalez S, et al. Benefits of chronic total coronary occlusion percutaneous intervention in patients with heart failure and reduced ejection fraction: insights from a cardiovascular magnetic resonance study. J Cardiovasc Magn Reson 2016;18:78.

8. Hoebers LP, Claessen BE, Elias J, Dangas GD, Mehran R, Henriques JP. Meta-analysis on the impact of percutaneous coronary intervention of chronic total occlusions on left ventricular function and clinical outcome. Int J Cardiol 2015;187:90-6.

9. Lee PH, Lee SW, Park HS, et al. Successful recanalization of native coronary chronic total occlusion is not associated with improved longterm survival. J Am Coll Cardiol Intv 2016;9: 530-8.

50

Impact of Routine Fractional Flow Reserve on Management Decision and 1-Year Clinical Outcome of Patients with Acute Coronary Syndromes

Ref.:Eric Van Belle, Sergio-Bravo Baptista, LuísRaposo, John Henderson, Gilles Rioufol, Lino Santos, Christophe Pouillot, Ruben Ramos, Thomas Cuisset, Rita Calé, Emmanuel Teiger, Elisabete Jorge, Loic Belle, Carina Machado, Didier Barreau, Marco Costa, Michel Hanssen, Eduardo Oliveira, Cyril Besnard, João Costa, Jean Dallongeville, JoãoPipa, Georgios Sideris, Nuno Fonseca, Christophe Bretelle, Jorge Guardado, Nicolas Lhoest, Bruno Silva, Pierre Barnay, Maria-João Sousa, Laurent Leborgne, João Carlos Silva, Flavien Vincent, Alberto Rodrigues, LuísSeca, Renato Fernandes and Patrick Dupouy for the PRIME-FFR Study Group.

Circulation: Cardiovascular Interventions. 2017;10:e004296, originally published June 14, 2017

Key Points

1. Although fractional flow reserve (FFR) has been shown to be of value in patients with stable coronary artery disease, with capacity to change the revascularization decision in up to 44% of patients and improve clinical outcomes and reduce costs, the same is unclear in patient with acute coronary syndrome (ACS).

2. By pooling two studies- R3F (French FFR Registry) and POST-IT (Portuguese Study on the Evaluation of FFR-Guided Treatment of Coronary Disease), management strategy based on angiography before performing FFR was prospectively defined in 533 patients with ACS. Final decision after FFR and 1-year clinical outcome were recorded.

3. Incorporating FFR into the decision-making process of ACS patients with obstructive coronary artery disease was associated with a high reclassification rate of treatment (38%) and was safe for outcomes assessed after 1 year.

Akshay Mehta

■ Introduction:

There are 2 issues concerning management decisions in patients with ACS. 1) More than 1 lesion suitable for revascularization and the difficulty of identification of the culprit lesion, particularly when stenoses are intermediate at angiography. 2) The reliability of FFR to guide PCI, which has been in doubt due to the potential for microcirculatory hypo-responsiveness that has been observed within the first days of the acute event.

Hence this hitherto largest prospective study ever to report on the use of FFR in patients with ACS undergoing angiography and its impact on treatment decisions and on clinical outcomes, assumes great importance.

Methods:

The R3F and the POST-IT were nationwide prospective studies that shared a common design and objective, dedicated to investigate the routine use of FFR at the time of diagnostic angiography and its impact on patient management decisions and on 1-year clinical outcome.

This PRIME-FFR joint international prospective study (POST-IT and R3F Integrated Multicenter Registries - Implementation of FFR in Routine Practice), a combination of the 2 FFR studies, aimed to assess the extent of treatment change by routine use of FFR in patients with ACS and the safety of reclassification as assessed by 1 year MACEand revascularization deferral as compared with stable patients.

Results:

The study showed that in the 533 ACS patients studied,

1. Reclassification rate of patient management strategy was as high in patients with ACS (38%) to the one observed in non-ACS.

2. PCI management based on this reclassification was safe, including deferral of PCI in FFR negative patients.

3. The diagnostic value of FFR was preserved in patients with single-vessel CADin whom the culprit vessel was the only one interrogated with FFR.

4. Disregarding the information derived from FFR was associated with adverse outcome in both groups, but more so in patients in ACS.

The study suggests that in patients with non-ST-segment-elevation ACS, microvascular dysfunction may be less marked, and the ability to achieve hyperemia likely is sufficient to maintain the diagnostic use of FFR, both in culprit and in non-culprit vessels, making FFR as useful in ACS patients as in non ACS patients.

Comments and Clinical Application:

This prospective, observational study of 533 ACS patients shows that the value of FFR is preserved in ACS patients as much as in stable patients. Decisions based on FFR, including the decision to defer PCI, are as safe as in stable patients and disregarding decisions based on FFR may be hazardous.

Large randomized trials, such as DEFINE-FLAIR 29 (Use of the Instantaneous Wave-Free Ratio or Fractional Flow Reserve in PCI) and iFR-SWEDEHEART30 (Evaluation of iFR vs FFR in Stable Angina or Acute Coronary Syndrome) powered for clinical outcomes, are awaited to further refine the role of FFR and of new physiological indexes, independent of inducible hyperemia, such as iFFR on patient management in this setting.

Till then, clinical practitioners can be assured that integrating FFR information to manage ACS patients is as safe and beneficial as it is in non ACS patients.

51

Procedural and Long Term Outcomes of Percutaneous Coronary Intervention for In-Stent CTO

Ref.: Iinterventions 2017;10(9):892-902

Key Points:
1. Prevalence rate of in-stent CTO (IS-CTO) is 12.3% of all CTOs.
2. Pocedural success rates are high and similar to those of de novo CTO.
3. IS-CTO is an independent marker of major adverse cardiac events (MACE) primarily driven by target vessel revascularization (TVR)

Dev Pahlajani

■ **Methods:**

The study enrolled consecutive patients from 3 participating centers from Italy, Canada and Spain who underwent CTO-PCI. Out of 899 patients 111 had IS-CTO while 788 underwent PCI for de novo CTO. Baseline clinical and angiographic characteristics, overall mean J-CTO score and mean PROGRESS CTO was similar in both types of CTO.

■ **Results:**

Procedural success rate was 86.5% in both the groups .

Use of Cross Boss was four times higher in the IS-CTO versus de novo CTO (26.1% versus 6.6%) (p=<0.001).

Less number of patients in IS-CTO received BVS and the total stent length was longer in IS-CTO.

Both types of CTOs had similar procedural complications.

The IS-CTO was an independent determinant of MACE. Post CABG status, eGFR ECS and number of diseased vessels and PROGRESS-CTO score were the other determinants of MACE.

Cases were followed up for a median period of 471 days.The adjusted 2 year survival free from MACE was lower in patients with IS-CTO versus de novo CTO which was primarily driven by TVR (Table).

Discussion:

About 5-25% patients with CTO who undergo PCI have been reported to have IS-CTO. The pathophysiology of IS-CTO is supposed to be in-stent restenosis with intimal hyperplasia due to neo intimal formation. However, other factors like stent thrombosis, neoatherosclerosis, stent fracture could be the other responsible factors.

Most of the patients can be tackled by antegrade technique with wire escalation. Newer technologies like Cross Boss have improved success rates.

Use of IVUS or OCT could guide as regards to the pathophysiology of IS-CTO and identify those patients who have either thrombus, malapposition. Appropriate delineation of pathophysiology would optimize results.

Table 1: Clinical outcomes on fellow-up

	Overall (N=807)	In-stent CTO (n=96)	De Novo CTO (n = 711)	P value
Major adverse cardiac events	119 (14.8)	20 (20.8)	99 (13.9)	0.07
Cardiac death	29 (3.6)	4 (4.2)	25 (3.5)	0.75
Target-vessel myocardial infarction	26 (3.2)	3 (3.1)	23 (3.2)	0.95
Ischemia-driven target-vessel revascularization	83 (10.3)	16 (16.7)	67 (9.4)	0.03
Value are n (%) CTO = chronic total occlusion				

▌ Suggested Readings

1. Abbas AE, Brewington SD, Dixon SR, Boura J, Grines CL, O'Neill WW. Success, safety, and mechanisms of failure of percutaneous coronary intervention for occlusive non-drug-eluting instent restenosis versus native artery total occlusion. Am J Cardiol 2005;95:1462-6.

2. Christopoulos G, Karmpaliotis D, Alaswad K, et al. The efficacy of "hybrid" percutaneous coronary intervention in chronic total occlusions caused by instent restenosis: Insights from a US multicenter registry. Catheter Cardiovasc Interv 2014;84:646-51.

3. Sianos G, Werner GS, Galassi AR, et al. Recanalisation of chronic total coronary occlusions: 2012 consensus document from the EuroCTO club. Euro Intervention 2012;8:139-45.

4. Morino Y, Abe M, Morimoto T, et al. Predicting successful guidewire crossing through chronic total occlusion of native coronary lesions within 30 minutes: the J-CTO (Multicenter CTO Registry in Japan) score as a difficulty grading and time assessment tool. J Am Coll Cardiol Intv 2011;4: 213-21.

5.. Christopoulos G, Kandzari DE, Yeh RW, et al. Development and validation of a novel scoring system for predicting technical success of chronic total occlusion percutaneous coronary interventions. J Am Coll Cardiol Intv 2016;9: 1-9.

6. Thygesen K, Alpert JS, Jaffe AS, et al. Third universal definition of myocardial infarction. Eur Heart J 2012;33:2551-67.

7. de la Torre Hernandez JM, Rumoroso JR, Subinas A, et al. Percutaneous intervention in chronic total coronary occlusions caused by in-stent restenosis. Procedural results and long term clinical outcomes in the TORO (Spanish registry of chronic total occlusion secondary to an occlusive in stent Resten Osis) multicenter registry.EuroIntervention 2016 Dec 20 [E-pub ahead of print].

8. Wilson WM, Walsh S, Hanratty C, et al. A novel approach to the management of occlusive in-stent restenosis (ISR). Euro Intervention 2014;9:1285-93.

9. Vaquerizo B, Barros A, Pujadas S, et al. Oneyear results of bioresorbable vascular scaffolds for coronary chronic total occlusions. Am J Cardiol 2016;117:906-17.

10. Hong SJ, Kim BK, Shin DH, et al. Usefulness of intravascular ultrasound guidance in percutaneous coronary intervention with second-generation drug-eluting stents for chronic total occlusions (from the Multicenter Korean-Chronic Total Occlusion Registry). Am J Cardiol 2014;114:534-40.

11. Azzalini L, Torregrossa G, Puskas JD, et al. Percutaneous revascularization of chronic total occlusions: rationale, indications, techniques, and the cardiac surgeon's point of view. Int J Cardiol 2017;231:90-6. 26.

52

Stress Perfusion CMR in Patients with Known and Suspected CAD

Ref.: Gabriella Vincenti, Pier Giorgio Ma sci, Pierre Monney, Tobias Rutz, Sarah Hugelshofer, Mirdita Gaxherri, Olivier Muller, Juan F. Iglesias, Eric Eeckhout, Valentina Lorenzoni, Cyril Pellaton, Christophe Sierro, Juerg Schwitter.
JACC: Cardiovascular Imaging May 2017, 10 (5) 526-537.

Key Points

1) To identify the ischemia threshold along with other prognostic factors that can identify patients who can be kept from revascularization intervention, stress-perfusion cardiac magnetic resonance (CMR) was used in a large cohort of all-comer patients with known or suspected coronary artery disease (CAD).
2) Out of a total of 1024 patients with known or suspected CAD, during a follow-up of 2.5 ± 1.0 years, an ischemia burden of ≥ 1.5 ischemic segments on stress-perfusion CMR was the strongest predictor of the primary and secondary endpoints. Age (≤ 67 years), left ventricular ejection fraction ($\geq 40\%$), and scar burden (LGE score ≥ 0.03) contributed significantly, but to a lesser extent to the prognosis.

Akshay Mehta

■ Introduction:

Based on landmark trials such as COURAGE and BARI 2 D, the American College of Cardiology Foundation/American Heart Association clinical practice guidelines for stable ischemic heart disease (SIHD) recommend prompt optimal medical treatment (OMT) for symptom reduction before embarking on an interventional strategy. Only when patients fail to reduce their symptoms or experience breakthrough ischemic symptoms should patients be referred for coronary revascularization. This is because of lack of mortality benefit or reduction in MI rates with invasive treatment in such patients as compared to OMT. However, stable IHD patients are a diverse group with differing levels of ischemia burden, LV function and scar burden. Would ischemia burden segregate SIHD patients into groups with diverse risks so as to identify the high risk group that may be benefitted with intervention?

Already, the COURAGE nuclear substudy and FAME II trials have hinted at some benefit of revascularization in stable IHD patients who have significant ischemia detected by SPECT perfusion or FFR respectively. Albeit, benefits in terms of mortality or MI reduction was not conclusively proven in these studies.

Cardiac magnetic resonance (CMR) has the advantages of producing high-resolution perfusion or cine imaging during pharmacological stress for myocardial infarction and ventricular function, without the need for ionizing radiation. Current practice guidelines in the United States and Europe recommend stress CMR imaging as a first-line procedure, with Class I and IIa indications for patients at intermediate pre-test risk who are unable to perform exercise stress testing or for those with an uninterpretable electrocardiography.

Study Protocol:

Between January 2012 and May 2015, 1024 patients from 1103 all-comer consecutive patients with known or suspected CAD referred to adenosine stress-perfusion CMR for assessment of myocardial ischemia were prospectively enrolled in a pre-defined registry at the CMR Center of the University Hospital Lausanne. The CMR examination included standard functional adenosine stress first-pass perfusion and late gadolinium enhancement (LGE) acquisitions. Presence of ischemia and ischemia burden (number of ischemic segments on a 16-segment model), and of scar and scar burden (number and transmurality of scar segments in a 17-segment model) were assessed. The primary endpoint was a composite of cardiac death, nonfatal myocardial infarction (MI), and late coronary revascularization (> 90 days post-CMR); the secondary endpoint was a composite of cardiac death and nonfatal MI.

Results and Conclusion:

During a follow-up of 2.5 ± 1.0 years, in multivariate Cox regression analyses of the entire population and of the subgroups, ischemia burden (threshold: ≥ 1.5 ischemic segments) was consistently the strongest predictor of the primary and secondary endpoints with hazard ratios (HRs) of 7.42 to 8.72 ($p < 0.001$), whereas age (≥ 67 years), left ventricular ejection fraction ($\leq 40\%$), and scar burden (LGE score ≥ 0.03) contributed significantly, but to a lesser extent.

Thus, patients with zero or 1 ischemic segment can be safely deferred from revascularizations. Age, LVEF, and scar burden contributed to a lesser extent to the outcome prediction.

Comments :

Even when the analysis was limited to hard endpoints (i.e., cardiac death and nonfatal MI), the study showed that an ischemic burden of ≥ 1.5 segments was independently associated with a nearly 9-fold increased risk during a mean follow-up of 2.5 years. This risk was same in patients with normal or reduced LVEF, with or without scar, or in patients with or without a history of coronary revascularization.

Interestingly, this CMR-based threshold (2 out of 17 segments) was close to the reported 12.5% for scintigraphic techniques. Although the risk was high in patients with 2 or more ischemic segments, the study cannot conclusively say that such patients did better with PCI intervention.

This is because this was an observational study which did not give details about the medical treatment, nor did it randomize patients into conservative therapy versus intervention. Hence all it shows is that in patients with < 1.5 ischemic segments, PCI can be safely deferred.

Although its wide spread application in practice can be hampered by problems of equipment availability, professional expertise etc, it validates the concept of an ischemic threshold which can define prognosis which in turn could help decide therapy.

53

Instantaneous Wave-Free Ratio versus Fractional Flow Reserve to Guide PCI

Ref.: MatthiasGötberg, M.D., Ph.D., Evald H. Christiansen, M.D., Ph.D., Ingibjörg J. Gudmundsdottir, M.D. et al.

LINK:N Engl J Med 2017; 376:1813-1823

Dev Pahlajani

Introduction:

Fractional flow reserve (FFR) guided PCI has been shown to be associated with better outcomes than the angiographic guided PCI. Conventionally most of the cardiac catheterization laboratories use FFR technique wherein maximum coronary dilatation is achieved by adenosine, papavarine or nicorandil. However, lately instant aneous wave free ratio (iIFR) has been used to assess the severity of coronary artery obstruction. While the use of iFR has been shown to match diagnostic accuracy of FFR, comparison of the clinical outcomes with these two different techniques are ill-defined. In the current study the investigators evaluated whether iFR is non-inferior to FFR and the clinical outcomes are comparable with both modalities of investigations.

Methods:

The current trial is a multi-center randomized open label clinical trial and enrolled 2037 patients with stable angina or acute coronary syndrome. Patients were randomly assigned to iIFR or FFR. The primary end point was composite of death from any cause, non-fatal MI or unplanned revascularization within 12 months. Of the 2037 patients, 1012 were assigned to FFR group and 1007 to FFR group. The primary end point occurred in 68 (6.7%) in the iFR group and 61 (6.1%) in the FFR group) (p=0.007 for non-inferiority). There was no difference in the rate of MI, target lesion revascularization, restenosis and stent thrombosis in both the groups. Patients evaluated with FFR more frequently complained of chest pain than the patients who underwent iFR.

Discussion:

iIFR isolates specific period for diastole which is wave free period when competing forces in the cardiac cycle are quiescent. During this period, the pressure and flow are linearly related and does not require the maximum vasodilation with adenosine that is required for measuring FFR. The procedure is performed very quickly in the cardiac catheterization laboratory and does not need elaborate measurement after injecting adenosine IV or through intra-coronary route. The iIFR could also be calculated on while withdrawal of the wire and one can plot the change of FFR or transient change throughout the vessel. Several studies like ADVISE that compared the FFR and iFR demonstrated that over a specific period in diastole microcirculatory resistance was lowest in the cardiac cycle. It was consistently reproduced in the left and right coronary arteries.

The current study has demonstrated the clinical validity of the test indicating non inferiority of the iFR versus conventional FFR.

However, there have been some concerns regarding the assumption that the minimum resting myocardial resistance through diastole is the same as the mean resistance during hyperemia. It has been shown that the blood flow primarily occurs in the coronary arteries during diastole and increases in both phases of the cardiac cycle and much more during diastole. Therefore, the values of iFR may not correlate with FFR. Nonetheless, the conclusions of the current study are quite compelling and there is ground for further large scale trials.

▍ Suggested Readings

1. Sen, Sayan :Development and Validation of a New Adenosine-Independent Index of Stenosis Severity From Coronary Wave-Intensity Analysis". Journal of the American College of Cardiology.2012: 59 (15): 1392-1402.

2. Nijjer, SS; Sen, S; Petraco, R; Escaned, J; Echavarria-Pinto, M; Broyd, C; Al-Lamee, R; Foin, N; Foale, RA; Malik, IS; Mikhail, GW; Sethi, AS; Al-Bustami, M; Kaprielian, RR; Khan, MA; Baker, CS; Bellamy, MF; Hughes, AD; Mayet, J; Francis, DP; Di Mario, C; Davies, JE: (December 2014). "Pre-angioplasty instantaneous wave-free ratio pullback provides virtual intervention and predicts hemodynamic outcome for serial lesions and diffuse coronary artery disease". JACC. Cardiovascular interventions. 2014, 7, 1386-96.

54

Biomarker-Based Risk Model to Predict Cardiovascular Mortality in Patients with Stable Coronary Disease

Ref.: Daniel Lindholm, Johan Lindbäck, Paul W. Armstrong, Andrzej Budaj, Christopher P. Cannon, Christopher B. Granger, Emil Hagström, Claes Held, Wolfgang Koenig, Ollie Östlund, Ralph A.H. Stewart, Joseph Soffer, Harvey D. White, Robbert J. de Winter, Philippe Gabriel Steg, Agneta Siegbahn, Marcus E. Kleber, Alexander Dressel, Tanja B. Grammer, Winfried März, Lars Wallentin

Journal of the American College of Cardiology

Vol. 70, Issue 7, August 2017.

Key Points

1) This study assessed the prognostic value of biomarkers and clinical variables to develop a biomarker-based prediction model in patients with stable CHD.

2) The 3 most important biomarkers were N-terminal pro-B-type natriuretic peptide (NT-proBNP), high-sensitivity cardiac troponin T (hs-cTnT), and low-density lipoprotein cholesterol. The final prediction model included age (A), biomarkers (B) (NT-proBNP, hs-cTnT, and low-density lipoprotein cholesterol), and clinical variables (C) (smoking, diabetes mellitus, and peripheral arterial disease), thus providing a robust tool for the prediction of CV death in patients with stable CHD.

Akshay Mehta

■ **Study Protocol:**

This was a biomarker substudy of the STABILITY (Stabilization of Atherosclerotic Plaque by Initiation of Darapladib Therapy) trial which compared darapladib, a selective inhibitor of Lp-PLA2, with placebo in 15,828 patients with stable CHD. A cohort of 13,164 patients with stable CHD, was analyzed for several candidate biomarkers and clinical variables and multivariable Cox regression used to develop a clinical prediction model based on the most important markers. Patients included in this trial either had a history of myocardial infarction, percutaneous coronary intervention, or coronary artery bypass grafting, or had angiographic evidence of multivessel obstructive coronary heart disease. The primary outcome was cardiovascular (CV) death, but model performance was also explored for other key outcomes. It was internally as well as externally validated in 1,547 patients in another study.

■ Results and Conclusions:

N-terminal pro-B-type natriuretic peptide (NT-proBNP) and cardiac troponin T measured with a high sensitivity assay (hs-cTnT) provided stronger prognostic information than any clinical variable and all other biomarkers concerning the endpoint of cardiovascular death. Adding 1 more biomarker (i.e., low-density lipoprotein cholesterol) and 4 clinical variables (i.e., age, diabetes mellitus, peripheral arterial disease, and smoking) modestly improved risk prediction Thus, an internally and externally validated biomarker-based model for the prediction of CV death in patients with stable CHD containing age (A), the biomarkers (B) NT-proBNP, hs-cTnT, and LDL-C, and the clinical variables (C) smoking, DM, and PAD was derived. The biomarker-based ABC-CHD model predicted not only the risk of CV death, but also the risk of most other important CV events, such as HF, MI, stroke, or composites of these events.

■ Comments :

The strength of the study was that a minimum number of easily measurable variables were derived from a cohort consisting of a contemporary large multinational multicenter population of patients with stable CHD which was also validated in another cohort of patients from another trial.

There was a possibility of selection bias as both cohorts consisted of high-risk subsets that may not be representative of patients with truly stable CHD.

NT-proBNP and hs-cTnT, are markers of increased myocardial stress and rate of cardiomyocyte turnover that may result in diffuse myocardial fibrosis, hypertrophy, and diastolic dysfunction. As these result in increased risk of heart failure, ventricular arrhythmias, and cardiovascular death, a strong association between them and these outcomes is not surprising and measures that are associated with decreased circulating concentrations of NT-proBNP and hs-cTnT may be beneficial.

Thus the ABC-CHD risk model score should probably not result in treatment with 1 specific drug for all patients, but rather prompt further cardiac evaluation to identify potential causes of biomarker elevation.

However, before it can become an established tool to guide decisions on more intense secondary prevention measures its broad validity and clinical utility should be tested in larger prospective clinical trials.

55

Cut off value and Long-Term Prediction of Clinical Events by FFR Measured Immediately After Implantation of a Drug - Eluting Stent in Patients with Coronary Artery Disease

1-3 Year Results from the DKCRUSH VII Registry

Ref.: Sui-Ji Li, MD, Zhen Ge, MD, Jing Kan, MBBS, Jun-Jie Zhang, PHD, Fei Ye, MD, Tak W. Kwan, MD, et al JACC Iinterventions 2017,10(10); 986 - 995

Key Points:

1. Following percutaneous coronary intervention (PCI) with drug eluting stents (DES) for bifurcations lesions FFR of ≤ 0.88 strongly correlates with target vessel failure (TVF)

2. For LAD bifurcation lesions post PCI FFR of ≤ 0.905 strongly predicts one year adverse outcome.

3. Stent length and diameter are independent determinants of lower post DES FFR.

4. The difference in outcomes is maintained up to 3 years follow up.

Dev Pahlajani

■ Introduction:

There has been significant reduction in the rate of post PCI in-stent restenosis following the wide spread use of DES. Fractional flow reserve (FFR) guided PCI has been used to appropriately select patients for PCI. Approximately 25-30% patients have bifurcation lesions which are tackled by various bifurcation PCI techniques. Despite achieving optimum angiographic results target vessel failure (TVF) has been reported in significant number of patients. Use of IVUS and FFR have been reported in some studies to optimize the results and predict outcomes. However ideal cut off value of FFR that would predict unfavorable outcomes has not been studied in great details. The current study aimed to ascertain the cut off value to predict adverse events following bifurcation PCI with DKCRUSH technique.

■ Methods:

Present study is a registry of bifurcation patients who underwent PCI by DKCRUSH technique. FFR was measured before and after PCI after having received single stent. PCI was performed in patients who had FFR of < 0.75 to 0.8. One year clinical follow up was available in 1,476 patients. Out of these, 478 patients had FFR of ≤ 0.88 whereas it was > 0.88 in 998 patients. Further 3 years follow up was available in both the groups. Post DES FFR value of < 0.88 had sensitivity of 83% and specificity of 78% for TVF.

Patients in the < 0.88 FFR group were more likely to be obese, taller, hyperlipidemic, diabetics with prior MI PCI than patients in FFR > 0.88. These patients also needed more medications before PCI. Total of 88 TVFs occurred in 40 patients (4%) in the FFR of > 0.88 group and 48 (10%) in the FFR of < 0.88 group (p=0.001). The TVF was mostly driven by greater number of cardiac deaths and TVR. At 3 years follow up TVF occurred in 119 patients. It occurred in 6.1% patients with FFR of > 0.88 and 12.3 % in the group of patients with FFR value of < 0.88 (p=0.002). Cardiac death was also higher in the lower FFR group versus higher FFR group (0.6% v/s 1. 9%). The TVR was higher in the lower FFR group.

However, the cut off point in case of LAD lesions was higher and post DES FFR of < 0.905 correlated strongly with 1 year TVF (Ref Fig A-F).

▌ Conclusions:

Post PCI FFR measurement following bifurcation stenting is a good clinical tool to identify patients who could be at greater risk of TVF. The data from the current study indicates that it is prudent to achieve FFR >0.88. Bifurcation lesions of LAD need careful attention since one must attempt to achieve higher cut off value of FFR as compared to the other vessels. The use of IVUS and OCT are excellent additional tools to achieve optimum results. Some of the earlier studies had reported cut off point of <0.9 to be associated with higher rates of adverse events.

While the current study is a registry which could have its inherent limitations, its findings are of great clinical value. Following bifurcation stenting mere angiographic impression may be misleading. Additional imaging tools like IVUS, OCT and physiological pressure measurements will help to improve medium and long terms results.

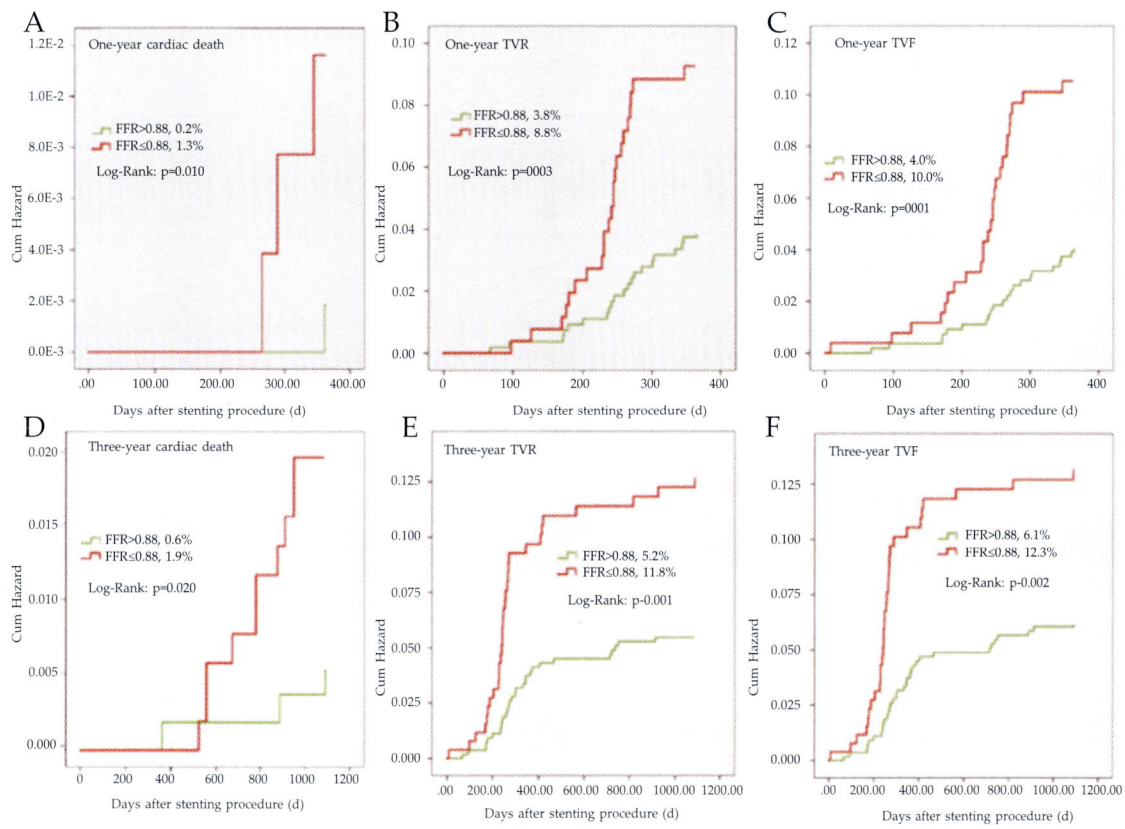

■ Suggested Readings

1. Chen SL, Xu B, Chen JB, et al. Diagnostic accuracy of quantitative angiographic and intravascular ultrasound parameters predicting the functional significance of single de novo lesions. Int J Cardiol 2013;168:1364-9.

2. Johnson NP, Toth GG, Lai D, et al. Prognostic value of fractional flow reserve: linking physiologic severity to clinical outcomes. J Am Coll Cardiol 2014;64:1641-54.

3. vanNunen LX, Zimmermann FM, Tonino PA, et al., FAME Study Investigators. Fractional flow reserve versus angiography for guidance of PCI in patients with multivessel coronary artery disease (FAME): 5-year follow-up of a randomized controlled trial. Lancet 2015;386:1853-60.

4. Pijls NH, Klauss V, Siebert U, et al. Coronary pressure measurement after stenting predicts adverse events at follow-up: a multicenter registry. Circulation 2002;105:2950-4.

5. Doh JH, Nam CW, Koo BK, et al. Clinical relevance of poststent fractional flow reserve after drug-eluting stent implantation. J Invasive Cardiol 2015;27:346-51.

6. Reith S, Battermann S, Hellmich M, Marx N, Burgmaier M. Correlation between OCT-derived intrastent dimensions and fractional flow reserve measurements after coronary stent implantation and impact on clinical outcome. J Invasive Cardiol 2015;27:222-8.

56

Predictors of Long-term Outcomes After Bypass Grafting Versus Drug-Eluting Stent Implantation for Left Main or Multivessel Coronary Artery Disease

Ref.: Mineok Chang MD, Cheol Whan Lee MD, PhD et al

Catheterization and cardiovascular Interventions Vol. 90, Issue 2, August 1, 2017, 177-185

Key Points

1) Predictors of long-term outcomes (approximately 5 years) after coronary artery bypass grafting (CABG) versus those after percutaneous coronary intervention (PCI) with drug-eluting stents (DES) in 3,230 patients with left main or multivessel coronary artery disease (CAD) were assessed by pooling data from BEST, PRECOMBAT, and SYNTAX trials.

2) Simple clinical variables and SYNTAX score differentially predict long-term outcomes after CABG versus those after PCI with DES for left main or multivessel CAD which might help to guide the choice of revascularization strategy in patients with left main or multi-vessel disease.

Akshay Mehta

▮ Introduction:

Protocol with pre-specified outcomes and a common set of baseline variables were determined by the principal investigators from BEST, PRECOMBAT, and SYNTAX trials. Data from 3,230 patients who had actually undergone either CABG (n = 1,538) or PCI with DES (n = 1,692) were merged at the coordinating institution (Asan Medical Center, Seoul, Korea). An independent clinical event committee blinded to the randomization adjudicated all end points in each study. Clinical outcomes were death from any cause; MI; stroke; and a composite of death from any cause, MI, or stroke. The Cox proportional hazards model was adopted to determine predictors of long-term outcomes.

▮ Results and Conclusions :

There were some predictors common to both PCI and CABG groups and some that impacted differently in the two groups.

Age, chronic kidney disease, chronic obstructive lung disease, left ventricular dysfunction (left ventricular ejection fraction < 40%), and peripheral artery disease were independent predictors of death from any cause in both groups.

Diabetes mellitus, previous MI, previous stroke, chronic kidney disease and the SYNTAX score impacted outcomes differently in the two groups as shown in the table.

Clinical variable	Impacted outcome
Diabetes mellitus, previous MI, and the SYNTAX score	long-term mortality after PCI with DES
Incomplete revascularization, Previous MI	MI after PCI with DES.
Age, previous stroke	Stroke after PCI with DES
Chronic kidney disease	A composite outcome of death, MI, or stroke after CABG
Age	MI after CABG
left ventricular dysfunction, hypertension, and PAD	Stroke after CABG

■ Comments and Clinical Application:

Selection of the optimal revascularization strategy for patients with left main or multivessel disease is a clinical challenge for which several risk models have been suggested, but difficult to use in real-world practice due to their perceived complexity. Current guideline recommendations are based on the extent of CAD or anatomical lesion complexity (the SYNTAX score) for selecting the revascularization strategy. The SYNTAX clinical score excludes diabetes as a determinant for revascularization strategy. This analysis is the first to identify simple common and differential clinical predictors along with the SYNTAX score for long-term outcomes after CABG and PCI with DES, in a similar patient population with left main or multivessel CAD.

The message from the analysis is that CABG may be preferred in patients with diabetes mellitus, previous MI, or high SYNTAX scores and can be considered a better strategy in patients with previous stroke and intermediate SYNTAX scores. On the other hand PCI with DES may be preferred for patients with low SYNTAX scores and a better strategy for those with chronic kidney disease.

Although this was a pooled analysis of data from only 3 trials - BEST, PRECOMBAT and SYNTAX, with conclusions based on indirect evidence,it suggests that simple clinical variables may be useful in decision-making for revascularization of patients with left main or multivessel disease.

■ Suggested Readings

1. Windecker S, Kolh P, Alfonso F, Collet JP, Cremer J, Falk V, Filippatos G, Hamm C, Head SJ, Jüni P, Kappetein AP, Kastrati A, Knuuti J, Landmesser U, Laufer G, Neumann FJ, Richter DJ, Schauerte P, Sousa Uva M, Stefanini GG, Taggart DP, Torracca L, Valgimigli M, Wijns W, Witkowski A. Authors/ Task Force members. 2014 ESC/EACTS guidelines on myocardial revascularization: The task force on myocardial revascularization of the European Society of Cardiology (ESC) and the European Association for Cardio-Thoracic Surgery (EACTS) developed with the special contribution of the European Association of Percutaneous Cardiovascular Interventions (EAPCI). Eur Heart J 2014;35:2541-2619.

2.	Mohr FW, Morice MC, Kappetein AP, Feldman TE, Ståhle E, Colombo A, Mack MJ, Holmes DR Jr, Morel MA, Van Dyck N, Houle VM, Dawkins KD, Serruys PW. Coronary artery bypass graft surgery versus percutaneous coronary intervention in patients with three-vessel disease and left main coronary disease: 5-Year follow-up of the randomised, clinical SYNTAX trial. Lancet 2013;381:629-638.

3.	Park SJ, Ahn JM, Kim YH, Park DW, Yun SC, Lee JY, Kang SJ, Lee SW, Lee CW, Park SW, Choo SJ, Chung CH, Lee JW, Cohen DJ, Yeung AC, Hur SH, Seung KB, Ahn TH, Kwon HM, Lim DS, Rha SW, Jeong MH, Lee BK, Tresukosol D, Fu GS, Ong TK, BEST Trial Investigators. Trial of everolimus-eluting stents or bypass surgery for coronary disease. N Engl J Med 2015;372:1204-1212.

4.	Roques F, Nashef SA, Michel P, Gauducheau E, de Vincentiis C, Baudet E, Cortina J, David M, Faichney A, Gabrielle F, Gams E, Harjula A, Jones MT, Pintor PP, Salamon R, Thulin L. Risk factors and outcome in European cardiac surgery: Analysis of the EuroSCORE multinational database of 19,030 patients. Eur J Cardiothorac Surg 1999;15:816-822.

β-blockers and Mortality After Acute Myocardial Infarction in Patients Without Heart Failure or Ventricular Dysfunction

Ref.: Tatendashe B. Dondo, MSC, Marlous Hall, PHD, Robert M. West, DPHIL, Tomas Jernberg, MD, PHD, et al.

LINK : JACC 2017;69(22):2710 - 2720

Key Points:

1. β-blockers did not provide mortality benefit to survivors of acute myocardial infarction (AMI) who did not have heart failure or left ventricular systolic dysfunction (LVSD).

2. Lack of benefit was observed in patients with STEMI as well as NSTEMI patients.

Dev Pahlajani

▮ Introduction:

β-blockers for long have been recommended to patients who survive AMI at the time of discharge. Earlier reports had indicated survival benefit for patients who were discharged from the hospital with β-blockers. However, some of the studies have failed to show this benefit among patients with preserved left ventricular function. The current study has been undertaken to assess whether post discharge beta blockers provide survival benefit to patients with MI without heart failure or LVSD.

▮ Material and Method:

The current study is a retrospective analysis of 179,810 patients with AMI who were prescribed β-blockers at discharge. Patients who were already on beta blockers prior to MI were excluded.

Results:

Amongst 179810 patients there were 91,895 patients with STEMI and 87,915 with NSTEMI. All of them had no heart failure or LVSD. 94.8% patients received β-blockers. Patients receiving β-blockers were younger, males with high ischemic risk including diabetes, chronic renal failure, COPD and cerebrovascular disease. Unadjusted 1 year mortality was significantly lower for patients who received β-blockers compared to those who did not (4.9% v/s 11.2% p =< 0.001). However, on balanced propensity score analysis 163,127 patients were removed from analysis leaving 16,683 patients for final analysis. At 1 month, 6 months and 1 year after hospitalization for AMI there was no significant difference in mortality among patients who received β-blockers v/s those who did not receive β-blockers. There was no significant treatment effect for the use of β-blockers at 1 month, 6 months and 1 year among patients with STEMI and NSTEMI.

■ Conclusion:

β-blockers failed to provide mortality benefit in survivors of AMI or NSTEMI without heart failure or LVSD.

■ Comments:

Earlier trials had shown that use of β-blockers in survivors of AMI was associated with decreased mortality as compared to patients who did not receive beta blockers. However these studies did not stratify these patients on the clinical basis of cardiac failure. Therefore the guidelines remained quiet on this issue. Further there has been a sea change in the management of AMI in last 2 decades. Several patients undergo primary angioplasty or CABG surgery that can salvage jeopardized myocardium. Patients also receive the guidelines recommended preventive treatment like antiplatelet drugs and statins along with good control of diabetes and hypertension. The US guidelines recommend β-blockers as Class I indication regardless of EF and heart failure as opposed to the European guidelines that give Class IIa for those without systolic dysfunction or heart failure. A meta-analysis reported significant reduction in the risk of death with the use of β-blockers. However, such studies included in the meta-analysis belong to the period prior to angioplasty or widespread use of CABG surgery. Another meta-analysis failed to show the advantage of routine administration of β-blockers to the survivors of β-blockers without LV dysfunction. Importantly only those trials where β-blockers were administered intravenously during MI and continued during the period of one month achieved survival benefit. With PCI and CABG greater amount of myocardial preservation occurs leading to smaller sized infarctions which are associated with better survival.

■ Clinical Implications:

Since β-blockers do have significant side effects , routine use in patients who survive MI or NSTEMI with normal EF or without LVD should be discouraged.

■ Suggested Readings

1. Timolol-induced reduction in mortality and reinfarction in patients surviving acute myocardial infarction. N Engl J Med 1981;304:801-7.

2. Chen Z, Pan H, Chen Y, et al. Early intravenous then oral metoprolol in 45,852 patients with acute myocardial infarction: randomisedplacebocontrolled trial. Lancet 2005;366:1622-32.

3. Roffi M, Patrono C, Collet JP, et al. 2015 ESC guidelines for the management of acute coronary syndromes in patients presenting without persistent ST-segment elevation: Task Force for the Management of Acute Coronary Syndromes in Patients Presenting without Persistent ST-Segment Elevation of the European Society of Cardiology (ESC). Eur Heart J 2016;37:267-315.

4. Amsterdam EA, Wenger NK, Brindis RG, et al. 2014 AHA/ACC guideline for the management of patients with non-ST-elevation acute coronary syndromes: a report of the American College of Cardiology/ American Heart Association Task Force on Practice Guidelines. J Am Coll Cardiol 2014;64: e1 39-228.

5. Huang B, Huang F, Zuo Z, et al. Meta-analysis of relation between oral b-blocker therapy and outcomes in patients with acute myocardial infarction who underwent percutaneous coronary intervention. Am J Cardiol 2015;115:1529-38.

6. Puymirat E, Riant E, Aissoui N, et al. β-Blockers and mortality after myocardial infarction in patients without heart failure: multicentre prospective cohort study. BMJ 2016;354:i4801.

58

Efficacy and Safety of a Pharmaco-Invasive Strategy with Half-Dose Alteplase Versus Primary Angioplasty in ST-Segment-Elevation Myocardial Infarction EARLY-MYO Trial (Early Routine Catheterization After Alteplase Fibrinolysis Versus Primary PCI in Acute ST-Segment-Elevation Myocardial Infarction)

Ref.: Jun Pu, MD Song Ding, MD Heng Ge, MD Yaling Han, MD JinchenGuo, MD Rong Lin, MD Xi Su, MD Heng Zhang, MD Lianglong Chen, MD Ben He, MD EARLY-MYO Investigator
Circulation. 2017;136:00-00.DOI:10.1161/Circulation AHA.117.030582

Key Points

1. The aim of this study was to compare the efficacy and safety of a pharmaco-invasive (PhI) strategy with half-dose fibrinolytic regimen versus primary PCI (PPCI) in patients with STEMI.

2. The EARLY-MYO trial showed that, in low risk STEMI patients presenting ≤ 6 hours after symptom onset and with an expected PCI-related delay, a PhI strategy with half-dose alteplase and timely PCI was noninferior (and even superior) to PPCI in terms of incidence of complete epicardial and myocardial reperfusion.

Akshay Mehta

▮ Study Protocol:

This was a prospective, multicenter, randomized, parallel-group, open-label noninferiority trial comparing a PhI strategy with half-dose alteplase versus PPCI in 344 patients with STEMI 18 to 75 years of age presenting ≤ 6 hours after symptom onset but with an expected PCI-related delay (from FMC to first balloon dilation ≥ 90 minutes and difference between the time of FMC to balloon dilation minus the time from FMC to start of fibrinolysis ≥ 60 minutes).

After random assignment, patients in the PhI group received half-dose alteplase (8-mg bolus followed by 42 mg in 90 minutes) and an unfractionated heparin bolus (60 U/kg to ≤ 4000 U followed by 12 U/kg/h to ≤ 1000 U/h). Eighteen-lead ECG was repeated every 30 minutes after start of fibrinolysis. Patients with persistent ST-segment elevation (i.e. < 50% resolution of ST-segment elevation) 90 minutes after start of alteplase with or without chest pain were considered as fibrinolysis failures and were referred for immediate rescue PCI. Other patients were recommended to undergo early routine catheterization within 3 to 24 hours after fibrinolysis and further undergo PCI of the presumed culprit lesion if the residual stenosis was ≥ 50%.

The primary end point of the study (available in 328 patients) was complete epicardial and myocardial reperfusion after PCI, defined as thrombolysis in myocardial infarction flow grade 3, thrombolysis in myocardial infarction myocardial perfusion grade 3, and ST segment resolution

≥ 70%. Also measured were infarct size and left ventricular ejection fraction with cardiac magnetic resonance done between day 4 and 7 and 30-day clinical and safety outcomes were also recorded.

▌ Results and Comment:

For patients with STEMI at low risk presenting ≤ 6 hours after symptom onset and for whom the expected PCI related delay was ≥ 60 minutes, a PhI strategy with half dose alteplase and timely PCI offered more complete epicardial and myocardial reperfusion when compared with PPCI. CMR-defined infarct size and LV function and the 30-day rate of clinical outcomes were similar. Bleeding rates were similar, except that minor bleedings seen more often in the PhI group. No intracranial hemorrhages were observed in either group.

The strengths of the trial are :

1. It is the first randomized trial comparing a PhI strategy with PPCI.

2. An ischemic time window of 6 hours (compared to 3 hours in the recent STREAM trial) which is more relevant to the situation in our population.

3. Use of half strength lytic drug for all patients, although below 75 years of age, thus completely preventing any episodes of intra cranial bleeds. Indeed, half-dose alteplase fibrinolytic regimen achieved a fibrinolysis success rate of 74.5% based on clinical criteria (i.e. STR ≥ 50% on ECG) and 75.2% based on angiographiccriteria (ie, TFG 2/3 on angiography).

Limitations of the study were lack of outcome data, small size, alteplase as the only fibrinolytic agent used and a relatively low risk East Asian population below age 75. All this makes its applicability to a wider population worth contemplating. Also, contrary to standard recommendations, some PhI patients received ticagrelor. There is no mention of its effect in PhI patients in the trial.

Apart from these limitations, this trial supports the concept (highlighted in recent similar trials) that such a PhI strategy is safe and effective for a large majority of patients with STEMI in all regions of the world who cannot or do not undergo timely PCI in an expert 24/7 facility. This option is not inferior and on occasion could even be superior-to PPCI.

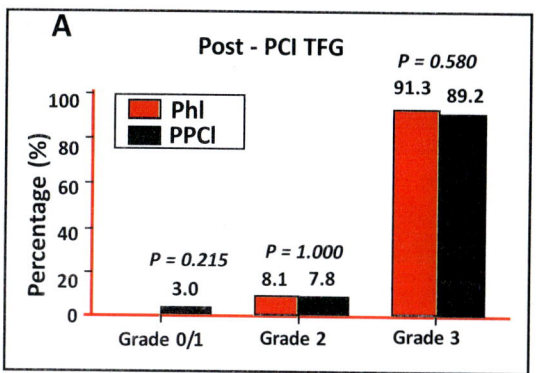

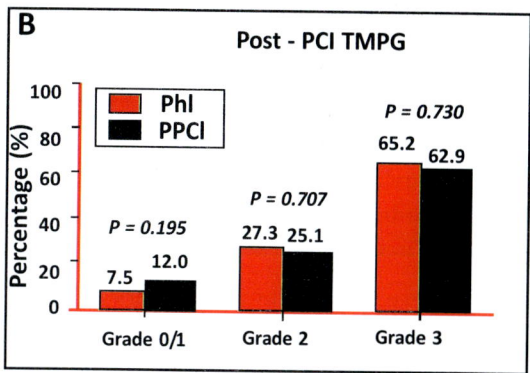

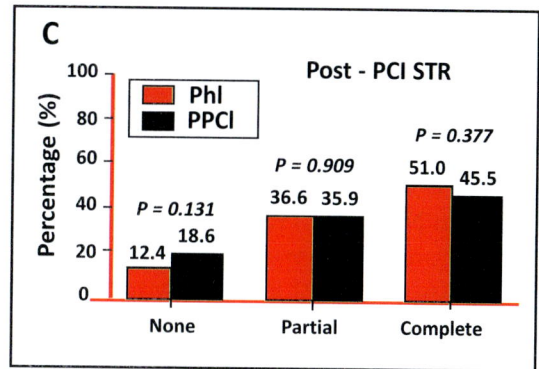

"Primary end points in the 2 treatment arms :

A, Postinterventional TFG. B, Postinterventional TMPG. C, Postinterventional STR. PCI indicates percutaneous coronary intervention; PI, pharmaco-invasive; PPCI, primary PCI; STR, ST segment resolution; TFG, TIMI flow grade; and TMPG, TIMI myocardial perfusion grade".

From : Jun Pu, MD Song Ding, MD Heng Ge, MD Yaling Han, MD JinchenGuo, MD Rong Lin, MD Xi Su, MD Heng Zhang, MD Lianglong Chen, MD Ben He, MD EARLY-MYO Investigators.

Efficacy and Safety of a Pharmaco-Invasive Strategy with Half-Dose Alteplase Versus Primary Angioplasty in ST-Segment-Elevation Myocardial Infarction EARLY-MYO Trial (Early Routine Catheterization After Alteplase Fibrinolysis Versus Primary PCI in Acute ST-Segment-Elevation Myocardial Infarction).

Circulation. 2017;136:00-00. DOI: 10.1161/CIRCULATIONAHA.117.030582.

❚ Suggested Readings

1. Danchin N, Coste P, Ferrières J, Steg PG, Cottin Y, Blanchard D, BelleL, Ritz B, Kirkorian G, Angioi M, Sans P, Charbonnier B, Eltchaninoff H, Guéret P, Khalife K, Asseman P, Puel J, Goldstein P, Cambou JP, SimonT; FAST-MI Investigators. Comparison of thrombolysis followed by broaduse of percutaneous coronary intervention with primary percutaneous coronary intervention for ST-segment-elevation acute myocardial infarction: data from the french registry on acute ST-elevation myocardial infarction (FAST-MI). Circulation.2008;118:268-276. doi: 10.1161/CIRCULATIONAHA 107.762765.

2. Sinnaeve PR, Armstrong PW, Gershlick AH, Goldstein P, Wilcox R, LambertY, Danays T, Soulat L, Halvorsen S, Ortiz FR, Vandenberghe K, RegelinA, Bluhmki E, Bogaerts K, Van de Werf F; STREAM Investigators. ST-segment-elevation myocardial infarction patients randomized to a pharmaco invasive strategy or primary percutaneous coronary intervention: Strategic Reperfusion Early After Myocardial Infarction (STREAM) 1-year mortality follow-up. Circulation. 2014;130:1139-1145.doi: 10.1161/CIRCULATIONAHA.114.009570.

3. O'Gara PT, Kushner FG, Ascheim DD, Casey DE Jr, Chung MK, de Lemos JA, Ettinger SM, Fang JC, Fesmire FM, Franklin BA, Granger CB, Krumholz HM, Linderbaum JA, Morrow DA, Newby LK, Ornato JP, Ou N, Radford MJ, Tamis-Holland JE, Tommaso CL, Tracy CM, Woo YJ, Zhao DX, Anderson JL, Jacobs AK, Halperin JL, Albert NM, Brindis RG, Creager MA, DeMets D, Guyton RA, Hochman JS, Kovacs RJ, Kushner FG, Ohman EM, Stevenson WG, Yancy CW; American College of Cardiology Foundation/American Heart Association Task Force on Practice Guidelines. 2013 ACCF/AHA guideline for the management of ST-elevation myocardial infarction: a report of the American College of Cardiology Foundation/ American Heart Association Task Force on Practice Guidelines. Circulation. 2013;127: e362-e425. doi: 10.1161/CIR.0b013e3182742cf6.

59

Impact of Collateral Circulation on Survival in ST-Segment Elevation Myocardial Infarction Patients including Primary Percutaneous Coronary Intervention with a Concomitant Chronic Total Occlusion

Ref.: Joëlle Elias, Loes P.C. Hoebers, Ivo M. van Dongen, Bimmer E.P.M. Claessen et al
LINK:JACC: Cardiovascular Interventions 2017; 10(9):906-914.

Key Points:

1. In patients with ST elevated Myocardial Infarction (STEMI), presence of well developed collaterals to chronic total occlusion (CTO) is associated with better survival as compared to poorly developed collaterals.

2. Poorly developed collaterals are observed in circumflex (Cx) CTO and patients with cardiogenic shock.

Dev Pahlajani

▌ Introduction:

Collateral circulation to CTO protects the ischemic myocardium in the area supplied by CTO vessel. Presence of well developed collaterals minimize the size of myocardial infarction and helps preserve LV function and reduce future adverse cardiac events.

Acute STEMI is a result of total occlusion of the infarct related vessel (IRV) with a thrombus. It has been documented that presence of collaterals distal to total occlusion in the IRV in STEMI is associated with better prognosis, decrease in myocardial infarction (MI) size and preservation of LV function. However, very little is known about the significance of collateral circulation from the IRV to the CTO in a setting of STEMI.

▌ Aims of the Study:

To evaluate long term clinical outcomes in STEMI patients with concomitant CTO with collaterals from the IRV to the CTO.

▌ Material and Methods:

The investigators included 413 patients with CTO in non IRV with collaterals from IRV. Patients were divided according to well developed versus poorly developed collaterals.

Results:

In 53% patients the collaterals to CTO were well developed. Patients with cardiogenic shock, CTO in Cx artery location, smaller diameter vessels of < 2.5 mm were determinants of poorly developed collaterals. Five year survival was better in patients with well developed collaterals versus poorly developed collaterals (74% versus 63% respectively, p=0.01).

Cardiogenic shock was present in 24% of patients.

Five years survival was 68.7%.

Of the 413 patients, close to 50% patients had well visible and developed collaterals whereas equal numbers had poorly developed collaterals.

CTO was more often located in the RCA in the well developed collateral group. The presence of well developed collaterals to CTO was an independent predictor for survival (Fig. 1).

Comments:

Collateral circulation develops as a result of pressure gradient between the donor and the totally occluded vessel. Further factors which help to develop collaterals are sheer stress on the collateral endothelium. Presence of collaterals protect the myocardium distal to CTO. Exercise, or chronic ischemia stimulate the recruitment of collaterals. Recruitment of collaterals has been noted in ischemic preconditioning and following repeated balloon inflation that leads to intermittent transient ischemia.

Clinical Relevance:

Further studies to stimulate formation of collaterals through physical exercise or granulocyte - monocyte stimulating factor could help in the development and growth of collaterals. Also presence of collateral circulation indicates viable muscle and every effort should be made to identify the presence of ischemic viable muscle that could benefit from revascularization.

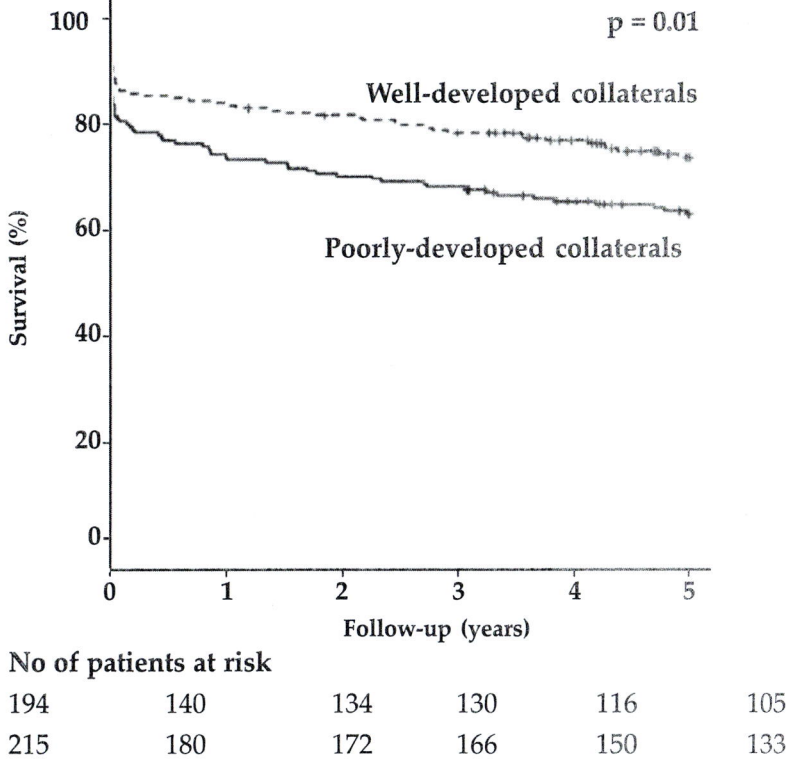

Fig. 1: *Survival in STEMI patients with poorly versus well-developed colateral to CTO*

No of patients at risk

194	140	134	130	116	105
215	180	172	166	150	133

▌ Suggested Readings

1. Meier P, Gloekler S, Zbinden R, et al. Beneficial effect of recruitable collaterals: a 10-year followup study in patients with stable coronary artery disease undergoing quantitative collateral measurements. Circulation 2007;116:975-83.

2. Kim EK, Choi JH, Song YB, et al. A protective role of early collateral blood flow in patients with ST-segment elevation myocardial infarction. Am Heart J 2016;171:56-63.

3. Choi JH, Chang SA, Choi JO, et al. Frequency of myocardial infarction and its relationship to angiographic collateral flow in territories supplied by chronically occluded coronary arteries. Circulation 2013;127:7039.

4. Claessen BE, Dangas GD, Weisz G, et al. Prognostic impact of a chronic total occlusion in a non-infarct-related artery in patients with ST-segment elevation myocardial infarction: 3-year results from the HORIZONS-AMI trial. Eur Heart J 2012;33:768-75.

5. Meier P, Hemingway H, Lansky AJ, Knapp G, Pitt B, Seiler C. The impact of the coronary collateral circulation on mortality: a meta-analysis. Eur Heart J 2012;33:614-21.

6. Meier P, Gloekler S, de Marchi SF, et al. Myocardial salvage through coronary collateral growth by granulocyte colony-stimulating factor in chronic coronary artery disease: a control led randomized trial. Circulation 2009;120:1355-63.

7. Froehlich G, Crake T, Meier P. Exercise training for refractory angina: improving the coronary collateral circulation. Cardiology 2012;123:78-9, author reply 80.

60

Disaster (Emergency) Management Processes Application to the Prevention and Treatment of Coronary Perforation

Akshay Mehta

Disaster (emergency) management core phases	PCI complications checklist: Coronary perforation
1. Prevention	**Prevention** - Is the guidewire in the right distal position? - Is the guidewire used for stent-delivery a soft-tip guidewire? - It the balloon/stent position appropriate? - Is the balloon/stent inflation too high? (awareness of nominal and rated pressure inflation)
2. Mitigation	**Detection** - Is there staining, suggesting distal vessel perforation? - Is there pulsusparadoxus developing? - Is the patient complaining of on unexplained chest pain or hemodynamic change? - Immediate angiography in case of balloon rupture
3. Preparedness	**Preparedness** - Equipment and procedures in place for a timely, efficient, successful response. - Are covered stents and coils available? - Is protamine-sulfate available for heparin reversal? - Cath lab team (techs, nurses, physicians) familiar with the use of equipment? - Annual complications simulation by cath lab staff

		Response and Treatment
4.	Response	- Immediate balloon inflation to occlude vessel (hemostasis) - "Block" - Intravenous fluids/pressors - STAT echocardiogram, pericardiocentesis - Type and screen, notify surgeons - Large vessel perforation: covered stent, prolonged balloon inflations - Distal vessel perforation: embolization (fat, coil, thrombin, etc) or covered stent over perforated branch origin - Anticoagulation reversal
		Recovery
5.	Recovery	- Should the patient be transferred to the intensive care unit? - Serial echocardiograms to assess for pericardial effusion? - Replace used equipment to ensure availability for subsequent cases - Case review, what went well? What went wrong? Morbidity and mortality conference, education

■ **Suggested Readings**

1. Yader Sandoval, MD and Emmanouil S. Brilakis, MD, PhD, Preventing and Treating Coronary Perforations: Lessons From Disaster Management, Cath CV Interventions. May 2017, Volume 89, Issue 6, pages 973-975.

61

Antithrombotic Therapy and First Myocardial Infarction in Patients with Atrial Fibrillation

Ref.: Christina J.Y. Lee, MD, Jannik L. Pallisgaard, MD, Jonas BjerringOlesen, MD, PHD, et al. LINK:JACC 2017;69:24 2901-2909.

Key Points:

1. Patients with atrial fibrillation (AF) without pre-existing coronary artery disease (CAD) have high incidence of myocardial infarction (MI).

2. Monotherapy with Vitamin K antagonist (VKA) is associated with lower risk of MI and stroke as compared to aspirin monotherapy.

3. Dual treatment with aspirin and VKA does not provide any greater benefit than monotherapy. Combination therapy is associated with greater risk of bleeding.

Dev Pahlajani

∎ Introduction:

Patients with AF carry an increased risk of stroke. Some of the earlier reports also indicate that AF is associated with higher risk of first MI. The pathophysiological factors responsible for AF and CAD are similar. Both of them are associated with older age, diabetes, hypertension and smoking. VKA have been used to decrease the risk of stroke in AF whereas antiplatelet drugs (AP) like aspirin has been recommended for prevention of CAD. Some of the studies have also investigated the role of combined treatment of VKA and aspirin and found an increased risk of bleeding with no additional benefit of preventing MI.

∎ Methods:

Current study enrolled 71959 patients from the Danish Nationwide administrative registry. These patients had AF without pre-existing CAD. Baseline treatment in these patients was :

a) VKA monotherapy

b) ASA monotherapy

c) VKA + ASA dual therapy

Primary outcome was first time MI and secondary outcomes were stroke and bleeding. Concomitant treatment with statins, renin angiotensin system, beta blockers, anti arrhythmic agents were also identified. Study period was 16 years and the mean age was 75 years with 47% females.

At baseline 37539 patients received VKA monotherapy, 25485 were treated with ASA monotherapy and 8962 were treated with VKA + ASA combination therapy. Patients who received monotherapy were more likely to be older, females and high CHA2DS2-VASc score. Patients with dual therapy had greater prevalence of heart failure, hypertension and diabetes.

▌ Results:

First MI developed in 2275 patients (3%) within a median time of 4 years. The incidence of MI was 8.0 per 1,000 patient years. VKA treated patients had significantlydecreased risk of MI as compared to ASA monotherapy or VKA + ASA dual therapy. As a matter of fact patients treated with dual therapy had greater risk of bleeding. Looking at the secondary end points, the risk of stroke was highest amongst the ASA monotherapy group. Surprisingly even the VKA + ASA dual therapy patients had a greater risk of stroke as compared to VKA monotherapy (Ref Fig).

▌ Conclusion:

Some of the earlier studies have shown an annual rate of MI ranging from 0.4 to 2.5% and reported that patients with AF developed MI twice as high as compared to the patients without AF. Significant number of patients today are treated with the novel oral anticoagulant (NOACS) like rivaroxaban, dabigatran or apixaban. It will be of greater interest to see whether these NOACS could have similar beneficial effect in preventing MI in patients with AF.

Fig. 1: Incidencerate and incidence rate ratios by Antithrombotic treatment for myocardial infaction, stroke and bleeding

Outcome	Events	Risk time (years)	Incidence rate		IRR Ref. = VKA
Myocardial infaction					
VKA	870	150188	0.58 (0.54 - 0.62)		1.00
ASA	1152	103017	1.12 (1.06 - 1.18)		1.54 (1.40 - 1.68)
ASA + VKA	253	32479	0.78 (0.69 - 0.88)		1.22 (1.06 - 1.40)
Stroke					
VKA	1768	144775	1.22 (1.17 - 1.28)		1.00
ASA	3180	99158	3.21 (3.10 - 3.32)		2.00 (1.88 - 2.12)
ASA + VKA	527	31617	1.67 (1.53 - 1.82)		1.30 (1.18 - 1.43)
Bleeding					
VKA	2684	133906	2.00 (1.93 - 2.08)		1.00
ASA	2141	87975	2.43 (2.33 - 2.54)		0.95 (0.90 - 1.01)
ASA + VKA	1244	27492	4.52 (4.28 - 4.78)		1.93 (1.81 - 2.07)

0.50   2.00   1.00   1.50

Incidence rate ratio (95% CI)

Suggested Readings

1. Soliman EZ, Safford MM, Muntner P, etal. Atrial fibrillation and the risk of myocardial infarction. JAMA Intern Med 2014;174:107-14.

2. Connolly S, Pogue J, Hart R, et al., for the ACTIVE writing group of the ACTIVE Investigators. Clopidogrel plus aspirin versus oral anticoagulation for atrial fibrillation in the Atrial fibrillation Clopidogrel Trial with Irbesartan for prevention of Vascular Events (ACTIVE W): a randomised controlled trial. Lancet 2006;367:1903-12.

3. Connolly SJ, Ezekowitz MD, Yusuf S, etal. Dabigatran versus warfarin in patients with atrial fibrillation. N Engl J Med 2009;361:1139-51.

4. Capodanno D, Capranzano P, Giacchi G, Calvi V, Tamburino C. Novel oral anticoagulants versus warfarin in non-valvular atrial fibrillation: a meta-analysis of 50,578 patients. Int J Cardiol 2013;167:1237-41.

Dual Antithrombotic Therapy with Dabigatran after PCI in Atrial Fibrillation

Ref.: Christopher P. Cannon, M.D., Deepak L. Bhatt, M.D., M.P.H., Jonas Oldgren, M.D., Ph.D., Gregory Y.H. Lip, M.D., Stephen G. Ellis, M.D., Takeshi Kimura, M.D., Michael Maeng, M.D., Ph.D., Bela Merkely, M.D., Uwe Zeymer, M.D., Savion Gropper, M.D., Ph.D., Matias Nordaby, M.D., Eva Kleine, M.Sc., Ruth Harper, Ph.D., Jenny Manassie, B.Med.Sc., James L. Januzzi, M.D., Jurrien M. ten Berg, M.D., Ph.D., P. Gabriel Steg, M.D., and Stefan H. Hohnloser, M.D., for the RE-DUAL PCI Steering Committee and Investigators
Link: NEJM August 27, 2017 DOI: 10.1056/NEJMoa1708454

Key Points
1) In patients with atrial fibrillation who had undergone PCI, the risk of bleeding was lower in those patients who received dual therapy with dabigatran and a P2Y12 inhibitor than in those who received triple therapy with warfarin, a P2Y12 inhibitor, and aspirin.
2) With respect to the risk of thromboembolic events, dual therapy was noninferior to triple therapy.

Akshay Mehta

▌ Introduction:

Although guideline directed standard of care after percutaneous coronary intervention (PCI) for patients with atrial fibrillation is triple antithrombotic therapy with warfarin plus two antiplatelet agents, it is associated with a high risk of bleeding. Hence, in recent years efforts are on to find an alternative that combines the reduced risk of bleeding with prevention of thrombo embolic and coronary stent thrombosis.

▌ Aims of the Study:

The RE-DUAL PCI trial (Randomized Evaluation of Dual Antithrombotic Therapy with Dabigatran versus Triple Therapy with Warfarin in Patients with Nonvalvular Atrial Fibrillation Undergoing Percutaneous Coronary Intervention) compared the use of two regimens of dual antithrombotic therapy that included dabigatran with the use of triple antithrombotic therapy that included warfarin in patients with atrial fibrillation who had undergone PCI.

▌ Material:

This was a multicenter trial in which 2725 patients with atrial fibrillation who had undergone PCI were randomly assigned to triple therapy with warfarin plus a P2Y12 inhibitor (clopidogrel or ticagrelor) and aspirin (for 1 to 3 months) (triple-therapy group) or dual therapy with dabigatran (110 mg or 150 mg twice daily) plus a P2Y12 inhibitor (clopidogrel or ticagrelor) and no aspirin (110-mg and 150-mg dual-therapy groups). The primary end point was a major or clinically relevant nonmajor bleeding event during follow-up (mean follow-up, 14 months). The trial also tested for the noninferiority of dual therapy with dabigatran (both doses combined) to triple therapy with warfarin with respect to the incidence of a composite efficacy end point of thromboembolic events (myocardial infarction, stroke, or systemic embolism), death, or unplanned revascularization.

▌ Results:

The mean age of patients was 70.8 years and the indication for PCI was an acute coronary syndrome in 50.5% of the patients. Drug-eluting stents alone were used in 82.6% of the patients. Most of the patients received clopidogrel; only 12.0% received ticagrelor. In the triple-therapy group, the mean percentage of time in the therapeutic INR range was 64%.

▌ Outcomes:

The incidence of the primary end point in the 110-mg dual-therapy as compared with the triple-therapy group was 15.4% versus 26.9% (hazard ratio, 0.52; 95% confidence interval [CI], 0.42 to 0.63), in the 150-mg dual-therapy group as compared with the triple-therapy group was 20.2% versus 25.7% (hazard ratio, 0.72; 95% CI, 0.58 to 0.88).

The incidence of the composite efficacy end point in the two dual-therapy groups combined as compared with the triple-therapy group was 13.7% versus 13.4%. (hazard ratio, 1.04; 95% CI, 0.84 to 1.29).

The rate of serious adverse events did not differ significantly among the groups.

▌ Conclusion:

The RE-DUAL PCI trial showed that, two different regimens of full-dose anticoagulation therapy with dabigatran (either 110 mg or 150 mg twice daily) plus a P2Y12 inhibitor (clopidogrel or ticagrelor) resulted in a risk of major or clinically relevant nonmajor bleeding events that was significantly lower than the risk with triple therapy with warfarin during 1 year of treatment. Also, dual therapy with dabigatran was noninferior to triple therapy with warfarin for the composite efficacy end point of thromboembolic events, death, or unplanned revascularization.

▌ Comments:

Some caveats of the trial were that the dual-therapy groups were combined for comparison of the composite efficacy end point, to give the analysis reasonable power. Also whether the bleeding benefits were due to dabigatran use or absence of aspirin in the dual therapy groups cannot be ascertained without a factorial 2 by 2 design.

▌ Clinical Relevance:

The trial offers new options in the treatment of AF patients who undergo PCI. Since the net clinical benefit of each of the two dual-therapy regimens differed slightly, clinicians could potentially select one of these two regimens on the basis of a patient's risk of bleeding and risk of thromboembolic events.

∎ Suggested Readings

1. Levine GN, Bates ER, Bittl JA, et al. 2016 ACC/AHA guideline focused update on duration of dual antiplatelet therapy in patients with coronary artery disease: a report of the American College of Cardiology/American Heart Association Task Force on Clinical Practice Guidelines: an update of the 2011 ACCF/AHA/SCAI guideline for percutaneous coronary intervention, 2011 ACCF/AHA guideline for coronary artery bypass graft Surgery, 2012 ACC/AHA/ACP/AATS/PCNA/SCAI/ STS guideline for the diagnosis and management of patients with stable ischemic heart disease, 2013 ACCF/AHA guideline for the management of ST-elevation myocardial infarction, 2014 AHA/ACC guideline for the management of patients with non-ST-elevation acute coronary syndromes, and 2014 ACC/AHA guideline on perioperative cardiovascular evaluation and management of patients undergoing noncardiac surgery. Circulation 2016; 134(10):e123-e155.

2. Steg PG, Bhatt DL. Viewpoint: a proposal for a simple algorithm for managing oral anticoagulation and antiplatelet therapy in patients with non-valvular atrial fibrillation and coronary stents. Eur Heart J Acute Cardiovasc Care 2017;6:93-7.

3. Lip GY, Windecker S, Huber K, et al. Management of antithrombotic therapy in atrial fibrillation patients presenting with acute coronary syndrome and/or undergoing percutaneous coronary or valve interventions: a joint consensus document of the European Society of Cardiology Working Group on Thrombosis, European Heart Rhythm Association (EHRA), European Association of Percutaneous Cardiovascular Interventions (EAPCI) and European Association of Acute Cardiac Care (ACCA) endorsed by the Heart Rhythm Society (HRS) and Asia-Pacific Heart Rhythm Society (APHRS). Eur Heart J 2014;35:3155-79.

4. January CT, Wann LS, Alpert JS, et al. 2014 AHA/ACC/HRS guideline for the management of patients with atrial fibrillation: executive summary: a report of the American College of Cardiology/American Heart Association Task Force on practice guidelines and the Heart Rhythm Society. Circulation 2014;130:2071-104.

5. Levine GN, Bates ER, Blankenship JC, et al. 2011 ACCF/AHA/SCAI guideline for percutaneous coronary intervention: executive summary: a report of the American College of Cardiology Foundation/American Heart Association Task Force on Practice Guidelines and the Society for Cardiovascular Angiography and Interventions. Circulation 2011;124:2574-609.

6. Windecker S, Kolh P, Alfonso F, et al. 2014 ESC/EACTS guidelines on myocardial revascularization: the Task Force on Myocardial Revascularization of the European Society of Cardiology (ESC) and the European Association for Cardio-Thoracic Surgery (EACTS) developed with the special contribution of the European Association of Percutaneous Cardiovascular Interventions (EAPCI). Eur Heart J 2014; 35:2541-619.

7. Dewilde WJ, Oirbans T, Verheugt FW,et al. Use of clopidogrel with or withoutaspirin inpatients taking oral anticoagulanttherapy and undergoing percutaneouscoronary intervention: an open-label, randomised, controlled trial. Lancet 2013; 381: 1107-15.

63

Heart Rate and Rhythm and the Benefit of Beta-Blockers in Patients with Heart Failure

Ref.: Dipak Kotecha, MBBS, PHD, Marcus D. Flather, MBBS, Douglas G. Altman, DSC et al.
LINK: JACC 2017;69(24):2885-2896.

Key Points:

1. Increased baseline heart rate is associated with higher all-cause mortality in patients with heart failure (HF) with sinus rhythm.

2. Reducing heart rate with beta-blockers (BB) in patients with sinus rhythm leads to decreased mortality.

3. Heart rate in patients with atrial fibrillation (AF) has no relationship to mortality.

4. Decreasing heart rate with BB does not reduce mortality in patients with AF.

Dev Pahlajani

▍ Introduction:

HF and reduced ejection fraction (EF) with increased sinus rate has been reported to be associated with increased mortality. Heart rate is considered as a marker of increased mortality in such patients. Earlier reports have also emphasized the importance of reducing heart rate with BB. The relationship between the mortality and heart rate in patients with HF with reduced EF in patients in sinus rhythm or AF is not well defined.

▍ Methods of investigation:

The investigators sought to ascertain the relationship between the heart rate and mortality and the effect of BB in patients with either sinus rhythm or AF. The study was taken by the Beta-blockers in heart failure collaborative group and performed meta-analysis of individual patient data from 11 double blind randomized control trials. After several exclusion criteria, the analysis was performed on 14313 patients in sinus rhythm and 3065 patients with AF.

▍ Results:

The primary outcome of the study was all cause mortality. Patients were analyzed after assigning to pre-specified groups according with heart rate of < 70, 70-90 and > 90 beats per minute. Median basal heart rate was 80 bpm in those with sinus rhythm and 81 in patients with AF. There were 2141 deaths among 14166 patients (15.1%) in sinus rhytm over mean follow up period of 1.5 ± 1.1 years. Increased heart rate at baseline was associated with higher all cause mortality in patients with sinus rhythm, whether the patients were assigned to placebo or beta-blockers. As opposed to sinus rhythm patients basal heart rate had no relationship to mortality in patients with AF. Amongst 3034 AF patients there were 609 deaths (20.1%) without any association between the baseline heart rate. Administration of beta-blockers reduced the heart rate by 11-12 bpm in both sinus rhythm and AF. Reduction of heart rate with beta-blockers in patients with sinus rhythm was associated with significantly reduced mortality as compared to placebo treated patients, with similar benefit for all three groups of baseline heart rate (p=<0.0001). Despite reduction in heart rate beta-blockers failed to reduce mortality in AF (Fig. 1 & 2).

▌ Conclusions and Clinical Implications:

Beneficial effects of BB in heart failure have been well described in some of the earlier trials. Carvedilol, bisoprolol and metoprolol have long been used to treat HF. Whether benefit of mortality reduction is by negative chronotropic action or negative ionotropic effect is not well understood. It has been l established that there are increased levels of epinephrine and norepinephrine in patients with cardiac failure. Blocking norepinephrine by BB would explain salutary effect of mortality reduction. However mechanism of action is not very clear since patients with AF did not show any benefit of treatment with beta-blockers irrespective of the baseline or the reduction in the heart rate. Failure of beta-blockers in AF could be attributed to other co-morbid conditions like diabetes, stroke, hypertension and chronic kidney disease that many patients of AF suffer from. The study strengthens the use of beta-blockers in patients with cardiac failure and sinus rhythm. However, whether the beta-blockers should be used routinely for mortality reduction in AF remains a matter to be investigated further.

A   Sinus rhythm

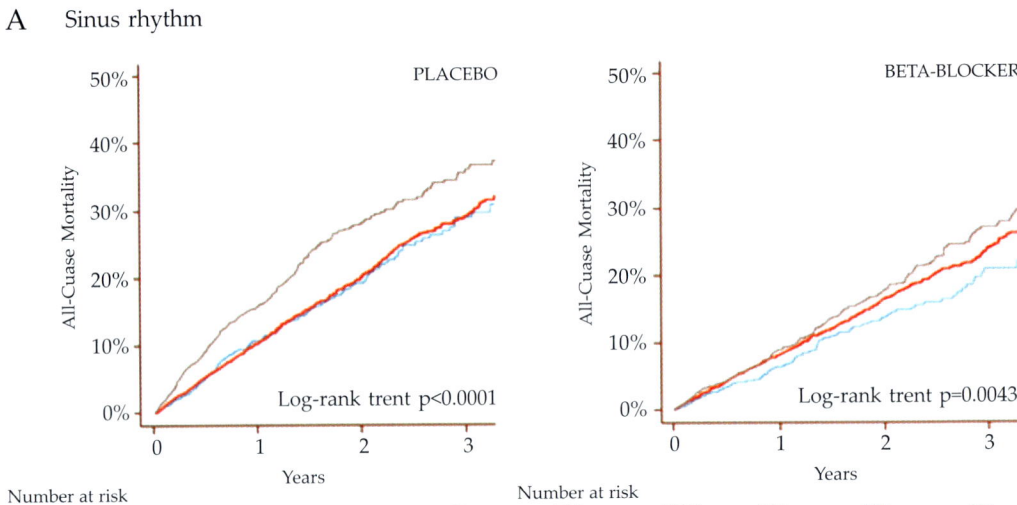

Number at risk					Number at risk				
< 70 bpm	1212	839	301	91	< 70 bpm	1208	883	335	111
70-90 bpm	4476	2946	963	350	70-90 bpm	4650	3101	1038	408
> 90 bpm	1318	818	266	120	> 90 bpm	1446	1028	423	202

B   Atrial fibrillation

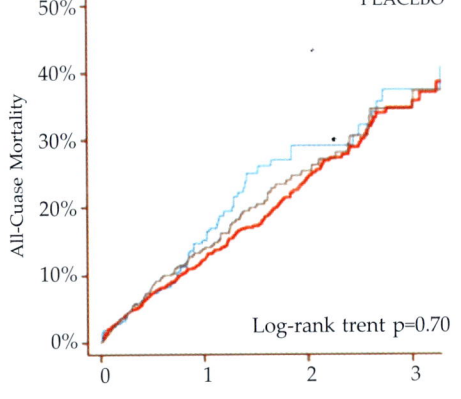
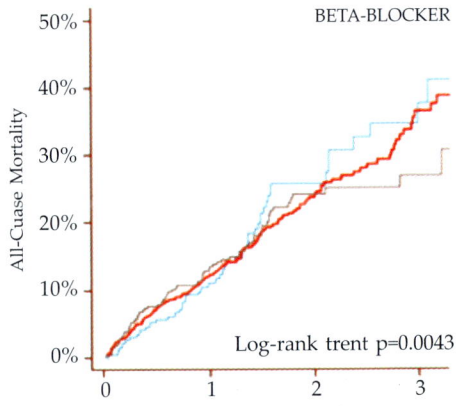

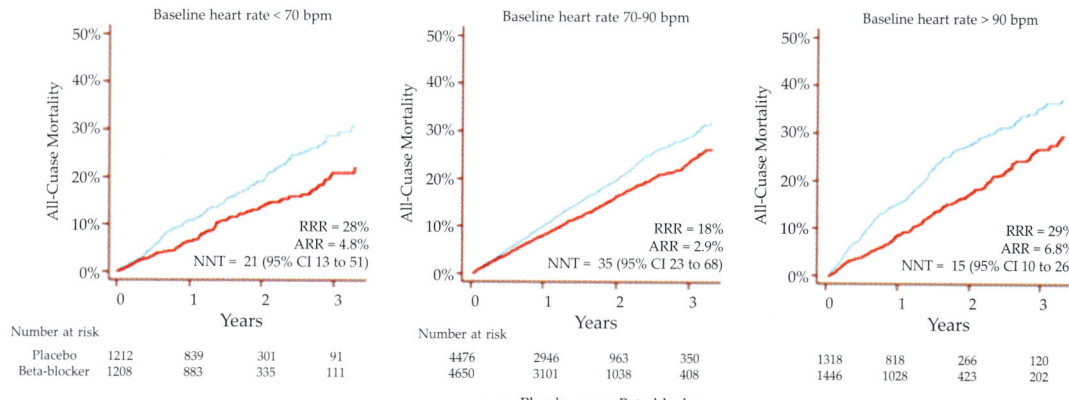

Fig. 2: *Mortality in patients randomly assighed to Placebo or Beta-Blocker according to baseline Heart*

■ Suggested Readings

1. Kotecha D, Holmes J, Krum H, et al., for the Beta-Blockers in Heart Failure Collaborative Group. Efficacy of b blockers in patients with heart failure plus atrial fibrillation: an individual patient data meta-analysis. Lancet 2014;384:2235-43.

2) Kotecha D, Manzano L, Krum H, et al., for the Beta-Blockers in Heart Failure Collaborative Group. Effect of age and sex on efficacy and tolerability of b blockers in patients with heart failure with reduced ejection fraction: individual patient-data meta-analysis. BMJ 2016;353:i1855.

3) Cullington D, Goode KM, Clark AL, Cleland JGF. Heart rate achieved or beta-blocker dose in patients with chronic heart failure: which is the better target? Eur J Heart Fail 2012;14:737-47.

4) Dargie HJ. Effect of carvedilol on outcome after myocardial infarction in patients with left-ventricular dysfunction: the CAPRICORN randomised trial. Lancet 2001;357:1385-90.

5) Floras JS, Ponikowski P. The sympathetic/parasympathetic imbalance in heart failure with reduced ejection fraction. Eur Heart J 2015;36:1974-1982.

6) Li SJ, Sartipy U, Lund LH, et al. Prognostic significance of resting heart rate and use of β-blockers in atrial fibrillation and sinus rhythm in patients with heart failure and reduced ejection fraction: findings from the Swedish Heart Failure Registry. Circ Heart Fail 2015;8:871-9.

7) Cullington D, Goode KM, Zhang J, Cleland JGF, Clark AL. Is heart rate important for patients with heart failure in atrial fibrillation? J Am CollCardiol HF 2014;2:213-20.

64

Clinical Outcomes of Deferred Lesions with Angiographically Insignificant Stenosis but Low Fractional Flow Reserve

Ref.: Joo Myung Lee, Bon-Kwon Koo, Eun-Seok Shin, Chang-Wook Nam, Joon-Hyung Doh, Xinyang Hu, Fei Ye, Shaoliang Chen, Junqing Yang, Jiyan Chen, Nobuhiro Tanaka, Hiroyoshi Yokoi, Hitoshi Matsuo, Hiroaki Takashima, Yasutsugu Shiono, Doyeon Hwang, Jonghanne Park, Kyung-Jin Kim, Takashi Akasaka, Jianan Wang

Journal of the American Heart Association. 2017;6:e006071

Originally published August 22, 2017

Key Points

1. Among angiographically insignificant stenosis, the lesions with low fractional flow reserve showed a higher risk of clinical events than those with high fractional flow reserve.
2. FFR was an independent predictor of future major adverse cardiovascular events in lesions with angiographically insignificant stenosis.

Akshay Mehta

■ **Introduction:**

Frequently, a discrepancy exists between angiographic stenosis severity and the presence of myocardial ischemia and angiography underestimates the functional significance of coronary artery stenosis.

For example, in the RIPCORD study, ≈16% of lesions with percentage of diameter stenosis (%DS) < 50% showed FFR < 0.80. There is a paucity of clinical outcome data for such lesions if deferred.

■ **Aims of the Study:**

To investigate the incidence and natural history of angiographically insignificant but functionally significant lesions in whom angioplasty was deferred.

■ **Material and methods:**

From a cohort of the 3V FFR-FRIENDS study, 2-year clinical outcome of 1024 patients with 2124 lesions with angiographically insignificant stenosis (percentage of diameter stenosis < 50%), in which revascularization was deferredwas analyzed. All lesions were classified according to FFR values, using a cutoff of 0.80 (high FFR > 0.80 versus low FFR ≤ 0.80). The primary end point was outcome of major adverse cardiovascular events (a composite of cardiac death, myocardial infarction, and ischemia-driven revascularization) at 2 years.

▌ Results:

Out of all lesions with angiographically insignificant (< 50% diameter) stenosis, 8.7% showed low FFR (185 lesions). The low-FFR group showed a significantly higher risk of major adverse cardiovascular events compared with the high FFR group at 2-year follow-up (3.3% versus 1.2%, hazard ratio: 3.371; 95% CI, 1.346-8.442; P=0.009). In multivariable analysis, low FFR was the most powerful independent predictor of future MACE in deferred lesions with angiographically insignificant stenosis (adjusted hazard ratio: 2.617; 95% CI, 1.026-6.679; P=0.044).

▌ Conclusion:

About 8.7% of lesions with angiographically insignificant stenosis, showed low FFR. These were observed without PCI and showed a significantly higher risk of MACE compared with those with high FFR. Low FFR was an independent predictor of MACE in deferred lesions with angiographically insignificant stenosis.

▌ Clinical Relevance:

The discrepancy between anatomic severity and presence of myocardial ischemiacan be classified into 2 categories, such as angiographically significant but functionally insignificant (mismatch) or functionally significant but angiographically insignificant (reverse mismatch).

Although evidence has shown favorable clinical outcomes for the former, information about the latter is scarce. Also, current guidelines do not recommend FFR measurement in stenosis with %DS 50%.

As per the results of this study, when clinically indicated, FFR measurement should be performed in patients with a lower degree of (<50% diameter) stenosis than those recommended in current guidelines.

Whether PCI should be attempted in such patients can only be ascertained by a study which randomizes such patients into PCI and OMT groups.

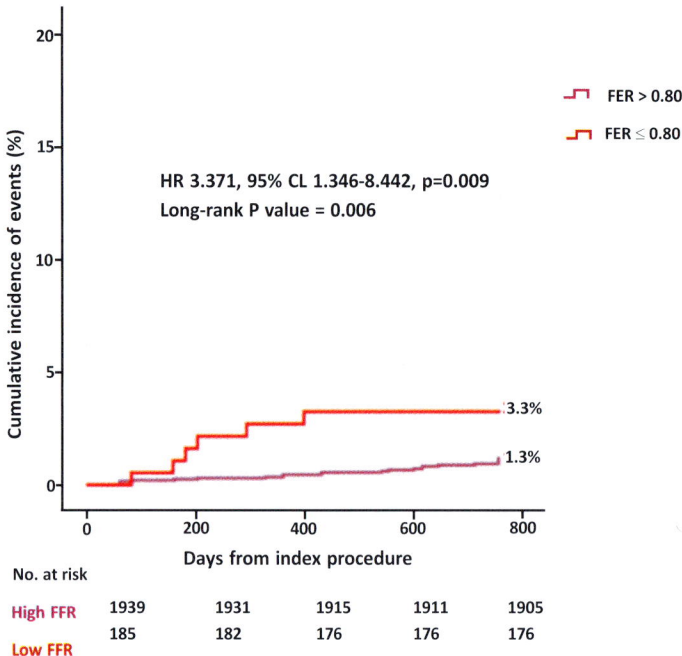

"Two year clinical outcomes of deferred angiographically insignificant lesions classified according to fractional flow reserve."

From : Joo Myung Lee, Bon-Kwon Koo, Eun-Seok Shin, Chang-Wook Nam, Joon-HyungDoh, Xinyang Hu, Fei Ye, Shaoliang Chen, Junqing Yang, Jiyan Chen, Nobuhiro Tanaka, Hiroyoshi Yokoi, Hitoshi Matsuo, Hiroaki Takashima, Yasutsugu Shiono, Doyeon Hwang, Jonghanne Park, Kyung-Jin Kim, Takashi Akasaka, Jianan Wang.

Journal of the American Heart Association. 2017;6:e006071.

Originally published August 22, 2017.

65

Temporal Trends, Complications and Predictors of Outcomes Among Nonagenarians Undergoing Percutaneous Coronary Intervention

Insights from the Veterans Affairs Clinical Assessment, Reporting, and Tracking Program

Ref.:Abhishek C. Sawant, MD, MPH, Kevin Josey, Mary E. Plomondon, PHD, Thomas M. Maddox, MD, MSC, et al.

JACC: Cardiovascular Iinterventions 2017; 10(13):1295 - 1303

Key Points:

1) There is progressive increase in number of nonagenarians who have been undergoing primary percutaneous coronary intervention (PCI) over last decade

2) Event rates in catheterization laboratory (cath lab) are similar to the those in younger population.

3) However 30 day and one year mortality is significantly higher in nonagenarians as compared to younger individuals.

Dev Pahlajani

∎ Introduction:

With increasing longevity it is expected that greater number of nonagenarians will be seeking percutaneous coronary interventional (PCI) treatment for coronary artery disease. Failure of optimum medical treatment leading to uncontrolled symptoms or acute coronary syndrome (ACS) or myocardial infarction will be the main drivers of PCI in this population. However, there is no adequate data on the outcomes following PCI in such patients. Also the predictors of mortality among these patients following PCI is not clearly defined.

∎ Aims and Treatment:

The aim was to study the temporal trends in the number of nonagenarians undergoing PCI, and also to study their clinical characteristics, cath lab complications and 30 day and one year mortality after PCI.

∎ Material and Methods:

The study enrolled patients from veteran hospitals who underwent PCI between 2008 and 2014. There were 67,148 patients who underwent PCI. Out of these 274 (0.4%) were nonagenarians. There was a temporal increase in the number of nonagenarians from 0.25% to 0.58% who underwent PCI over 6 years period.

Results:

Nonagenarians had higher risk for acute cardiogenic shock post procedure (0.73% versus 0.12% p=0.04). As compared to younger patients they also had greater risk of no reflow. Nonagenarians had 8 times greater 30 day mortality as compared to younger patients (10.6% v/s 1.4%) (p=<0.0001). Even one year undadjusted and adjusted mortality was 4 times greater than the younger individuals. Amongst the associated clinical characteristics nonagenarians had lower BMI, were less likely to be smokers and diabetics. However, they had greater incidence of hypertension, systolic heart failure, cardiovascular disease and chronic kidney diseases as compared to younger and new patients (Fig 1 & 2) (Table).

Conclusion:

The study indicates that a busy cardiac catheterization laboratory should be ready and well equipped to receive patients who are elderly, in the 90s . These patients would have higher co-morbidities and significantly higher 30 day and one year mortality. The contributing factors to the mortality could be post procedural complications like acute kidney injury, bleeding and stroke. Age is a strong predictor for excessive bleeding and stroke . While the success rate has been reported to be comparable to the younger patients the later outcomes could be worse than the younger individuals. The study calls for identifying patients who are at the higher risk of adverse outcomes like chronic kidney disease, carotid artery obstruction and high bleeding risk.

Table 1. Procedural characteristics among Nonagenarians and Younger patients

	Age < 90 Years (n = 66,874)	Age ≥ 90 Years (n = 274)	All Patients (N = 67,148)	p Value
PCI indication				< 0.0001
STEMI	4,599 6.9)	40 (14.6)	4,639 (6.9)	
NSTEMI	12,921, (19.3)	107 (39.1)	13,028 (19.4)	
Other	49,354 (73.8)	127 (46.4)	49,481 (73.7)	
Access site				0.385
Brachial	312 (0.5)	1 (0.4)	313 (0.5)	
Femoral	57,363 (85.8)	245 (89.4)	57,608 (85.9)	
Radial	7,896 (11.8)	25 (9.1)	7,921 (11.8)	
Unknown	1,258 (1.9)	3 (1.1)	1,261 (1.9)	
Fractional flow reserve performed	4,473 (6.7)	10 (3.6)	4,483 (6.7)	0.059
Lesions				0.338
1-vessel PCI	45,205 (67.6)	177 (64.6)	45,382 (67.6)	
2-vessel PCI	15,922 (23.8)	67 (24.5)	15,989 (23.8	
≥ 3-vessel PCI	5,747 (8.6)	30 (10.9)	5,777 (8.6)	

Values are n (%)
NSTEMI = non-ST-segment elevation myocardial infarction; PCI = percutaneous coronary intervention; STEMI = ST-segment elevation myocardia infarction.

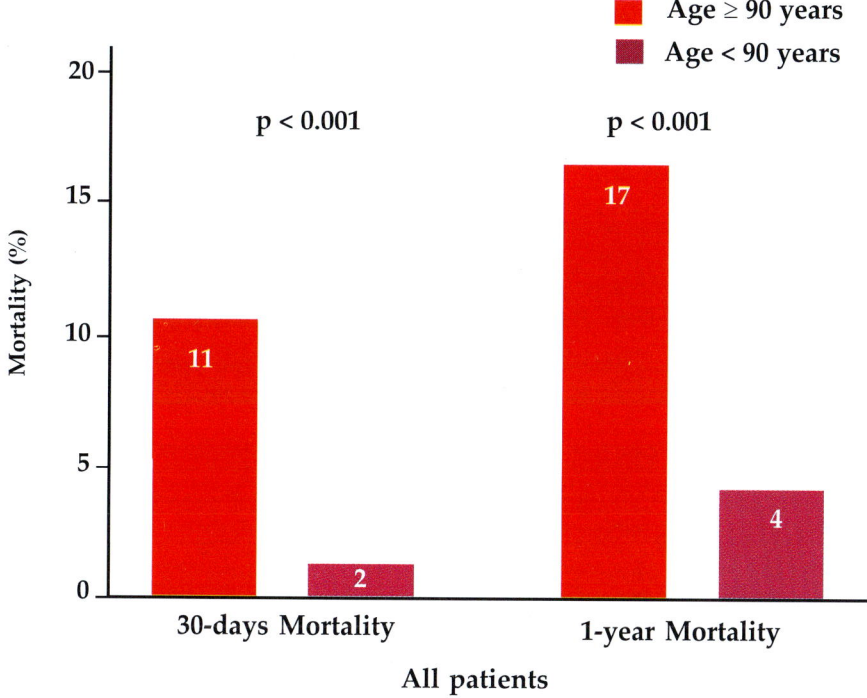

Fig. 1: *Comparison of short-term (30-day) and long-term (1-year) unadjusted mortality post-percutaneous coronary intervention among nonagenarians and younger patients*

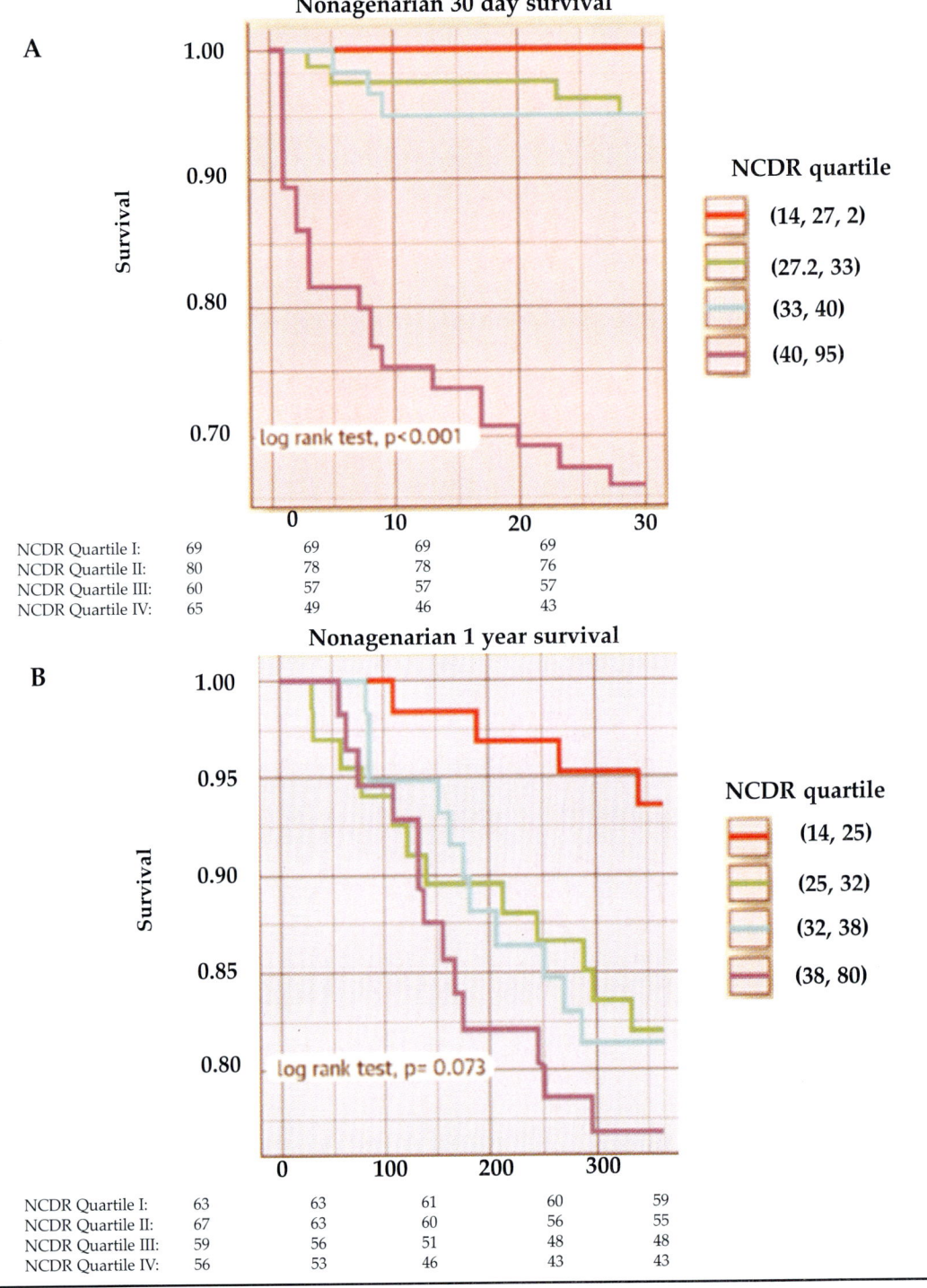

Fig. 2: *Survival among nonagenarian only post-percutaneous coronary intervention stratified by national cardiovascular data registry risk score quartiles*

Nonagenarian 30 day survival

A

NCDR Quartile I:	69	69	69	69
NCDR Quartile II:	80	78	78	76
NCDR Quartile III:	60	57	57	57
NCDR Quartile IV:	65	49	46	43

Nonagenarian 1 year survival

B

NCDR Quartile I:	63	63	61	60	59
NCDR Quartile II:	67	63	60	56	55
NCDR Quartile III:	59	56	51	48	48
NCDR Quartile IV:	56	53	46	43	43

Suggested Readings

1. From AM, Rihal CS, Lennon RJ, Holmes DR Jr., Prasad A. Temporal trends and improved outcomes of percutaneous coronary revascularization in nonagenarians. J Am Coll Cardiol Intv 2008;1:692-8

2. Kim JY, Jeong MH, Choi YW, et al. Temporal trends and in-hospital outcomes of primary percutaneous coronary intervention in nonagenarians with ST-segment elevation myocardial infarction. Korean J Intern Med 2015;30:821-8.

3. Khera S, Kolte D, Palaniswamy C, et al. ST-elevation myocardial infarction in the elderly-temporal trends in incidence, utilization of percutaneous coronary intervention and outcomes in the United States. Int J Cardiol 2013;168:3683-90.

4. Schoenenberger AW, Radovanovic D, Windecker S, et al. Temporal trends in the treatment and outcomes of elderly patients with acute coronary syndrome. Eur Heart J 2016;37:1304-11.

5. Shanmugasundaram M. Percutaneous coronary intervention in elderly patients: is it beneficial? Tex Heart Inst J 2011;38:398-403.

6. Petroni T, Zaman A, Georges JL, et al. Primary percutaneous coronary intervention for ST elevation myocardial infarction in nonagenarians. Heart 2016;102:1648-54.

7. Skolnick AH, Alexander KP, Chen AY, et al. Characteristics, management, and outcomes of 5,557 patients age $90 years with acute coronary syndromes: results from the CRUSADE initiative. J Am Coll Cardiol 2007;49:1790-7.

8. Presutti DG, D'Ascenzo F, Omede P, et al. Percutaneous coronary intervention in nonagenarian: a meta-analysis of observational studies. J Cardiovasc Med (Hagerstown) 2013;14:773.

66

Rivaroxaban with or without Aspirin in Stable Cardiovascular Disease COMPASS Trial and PAD Subgroup Analysis

Ref.: John W. Eikelboom, M.B., B.S., Stuart J. Connolly, M.D., et al for the COMPASS Investigators NEJM August 27, 2017 DOI: 10.1056/NEJMoa1709118

Key Point

In patients with stable atherosclerotic vascular disease, the risk of major adverse cardiovascular events was significantly lower with the combination of rivaroxaban plus aspirin than with aspirin alone, with significantly higher risk of major bleeding. Rivaroxaban alone did not result in a significantly lower risk of major adverse cardiovascular events compared to aspirin alone and resulted in a significantly higher risk of major bleeding.

Akshay Mehta

▌ Introduction:

Till now aspirin (or clopidogrel, if aspirin is not tolerated) is the only anti thrombotic used in the secondary prevention of stable atherosclerotic vascular disease. Addition of Vit K antagonists in stable post MI patients have produced benefits but at the expense of more bleeding. Rivaroxaban is a selective direct factor Xa inhibitor that has lesser propensity for bleeding and hence could be beneficial when added to aspirin in low doses in stable patients.

▌ Aims of the Study:

To check whether rivaroxaban in combination with aspirin or given alone is more effective than aspirin alone in preventing recurrent cardiovascular events, with acceptable safety, in patients with stable atherosclerotic vascular disease.

▌ Material and Methods:

For the COMPASS trial, 27,395 patients with stable atherosclerotic vascular disease (coronary artery disease or peripheral arterial disease [PAD]) were randomized to one of three groups: rivaroxaban 2.5 mg twice daily plus aspirin 100 mg daily; rivaroxaban 5 mg twice daily alone; or aspirin 100 mg daily alone. The primary end point was a composite of cardiovascular death, stroke, or MI.

The main safety outcome was a modification of the International Society on Thrombosis and Haemostasis (ISTH) criteria for major bleeding. Three secondary efficacy outcomes and tertiary efficacy outcomes were also specified.

Results:

After a mean follow up of 23 months the trial was stopped prematurely due to significant reductions in the composite primary end point by 1.3% (Absolute risk reduction-ARR). In addition, the rivaroxaban-plus-ASA combination reduced two other key composite secondary end points by 1.3% and 1.4% respectively, as well as lowering all-cause death by 0.7%. Although major bleeding was higher with rivaroxaban/aspirin, by 1.2%, fatal bleeding did not differ.

The rivaroxaban-plus-ASA combination reduced the net-benefit surrogate of cardiovascular death, stroke, MI, fatal bleeding, or symptomatic bleeding into a critical organ by 1.2%.

Conclusion:

Among patients with stable atherosclerotic vascular disease, a high proportion of whom were receiving proven secondary prevention therapies, the rate of the primary outcome (a composite of cardiovascular death, stroke, or myocardial infarction) was lower by 24% (RRR) with rivaroxaban (2.5 mg twice daily) plus aspirin than with aspirin alone (4.1% vs. 5.4%), but the rate of major bleeding was higher by 70% (3.1% vs. 1.9%). The rate of the net-clinical-benefit outcome was lower by 20% with rivaroxaban plus aspirin than with aspirin alone (4.7% vs. 5.9%). Rivaroxaban (5 mg twice daily) alone as compared to aspirin alone did not show a significant difference in the primary outcome or the net-clinical-benefit outcome, but the rate of major bleeding was higher.

Clinical Relevance:

Patients with stable atherosclerotic disease are already at low risk, especially with optimal medical treatment with statins, aspirin, RAAS blockers etc. To show mortality benefit on top of these treatments says something about this trial with Rivaroxaban. Of course, major bleeding was a price to pay for the benefit, which is understandable with the use of any oral anticoagulant.

PAD Subgroup Analysis :

The COMPASS trial included 7470 PAD patients - 4129 with symptomatic PAD limbs, 1919 with carotid disease, and 1422 with CAD and low ankle-brachial index (< 0.90).

Results from the PAD subgroup were presented at the European Society of Cardiology (ESC) 2017 Congress, and are slated to be published in Lancet.

Results showed that the combination of low-dose (2.5 mg twice daily) rivaroxaban plus aspirin 100 mg daily showed significant reductions in both major cardiovascular and limb events, including amputations, in patients with peripheral arterial disease (PAD).

Besides reducing the primary outcome of a composite of CV death/stroke/MI by 30%, the combination treatment reduced major adverse limb events by 50 % and major amputation by 70% - results which can be described as spectacular.

The combination also increased the risk of major bleeding by 60% but did not increase the risk of fatal or critical organ bleeding, and most major bleeds were reversible.

Thus, we now have a truly effective treatment for PAD which shows not only a reduction in cardiovascular events but also a substantial reduction in limb events.

To incorporate the benefits of adding Rivaroxaban in small doses to aspirin in clinical practice, the main objective will be to select patients after balancing bleeding risk and benefits.

▮ Suggested Readings

1. Eikelboom JW, Connolly S J, Bosch J, et al. Rivaroxaban with or without aspirin in stable cardiovascular disease. N Engl J Med 2017; DOI:10.1056/NEJMoa1709118.

2. Braunwald E. An important step for thrombocardiology. N Engl J Med 2017; DOI:10.1056/NEJMe1710241.

3. Anand S et al. COMPASS PAD: Cardiovascular Outcomes for People Using Anticoagulation Strategies trial: Results in patients with peripheral artery disease. European Society of Cardiology 2017 Congress. August 27, 2017; Barcelona, Spain.

4. Antithrombotic Trialists' (ATT) Collaboration. Aspirin in the primary and secondary prevention of vascular disease: collaborative meta-analysis of individual participant data from randomised trials. Lancet 2009;373:1849-1860.

5. Anand SS, Yusuf S. Oral anticoagulants in patients with coronary artery disease. J Am CollCardiol 2003;41:Suppl S:62S-69S.

6. Mega JL, Braunwald E, Wiviott SD, et al. Rivaroxaban in patients with a recent acute coronary syndrome. N Engl J Med 2012;366:9-19.

67

The Relationship of Body Mass Index to Percutaneous Coronary Intervention Outcomes

Does the Obesity Paradox Exist in Contemporary Percutaneous Coronary Intervention Cohorts? Insights from the British Cardiovascular Intervention Society Registry

Ref.: Eric W. Holroyd, MD, Alex Sirker, MB, BCHIR, PHD, Chun Shing Kwok, MBBS, BSC, MSC, Evangelos Kontopantelis, PHD, Peter F. Ludman, MD, Mark A. De Belder, MD, Robert Butler, MBCHB, MD, James Cotton, MBBS, MD, Azfar Zaman, MBCHB, MD, Mamas A. Mamas, BMBCH, DPHIL, on behalf of the British Cardiovascular Intervention Society and National Institute of Cardiovascular Outcomes Research
LINK: JACC INTV 2017;10(13):1283-92

Key Points:

1) There exists obesity paradox regarding outcomes following percutaneous coronary intervention (PCI).

2) There is significantly lower mortality in patients with high body mass index (BMIs) as compared to low BMI.

3) Obesity advantage for mortality and adverse outcomes is observed at 30 days, one year and 5 years post PCI.

4) Obesity advantage is independent of other co-founders.

Dev Pahlajani

▮ Introduction:

Obese individuals have high incidence of coronary artery disease, hypertension, diabetes, premature death and decreased life expectancy as compared to normal weight individuals. However, several studies have pointed out that mortality amongst individuals undergoing coronary artery bypass grafting (CABG) or PCI is lower in patients with high BMI as compared to those withnormal or low BMI. Current study analyzes the relationship between BMI and clinical outcomes following PCI. The study also analyzes the relationship of different clinical presentations, mortality and BMI.

▮ Methods:

Patients in the study were enrolled from British Cardiovascular Intervention Society registry. It analyzed the outcomes in 345192 patients in the relationship to the various BMI that was classified as <18.5, 18.5 - 24.9, 25 - 30 and >30 kgs/m^2. The outcome of death and MACE was determined at 30 day, one year andfurther followed upto 5 years. MACE was defined as the composite of in-hospital reinfarction, repeat PCI, emergency CABG and in-hospital mortality.

Results:

Lean patients were significantly older, less likely to be males and tended to have poor left ventricular function. As opposed to this obese patients were significantly younger, smokers, had features of metabolic syndrome, hypertension, high cholesterol and diabetes. Thirty days mortality was 1% in obese patients compared to 2% in those with normal BMI and 4% in lean patients. At one year and 5 years the difference in mortality was maintained with lean and the normal BMI patients having more than twice the mortality as compared to obese patients. Better survival in obese patients were irrespective of other co-morbid conditions (Fig.1).

Some of the earlier meta-analysis have shown favorable outcomes in patients who are obese and high BMI not only after PCI but CABG surgery as well.

Conclusion:

Lean patients as well as patients with normal BMI need a careful assessment of the associated risk factors and careful monitoring to achieve comparable results.

Fig. 1: *Adjusted odds ratio for 30 days Mortality according to BMI groups*

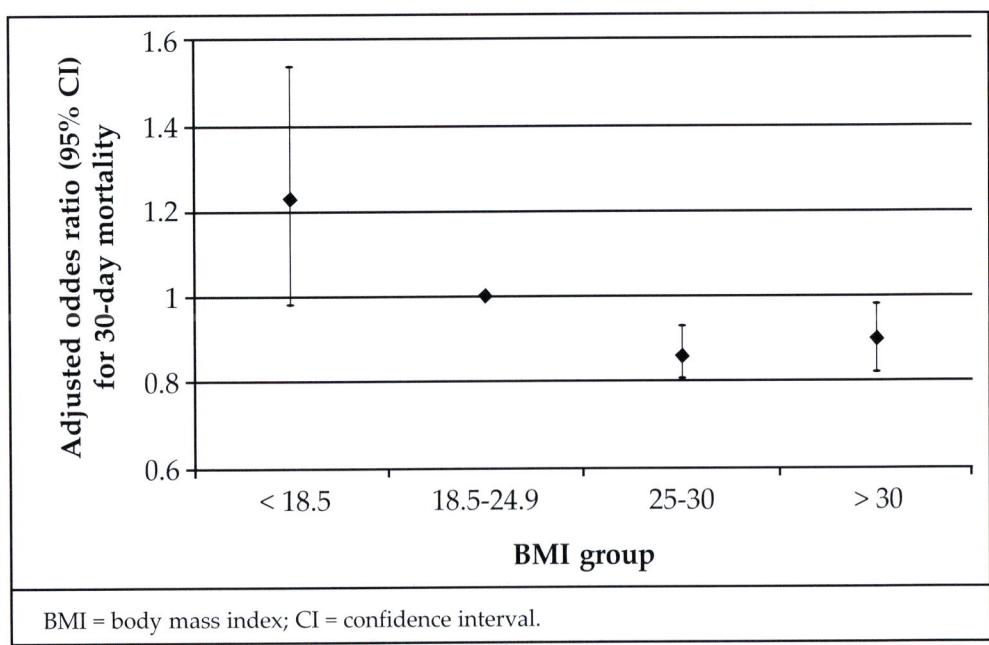

BMI = body mass index; CI = confidence interval.

▌ Suggested Readings

1. Manson JE, Willett WC, Stampfer MJ, et al. Body weight and mortality among women. N Engl J Med 1995;333:677-85.

2. Garrison RJ, Castelli WP. Weight and thirty-year mortality of men in the Framingham Study. Ann Intern Med 1985;103:1006-9.

3. Peeters A, Barendregt JJ, Willekens F, Mackenbach JP, Al Mamun A, Bonneux L. Obesity in adulthood and its consequences for life expectancy: a life-table analysis. Ann Intern Med 2003; 138:24-32.

4. Romero-Corral A, Montori VM, Somers VK, et al. Association of bodyweight with total mortality and with cardiovascular events in coronary artery disease: a systematic review of cohort studies. Lancet 2006;368:666-78.

5. Ellis SG, Elliott J, Horrigan M, Rayomnd RE, Howell G. Low-normal or excessive body mass index: newly identified and powerful risk factors for death and other complications with percutaneous coronary intervention. Am J Cardiol 1996; 78:642-6.

6. Gruberg L, Weissman NJ, Waksman R, et al. The impact of obesity on the short-term and long-term outcomes after percutaneous coronary intervention: the obesity paradox? J Am CollCardiol 2002;39:578 84.

7. Buschur ME, Smith D, Share D, et al. The burgeoning epidemic of morbid obesity in patients undergoing percutaneous coronary intervention. J Am CollCardiol 2013;62:685-91.

8. Oreopoulos A, Padwal R, Norris CM, Mullen JC, Pretorius V, Kalantar-Zadeh K. Effect of obesity on short- and long-term mortality postcoronary revascularization: a meta-analysis. Obesity 2008; 16:442-50.

9. Akin I, Tölg R, Hochadel M, et al. No evidence of "obesity paradox" after treatment with drug eluting stents in a routine clinical practice: results from the prospective multicenter German DES.DE (German Drug-Eluting Stent) registry. J Am CollCardiolIntv 2012;5:162-9.

10. Das SR, Alesander KP, Chen AY, et al. Impact of body weight and extreme obesity on the presentation, treatment and in-hospital outcomes of 50, 149 patients with ST-segment elevation myocardial infarction. J Am CollCardiol 2011;59:2642-50.

11. Bundhun PK, Li N, Chen MH. Does an obesity paradox really exist after cardiovascular intervention? A systematic review and meta-analysis of randomized controlled trials and observational studies. Medicine 2015;94:e1910.

12. Tan XF, Shi JX, Chen AM. Prolonged and intensive medication use are associated with the obesity paradox after percutaneous coronary intervention: a systematic review and metaanalysis of 12 studies. BMC CardiovascDisord 2016;16:125.

13. Wang ZJ, Zhou YJ, Galper BZ, Gao F, Yeh RW, Mauri L. Association of body mass index with mortality and cardiovascular events for patients with coronary artery disease: a systematic review and meta-analysis. Heart 2015;101:1631-8.

14. Sharma A, Vallakati A, Einstein AJ, et al. Relationship of body mass index with total mortality, cardiovascular mortality, myocardial infarction after coronary revascularization: evidence from a meta-analysis. Mayo ClinProc 2014; 89:364-71.

68

Benefit of Switching Dual Antiplatelet Therapy After Acute Coronary Syndrome: The TOPIC (Timing of Platelet Inhibition After Acute Coronary Syndrome) Randomized Study

Ref.: Thomas Cuisset Pierre Deharo Jacques Quilici Thomas W. Johnson Stéphanie Deffarges Clémence Bassez Guillaume Bonnet Laurent Fourcade Jean Philippe Mouret Marc Lambert Valentine Verdier Pierre Emmanuel Morange Marie Christine Alessi Jean Louis Bonnet

European Heart Journal, ehx175, https://doi.org/10.1093/eurheartj/ehx175

Published: 16 May 2017

Key Point

Switching dual antiplatelet therapy (DAPT) from aspirin plus a newer P2Y12 blocker to aspirin plus clopidogrel 1-month after ACS was effective in preventing bleeding complications without increasing ischaemic events following ACS.

Akshay Mehta

▌ Study Objective:

To evaluate the benefit of switching dual antiplatelet therapy (DAPT) from aspirin plus a newer P2Y12 blocker to a fixed dose combination of aspirin plus clopidogrel 1month after ACS.

▌ Study Protocol:

In this open-label, single center, randomized trial, 645 patients with ACS requiring coronary intervention, on aspirin and a newer P2Y12 blocker and without adverse event at 1-month, were randomized after 1 month to aspirin and clopidogrel (switched DAPT-322 patients) in a fixed dose combination (FDC) or continued with their drug regimen (unchanged DAPT-323 patients). While switching, the clopidogrel dose in the FDC was 75 mg.

The primary outcome was a composite of cardiovascular death, urgent revascularization, stroke and bleeding as defined by the Bleeding Academic Research Consortium (BARC) classification ≥2 at 1 year post ACS.

▌ Results:

The primary endpoint occurred in 43 (13.4%) patients in the switched DAPT group and in 85 (26.3%) patients in the unchanged DAPT (HR 95% CI 0.48 (0.34-0.68), P < 0.01). No significant differences were reported on ischaemic endpoints, while BARC ≥ 2 bleeding occurred in 13 (4.0%)

patients in the switched DAPT and in 48 (14.9%) in the unchanged DAPT group (HR 95%CI 0.30 (0.18-0.50), P < 0.01).

■ Conclusion:

Changing DAPT from a newer P2Y12 blocker plus aspirin to a fixed dose combination of aspirin and clopidogrel, 1-month after an ACS, was associated with a net clinical benefit mainly driven by a significant reduction in bleeding complications, while the risk of recurrent ischaemic events was not different.

■ Comment and Clinical Application:

The study was based on the observation that in PLATO and TRITON TIMI trials, the greatest ischaemic benefit was observed during the earliest phase after ACS,which was followed by a dynamic and time-dependent risk reduction in ischemic events after that. On the other hand, the heightened bleeding risk with the new P2Y12 inhibitors continued throughout the year after PCI. Bleeding is the most frequent non-cardiac complication after PCI, with an adverse prognostic impact comparable with that of ischaemic events.

The trial utilized the anti thrombotic benefit of newer P2Y12 inhibitors for the first month and showed that switching to clopidogrel after 1-month is an effective strategy that allows a significant reduction of the bleeding risk with no increase in ischaemic complications.

The results were same for NSTE ACS as well as STEMI.

This has great advantages in practice, given the cost of new P2Y12 inhibitors (especially Ticagrelor) and a relatively cheap and convenient once daily dosing of aspirin plus clopidogrel.

Although this was an open label study, all events for which medical attention was sought were adjudicated by a blinded critical events committee. Despite the small sample size of the present study, the between group differences in end points were robust.

In real life, this kind of switch has already been common in practice, although without scientific support. This study appears to provide that support.

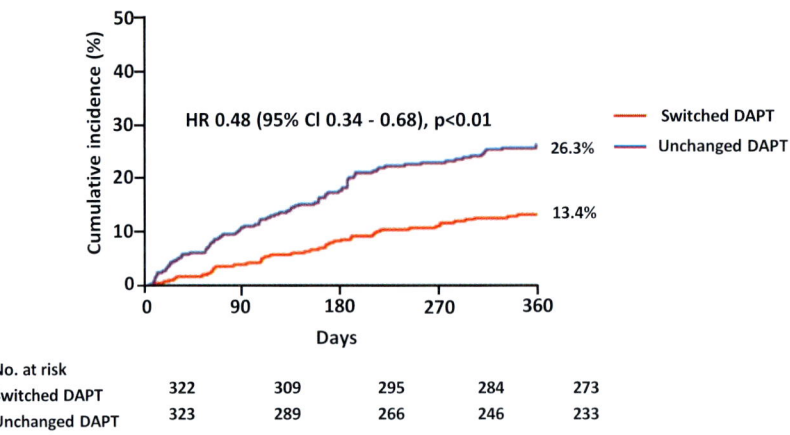

"Incidence of net clinical benefit at 1 year".

From: Thomas Cuisset Pierre Deharo Jacques Quilici Thomas W. Johnson Stéphanie Deffarges Clémence Bassez Guillaume Bonnet Laurent Fourcade Jean Philippe Mouret Marc Lambert.

Benefit of switching dual antiplatelet therapy after acute coronary syndrome: the TOPIC (timing of platelet inhibition after acute coronary syndrome) randomized study.

European Heart Journal, Volume 38, Issue 41, 1 November 2017, Pages 3070-3078.

▮ Suggested Readings

1. Wiviott SD, Braunwald E, McCabe CH, Montalescot G, Ruzyllo W, Gottlieb S, Neumann FJ, Ardissino D, De Servi S, Murphy SA, Riesmeyer J, Weerakkody G, Gibson CM, Antman EM; TRITON-TIMI 38 Investigators. Prasugrel versus clopidogrel in patients with acute coronary syndromes. N Engl J Med 2007; 357:2001-2015.

2. Lars Wallentin, M.D., Ph.D., Richard C. Becker, M.D., Andrzej Budaj, M.D., Ph.D., Christopher P. Cannon, M.D., HåkanEmanuelsson, M.D., Ph.D., Claes Held, M.D., Ph.D., Jay Horrow, M.D., Steen Husted, M.D., D.Sc., Stefan James, M.D., Ph.D., Hugo Katus, M.D., Kenneth W. Mahaffey, M.D., Benjamin M. Scirica, M.D., M.P.H., Allan Skene, Ph.D., Philippe Gabriel Steg, M.D., Robert F. Storey, M.D., D.M., and Robert A. Harrington, M.D., for the PLATO Investigators*

   Ticagrelor versus Clopidogrel in Patients with Acute Coronary Syndromes. N Engl J Med 2009; 361: 1045-1057.

3. Deharo P, Quilici J, Bonnet G, Pankert M, Verdier V, Morange P, Alessi MC, Bonnet JL, Cuisset T. Fixed-dose aspirin-clopidogrel combination enhances compliance to aspirin after acute coronary syndrome. Int J Cardiol 2014;172:e1-e2.

69

Effects of Successful Percutaneous Coronary Intervention of Chronic Total Occlusions on Myocardial Perfusion and Left Ventricular Function

Ref.: Wijnand J. Stuijfzand, MD; P. Stefan Biesbroek, MD; Pieter G. Raijmakers, MD, PhD; et al
Euro intervention 2017;13:345-354

Key Points:

1. Successful percutaneous coronary intervention of chronic total occlusion (PCI-CTO) is associated with

   - Improvement in stress myocardial blood flow (MBF) in the CTO area.

   - Significant increase in the stress MBF in the remote area as compared to the baseline MBF.

   - Minimal improvement in the left ventricular ejection fraction (LVEF)

   - Improvement in overall ischemic burden

Dev Pahlajani

∎ Introduction:

CTO is observed in approximately 30% patients who undergo coronary angiography. However, only about 15-20 % of them undergo PCI. Some of the reasons are:

a) Collaterals are assumed to be adequate to maintain perfusion and prevent myocardial infarction

b) Low success rates of CTO PCI in inexperienced hands

c) Conflicting reports of benefits of CTO PCI.

∎ Methods:

The current study was undertaken to ascertain whether successful CTO PCI achieves improvement in MBF and leads to functional recovery. The study prospectively enrolled 69 consecutive patients with CTO. All of them underwent cardiac positron emission tomography (PET) and cardiac MTI (CMR) prior to PCI and atleast 12 weeks following successful CTO PCI. Fifty nine patients had PCI for the CTO only while 10 had additional PCI for the non CTO diseased vessel.

∎ Results:

The MBF during rest and stress at baseline were significantly lower in the CTO territory when compared myocardium in the remote area (p = < 0.001). PCI was associated with significantly increase in the MBF during stress by 1.18 ± 0.79 and 0.19 ± 0.58 ml.min-1g-1 in CTO and remote territories respectively. While the MBF increased, the LV end diastolic volume as well as mean LV end systolic volume decreased but not significantly. The effect on the LV function was modest (Table 1).

The data from some of the earlier studies have given conflicting results as regards to the effect of CTO PCI on LVEF. This could be due to the differences in the patient population, associated co-morbidities and angiographic patterns and the degree of viability in the CTO areas. The LVEF is governed by the degree and size of MI and therefore one would assume that larger the infarct pre PCI smaller will be the improvement in the LV function.

▌ Clinical Implications:

Since the study indicates a significant improvement in MBF and decrease in the ischemic burden, carefully selected patients with myocardial viability would certainly be expected to benefit from the CTO PCI. However, the real clinical benefit should be wothwhile the procedure if long term follow up demonstrates decrease in the hard end points like death, MI, target vessel revascularisation. The study does not comment on the improvement in the symptomatic status and its correlation with improved MBF and decreased ischemic burden.

Table 1. Left ventricular function and volumes

	Basdeline	Follow-up	*p*-Value
All patients (n = 69)			
LVEDV (mL)	199 ± 64	193 ± 61	0.03
LVESV (mL)	112 ± 60	106 ± 59	< 0.01
LVEF (%)	46.4 ± 11.0	47.5 ± 11.4	0.01
LV Stroke volume (mL)	87 ± 20	87 ± 19	0.66
SWT CTO area (%)	53.8 ± 22.4	56.4 ± 25.4	0.18

CTO: chronic total occlusion; LV: left ventricle; LVEDV: left ventricular end-diastolic volume; LVEF: left ventricular ejection fraction; LVESV: left ventricular end-systolic volume; SWT: segmental systolic wall thickning

▌ Suggested Readings

1. Stuijfzand WJ, Raijmakers PG, Driessen RS, van Royen N, Nap A, van Rossum AC, Knaapen P. Value of Hybrid Imaging with PET/CT to Guide Percutaneous Revascularization of Chronic Total Coronary Occlusion. Curr Cardiovasc Imaging Rep. 2015;8:26.

2. Stuijfzand WJ, Driessen RS, Raijmakers PG, Rijnierse MT, Maeremans J, Hollander MR, Lammertsma AA, van Rossum AC, Dens J, Nap A, van Royen N, Knaapen P. Prevalence of ischaemia in patients with a chronic total occlusion and preserved left ventricular ejection fraction. Eur Heart J Cardiovasc Imaging.2016 Sep 1.[Epub ahead of print].

3. Simonsen JA, Johansen A, Gerke O, Mickley H, Thomassen A, Hess S, Rask CK, Tamadoni M, Jensen LO, Hallas J, Vach W, Hoilund-Carlsen PF. Outcome with invasive versus medical treatment of stable coronary artery disease: influence of perfusion defect size, ischaemia, and ejection fraction. Euro Intervention. 2016;11:1118-24.

4. Pujadas S, Martin V, Rossello X, Carreras F, Barros A, Leta R, Alomar X, Cinca J, Sabate M, Pons-Llado G. Improvement of myocardial function and perfusion after successful percutaneous revascularization in patients with chronic total coronary occlusion. Int J Cardiol. 2013;169:147-52.

70

Metoprolol Reduces Hemodynamic and Metabolic Overload in Asymptomatic Aortic Valve Stenosis Patients

Ref.: Nils Henrik Hansson, Jens Sörensen, Hendrik Johannes Harms, Won Yong Kim, Roni Nielsen, Lars Poulsen Tolbod, Jørgen Frøkiær, Kirsten Bouchelouche, Karen Kaae Dodt, Inger Sihm, Steen Hvitfeldt Poulsen, Henrik Wiggers

Circulation: Cardiovascular Imaging. 2017;10:e006557, Originally published September 27, 2017

Key Points

1. In patients with asymptomatic AS, metoprolol displays favorable hemodynamic and metabolic effects by increasing systolic ejection time and reducing aortic valve gradients, global afterload, and myocardial oxygen requirements.
2. Thus, metoprolol could postpone or prevent the need for aortic valve replacement in patients with asymptomatic AS.

Akshay Mehta

▐ Introduction:

The treatment of symptomatic severe valvular aortic stenosis is valve replacement. However, what to do with asymptomatic valvular aortic stenosis ? Is there a medical treatment regimen which can keep the patient stable and possibly postpone surgery?

▐ Objectives :

The purpose of this trial was to find whether metoprolol reduces the hemodynamic and metabolic burden imposed by AS.

▐ Methods :

This was a randomized, double-blind, placebo-controlled trial. Forty patients with asymptomatic AS (aortic valve area, 0.5 ± 0.1 cm^2/m^2; peak gradient, 53 ± 19 mm Hg) were randomly assigned to receive either extended-release metoprolol or placebo (1:1) once daily for 22 weeks the target dose being 50 - 200 mg titrated over 6 weeks based on telephone interviews with home blood pressure and HR readings 2 and 4 weeks after initiation of treatment. Patients were evaluated by echocardiography, cardiovascular magnetic resonance, 11C-acetate positron emission tomography and 6 minute walk test at baseline and after 22 weeks.

Results :

Extended-release metoprolol compared with placebo, in a dose of 100 ± 53 mg/d decreased heart rate, increased ejection time, reduced aortic valve peak gradients, without affecting stroke volume. Also, valvuloarterial impedance (ie, global afterload) and myocardial oxygen consumption were reduced with improved myocardial efficiency defined as stroke work/myocardial oxygen consumption.

There were 2 cardiovascular adverse events in the placebo group (hypertension and anemia) compared with 4 in the metoprolol group (dizziness, cold hands/feet, bradycardia, and fatigue).

All adverse reactions ceased after a reduction in dose or discontinuation of the treatment, except for the patients who experienced congestion and atypical chest pain. Both patients were stabilized with AVR.

A small increase in NT-proBNP was observed in patients who were treated with metoprolol, a finding which is a well-known phenomenon when initiating ?-blocker treatment in patients with a normal or near-normal NT-proBNP.

Severe reduction in HR (e.g., > -20 minute^{-1}) may inhibit the compensatory increase in SV and reduce cardiac index, which may diminish any favorable effect achieved by metoprolol and increase the risk of adverse effects.

Conclusion:

In patients with asymptomatic AS, metoprolol treatment :

1) Unloaded the LV by reducing afterload (i.e., aortic valve gradients and valvulo arterial impedence-Zva); and

2) Lowered myocardial oxygen requirements.

Comment:

In this first of its kind study, it was shown that metoprolol in asymptomatic AS patients increases systolic ejection time and decreases aortic valve gradients and valvuloarterial impedance, without reducing SV. Consequently, it decreases stroke work and myocardial oxygen requirement.

It has been known that unloading the LV by decreasing aortic valve gradients and Zva are both strong predictors of LV function and survival in patients with AS.

Hence metoprolol can postpone or prevent the need for AVR in patients with asymptomatic AS.

Metoprolol would also benefit if there is associated CAD, AF or HF.

In addition, some patients with bicuspid AV may have dilated aortic roots (bicuspid aortopathy) where beta blockade (though not proven) may be of additional help in reducing the stress on aorta.

As the study shows, if care is taken while up-titrating the dose to prevent excessive bradycardia or congestion, this therapeutic intervention may represent an important breakthrough which can improve prognosis in the large population of patients with asymptomatic AS.

▌ Suggested Readings

1. Rossi A, Temporelli PL, Cicoira M, Gaibazzi N, Cioffi G, Nistri S, Magatelli M, Tavazzi L, Faggiano P. Beta-blockers can improve survival in medically-treated patients with severe symptomatic aortic stenosis. Int J Cardiol. 2015;190:15-17.

2. Beanlands RS, Nahmias C, Gordon E, Coates G, deKemp R, Firnau G, Fallen E. The effects of beta(1)-blockade on oxidative metabolism and the metabolic cost of ventricular work in patients with left ventricular dysfunction: a double-blind, placebo-controlled, positron-emission tomography study. Circulation. 2000;102:2070-2075.

3. Hachicha Z, Dumesnil JG, Pibarot P. Usefulness of the valvuloarterial impedance to predict adverse outcome in asymptomatic aortic stenosis. J Am Coll Cardiol. 2009;54:1003-1011.

4. Lancellotti P, Donal E, Magne J, Moonen M, O'Connor K, Daubert JC, Pierard LA. Risk stratification in asymptomatic moderate to severe aortic stenosis: the importance of the valvular, arterial and ventricular interplay. Heart. 2010;96:1364-1371.

5. Rosenhek R, Zilberszac R, Schemper M, Czerny M, Mundigler G, Graf S, Bergler-Klein J, Grimm M, Gabriel H, Maurer G. Natural history of very severe aortic stenosis. Circulation. 2010;121:151-156.

71

Impact of Stent Overlapping on Long-Term Clinical Outcomes in Patients with ST-Segment Elevation Myocardial Infarction: Insights from the Five-Year Follow-Up of the EXAMINATION Trial

Ref.: Luis Ortega-Paz1, MD; Salvatore Brugaletta1*, MD, PhD; Giuseppe Giacchi1, MD; Kohki Ishida1, MD et al on behalf of the EXAMINATION investigators

LINK: Eurointervention 2017;13:e557-e563

Key Points:

1. Overlapping and non overlapping stents in patients with STEMI have similar outcomes.

2. Five year outcomes in patients who receive bare metal stents (BMS) have greater rate of adverse cardiac events as compared to everolimus eluting stent (EES).

3. There was a trend towards higher rate of definite / probable stent thrombosis in overlapping stent group as compared to no overlapping group.

Dev Pahlajani

❚ Introduction:

About 30% patients who undergo percutaneous coronary intervention (PCI) receive overlapping stents. Overlap is usually done either for long lesions or to cover dissection occurring during PCI procedure. Data regarding outcome following overlapping stents in drug eluting stent era is limited.

❚ Aims of the Study:

To compare long term outcomes of overlapping stents versus non overlapping stents in STEMI patients who undergo PCI.

❚ Material:

Patients in the study were enrolled from EXAMINATION trial which was a prospective randomized multicentre trial of all comers STEMI patients.

In the trial 1498 patients were randomized to undergo PCI with EES versus cobalt chromium BMS.

❚ Results:

Amongst enrolled patients 404 (27%) received overlapping stents whereas 1094 (73%) had non overlapping stents. Dissection was the reason for overlapping in 10.6% patients with EES and 7.9% in patients treated with BMS. Rest of them had overlapping due to non coverage of the lesions.

■ **Ootcomes:**

At 1 and 5 years, there was no difference in outcomes between the overlapping versus no overlapping group (14.9% v/s 12.4%) (p=0.47). Five years follow up showed that there was a trend towards higher rate of patient oriented end points of all cause death, myocardial infarction (MI) and repeat revascularization in BMS treated group as compared to EES treated group. There was also higher rate of definite / probable stent thrombosis in the overlap group versus non overlap group (2.2% versus 1.6% at one year) which was statistically nosignificant. It was mainly driven by the higher rate in BMS treated patients (4.4% versus 0%) (Fig.1 & Table 1).

■ **Conclusion:**

With second generation EES deployment of overlapping stents appears to be quite safe and associated with low patient oriented cardiac events when compared to no overlap.

■ **Clinical Relevance:**

In patients with STEMI who undergo primary or pharmaco-invasive PCI one should not hesitate to deploy overlapping stents since the event rates are quite low. The results are in confirmation with the earlier trials. Earlier concerns of restenosis or stent thrombosis following overlapping stents are not relevant in the contemporary PCI practice since more often than not second generation stents are deployed by default strategy. Second generation stents like EES have newer design, low strut thickness and coated with non inflammatory or absorbable polymer.

Fig. 1: *Time to event and landmark analysis of DoCE*

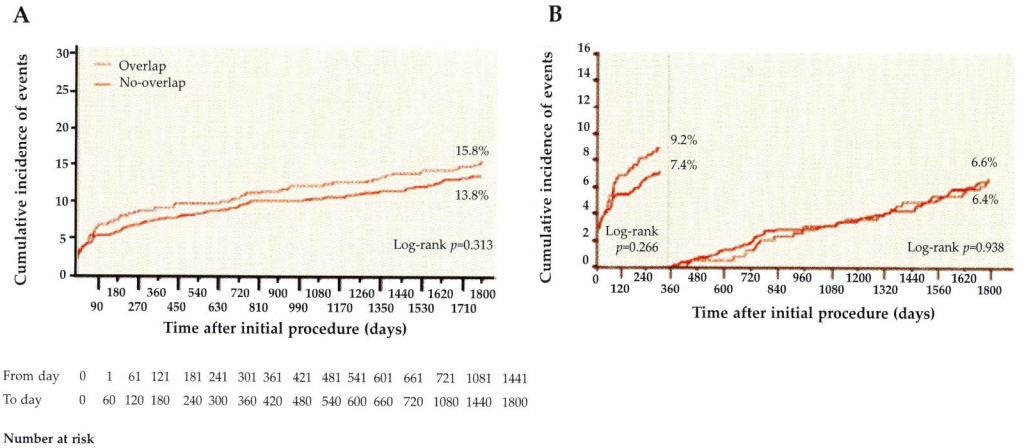

Fig. 2: *Definite probable stent thrombosis*

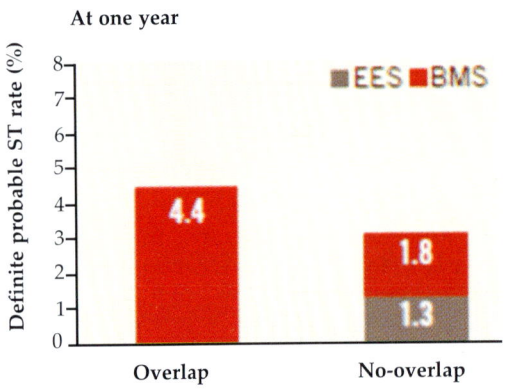

At one year

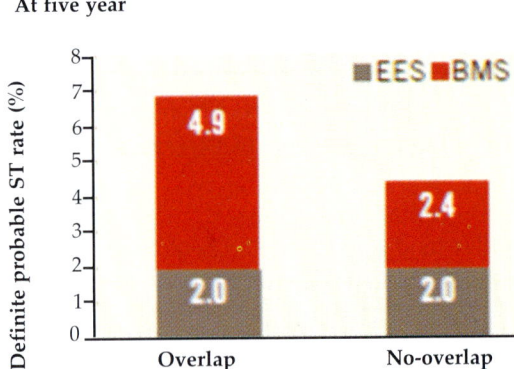

At five year

▌ Suggested Readings

1. Räber L, Jüni P, Löffel L, Wandel S, Cook S, Wenaweser P, Togni M, Vogel R, Seiler C, Eberli F, Luscher T, Meier B, Windecker S. Impact of stent overlap on angiographic and longterm clinical outcome in patients undergoing drug-eluting stent implantation. J Am CollCardiol. 2010;55:1178-88.

2. O'Sullivan CJ, Stefanini GG, Räber L, Heg D, Taniwaki M, Kalesan B, Pilgrim T, Zanchin T, Moschovitis A, Bullesfeld L, Khattab AA, Meier B, Wenaweser P, Jüni P, Windecker S. Impact of stent overlap on long-term clinical outcomes in patients treated with newer-generation drug-eluting stents. Euro Intervention. 2014;9:1076-84.

3. Farooq V, Vranckx P, Mauri L, Cutlip DE, Belardi J, Silber S, Widimsky P, Leon M, Windecker S, Meredith I, Negoita M, van Leeuwen F, Neumann FJ, Yeung AC, Garcia-Garcia HM, Serruys PW. Impact of overlapping newer generation drug-eluting stents on clinical and angiographic outcomes: pooled analysis of five trials from the international Global RESOLUTE Program. Heart. 2013;99:626-33.

4. Sabaté M, Cequier A, Iniguez A, Serra A, Hernandez Antolin R, Mainar V, Valgimigli M, Tespili M, den Heijer P, Bethencourt A, Vazquez N, Brugaletta S, Backx B, Serruys P. Rationale and design of the EXAMINATION trial: a randomised comparison between everolimus-eluting stents and cobalt-chromium bare-metal stents in ST-elevation myocardial infarction. Euro Intervention. 2011;7:977-84.

5. Sabaté M, Brugaletta S, Cequier A, Iniguez A, Serra A, Jiménez-Quevedo P, Mainar V, Campo G, Tespili M, den Heijer P, Bethencourt A, Vazquez N, van Es GA, Backx B, Valgimigli M, Serruys PW. Clinical outcomes in patients with ST-segment elevation myocardial infarction treated with everolimus-eluting stents versus bare-metal stents (EXAMINATION): 5-year results of a randomised trial. Lancet. 2016;387:357-66. 9. Brugaletta S, Sabate M, Martin-Yus.

72

Relationships Between Baseline Q Waves, Time from Symptom Onset, and Clinical Outcomes in ST-Segment-Elevation Myocardial Infarction Patients

Insights from the Vital Heart Response Registry

Ref.: Yinggan Zheng, Kevin R. Bainey, Benjamin D. Tyrrell, Neil, Brass, Paul W. Armstrong, Robert C. Welsh.

Link: https://doi.org/10.1161/Circular Iinterventions .117.005399

Circulation: Cardiovascular Interventions. 2017;10:e005399

Originally published November 16, 2017

Key Points

1. In a registry of consecutive STEMI patients, the presence of baseline Q waves was independently associated with adverse clinical events, whereas the time from symptom onset to reperfusion was not.
2. The absence of a baseline Q wave was associated with improved reperfusion success across all 3 time periods of symptom onset to treatment (<3, 3-6, and >6 hours).
3. This may be important for decision making regarding delivery of reperfusion therapy in late comers without Q waves.

Akshay Mehta

∎ Introduction:

In clinical trialsof ST-segment-elevation myocardial infarction (STEMI), the presence of baseline Q waves has been associated with increased adverse clinical events.Symptom duration also is critical in such patients because of its direct relationship between duration of coronary occlusion, myocardial necrosis, and clinical outcomes. The relationship between the presence of baseline Q waves and time from symptom onset to treatment on in-hospital clinical outcomes with primary PCI, fibrinolysis or no reperfusion has not been studied so far.

∎ Aims:

A STEMI registry was used to evaluate the relationship between the presence of baseline Q waves and time from symptom onset to treatment on in-hospital clinical outcomes and whether the applied reperfusion strategy (i.e, pharmacological reperfusion, mechanical reperfusion, or no reperfusion) modifies these relationships.

Methods:

Out of all consecutive patients with a STEMI admitted to hospital in Edmonton, Alberta, Canada from October 2006 to October 2011, 2290 patients were divided into 3 groups according to the reperfusion strategy they received: primary PCI, fibrinolytic treated, and no acute reperfusion. Time to treatment was defined from symptom onset to the first intervention device in the primary PCI group and from symptom onset to time of fibrinolysis administration in the fibrinolytic-treated group.

End Points:

The primary clinical end point included in this study was the composite of death, congestive heart failure, cardiogenic shock, and reinfarction within the index hospitalization.

Results:

Among 2290 ST-segment-elevation myocardial infarction patients, 36.9% had Q waves on their baseline ECG. Patients with Q waves were older, more often males, had higher heart rate, had higher Global Registry of Acute Coronary Events risk score and were with longer time to reperfusion. They also had higher composite end points for all time points from symptom onset to presentation.(15.4% versus 9.9% ≤ 3 hours; 18.5% versus 8.9% >3 to ≤6 hours; 15.9% versus 11.3% >6 hours; Q and no Q, respectively).

Conclusion:

Baseline Q waves, but not time to reperfusion, were associated with an increased risk of the composite end point of death, congestive heart failure, cardiogenic shock, and reinfarction. Presence or type of reperfusion did not modify the association of baseline Q waves and in-hospital outcomes.

Strengths and Weaknesses :

Besides supporting previous data showing that the presence of baseline Q waves was associated with worse clinical outcomes in STEMI patients, this study for the first time compares the prognostic impact of baseline Q waves with ischemic times in STEMI patients with different types of reperfusion therapies.

Limitations of the study were that :

1. Itwas based on registry data which has the inherent limitations of an observational study.

2. Reperfusion therapy was individualized

3. Only in-hospital clinical outcomes were assessed and not longer-term clinical outcomes.

Clinical Implications:

Although total ischemic time is an important determinant of prognosis, in many STEMI patients symptom duration is a subjective ascertainment and is therefore a suboptimal metric.

Presence or absence of admission Q waves can thus add to and refine prognostication of such patients.

Although Q waves predict adverse clinical outcomes, the study, like prior studies shows benefit of reperfusion in these patients too.

Of greater import, absence of Q waves in late comers show substantial benefit with reperfusion therapy and has implications for clinical practice.

▌ Suggested Readings

1. McDonald MA, Fu Y, Zeymer U, Wagner G, Goodman SG, Ross A, Granger CB, Van de Werf F, Armstrong PW; ASSENT-4 PCI Investigators. Adverse outcomes in fibrinolytic-based facilitated percutaneous coronary intervention: insights from the ASSENT-4 PCI electrocardiographic substudy. Eur Heart J. 2008;29:871-879. doi: 10.1093/eurheartj/ehn078.

2. Armstrong PW, Fu Y, Westerhout CM, Hudson MP, Mahaffey KW, White HD, Todaro TG, Adams PX, Aylward PE, Granger CB. Baseline Q-wave surpasses time from symptom onset as a prognostic marker in ST-segment elevation myocardial infarction patients treated with primary percutaneous coronary intervention. J Am CollCardiol. 2009;53:1503-1509. doi: 10.1016/j.jacc.2009.01.046.

3. Siha H, Das D, Fu Y, Zheng Y, Westerhout CM, Storey RF, James S, Wallentin L, Armstrong PW. Baseline Q waves as a prognostic modulator in patients with ST-segment elevation: insights from the PLATO trial. CMAJ. 2012;184:1135-1142. doi: 10.1503/cmaj.111683

4. Topal DG, Lønborg J, Ahtarovski KA, Nepper-Christensen L, Helqvist S, Holmvang L, Pedersen F, Clemmensen P, Saünamaki K, Jørgensen E, Kyhl K, Ghotbi A, Schoos MM, Göransson C, Bertelsen L, Høfsten D, Køber L, Kelbæk H, Vejlstrup N, Engstrøm T. Association between early Q waves and reperfusion success in patients with ST-segment elevation myocardial infarction treated with primary percutaneous coronary intervention: A cardiac magnetic resonance imaging study. CircCardiovas Interv. 2017;10:e004467. doi: 10.1161/Circ Interventions .116.004467.

73

Impact of Aspirin and Clopidogrel Hyporesponsiveness in Patients Treated with Drug-Eluting Stents

2-Year Results of a Prospective, Multicenter Registry Study

Ref.: Thomas D. Stuckey, Ajay j. Kirtane, Bruce R. Brodie,Bernhard Witzenbichler, Claire Litherland etc all.
REVIEWED BY: Dr. D.B. Pahlajani
LINK: JACC Cardiovascular Iinterventions 2017;10:16, 1607-1617

Key Points
1. Aspirin hypo responsiveness is not associated with late or very late stent thrombosis.

2. Clopidogrel hypo responsiveness has strong and independent association with ischemic events and inverse relationship to bleeding

Dev Pahlajani

▌ Background:

Dual antiplatelet therapy (DAPT) is considered the standard of care in patients with acute coronary syndrome (ACS) and following DES implantation.

Incidence of aspirin and or Clopidogrel resistance is reported in 5-25% of patients.

Whether high residual platelet reactivity (HRP) to either aspirin or Clopidogrel is associated with long term adverse events has not been adequately reported.

▌ Aims:

To study the relationship between HPR to aspirin and Clopidogrel and its long term outcomes.

▌ Material and methods:

Study enrolled 8582 from DAPT-DES which is a multi center registry of patients who underwent DES implantation. Amongst these 46.3% patients continued DAPT for over 2 years.

▌ End points:

Definite or probable stent thrombosis (ST) all cause mortality, myocardial infarction (MI) and clinically relevant bleeding.

Results:

At 2 years ST occurred in 92 (1.07%) patients.HPR was independently associated with probable or definite ST (HR 2.6 p=0.003), MI (HR 1.35 p=0.02), freedom from bleeding (HR 0.74 p=0.002), and all cause mortality (HR 1.36 p=0.04). Majority of events occurred in first year.

While aspirin mono therapy was not associated with early, late or very late stent thrombosis, there was strong relationship with residual HPR to Clopidogrel upto 1 year (See Fig.1 and Table 1).

The study could suggest that platelet reactivity should be measured to identify patients on residual HPR to Clopidogrel. Alternate P2Y12 inhibitor could be administered to further reduce the risk of ST in the first year.

Fig. 1: *Time to First Stent Thrombosis to 2 Years*

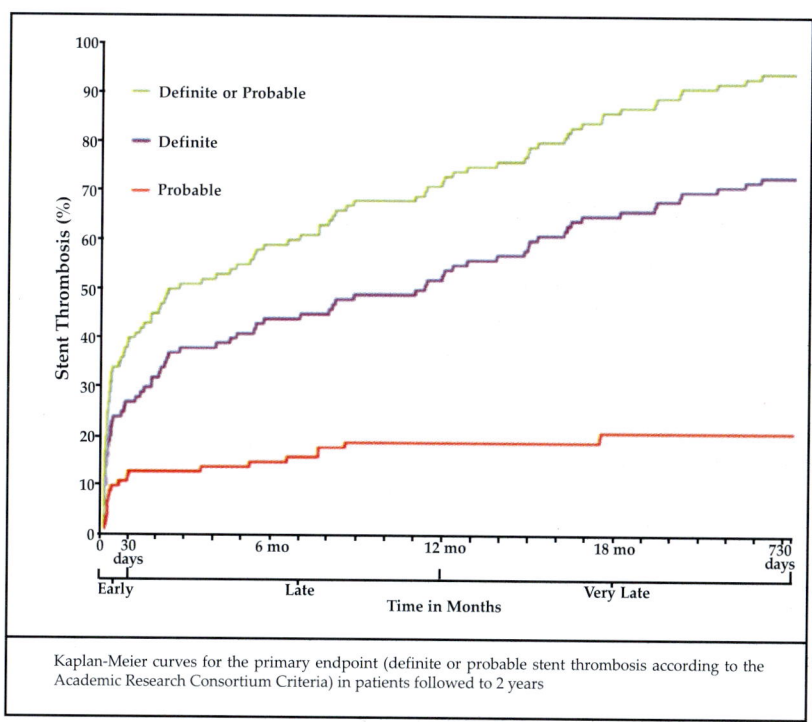

Kaplan-Meier curves for the primary endpoint (definite or probable stent thrombosis according to the Academic Research Consortium Criteria) in patients followed to 2 years

Table 1: Relationship between Platelet Reactivity and subsequent Definite or Probable ST in Patients on DAPT through 2 year Follow-up.

	ST (n = 69)	No ST (n = 4,138)	HR (95% CI)	p Value
ARU	420 ± 52	423 ± 58	-	0.62
> 550	3/68 (4.4)	274/4,138 (6.7)	0.66 (0.21-2.10)	0.48
PRU	224 ± 101	192 ± 95	-	0.01
> 208	44/69 (63.8)	1,832/4,138 (44.3	2.22 (1.36-3.63)	0.0001

Values are mean ± SD or n/N (%)

ST = Stent thrombosis

▌ Suggested Readings

1. Levine GN, Bates ER, Bittl JA, et al. 2016 ACC/ AHA guideline focused update on duration of dual antiplatelet therapy in patients with coronary artery disease: a report of the American College of Cardiology/American Heart Association Task Force on Clinical Practice Guidelines. J Am Coll Cardiol 2016;68:1082-115.

2. Gilard M, Barragan P, Noryani AA, et al. 6- versus 24-month dual antiplatelet therapy after implantation of drug eluting stents in patients nonresistant to aspirin: the randomized, multicenter ITALIC trial. J Am Coll Cardiol 2015;65: 777-86.

3. Chen WH, Lee PY, Ng W, Tse HF, Lau CP. Aspirin resistance is associated with a high incidence of myonecrosis after non-urgent percutaneous coronary intervention despite clopidogrel pretreatment. J Am Coll Cardiol 2004;43:1122-6.

4. Yeh RW, Kereiakes DJ, Steg PG, et al. Benefits and risks of extended duration dual antiplatelet therapy after PCI in patients with and without acute myocardial infarction. J Am Coll Cardiol 2015;65:2211-21.

5. Yeh RW, Secemsky EA, Kereiakes DJ, et al. Development and validation of a prediction rule for benefit and harm of dual antiplatelet therapy beyond 1 year after percutaneous coronary intervention. JAMA 2016;315:1735-49

6. Cayla G, Cuisett T, Silvain J, et al. Platelet function monitoring to adjust antiplatelet therapy in elderly patients stented for an acute coronary syndrome (ANTARCTIC): an open-label, blinded endpoint, randomized controlled superiority trial. Lancet 2016;388:2015-22.

7. Nuhrenberg TG, Stratz C, Leggewie S, et al. Temporal variability in the antiplatelet effects of clopidogrel and aspirin after elective drug-eluting stent implantation. An ADAPT-DES substudy. Thromb Haemost 2015;114:1020-7.

74

Walk Fast, Especially if your BMI is Low !

Association of Walking Pace and Handgrip Strength with all-Cause, Cardiovascular, and Cancer Mortality: A UK BioBank Observational Study

Ref.: Thomas Yates Francesco Zaccardi Nafeesa N Dhalwani Melanie J Davies Kishan Bakrania Carlos A Celis-Morales Jason M R Gill Paul W Franks Kamlesh Khunti

Link: European Heart Journal, Volume 38, Issue 43, 14 November 2017

Key Point

In a population of 420727 men and women free of cancer and CVD, self-reported measure of walking pace correlated with aerobic fitness and all-cause and cardiovascular mortality.

Akshay Mehta

❚ Study protocol:

In 230670 women and 190057 men free from prevalent cancer and cardiovascular disease from UK Biobank, walking pace was assessed by the following single item question: 'How would you describe your usual walking pace?

i)   Slow pace,

ii) Steady/average pace, and

iii) Brisk pace'.

Handgrip strength was assessed through the use of a hydraulic hand dynamometer while sitting and squeezing the handle of the dynamometer as hard as they could for 3s. Both left and right hand strengths were measured. The values for the right and left hand were summed and divided by 2 to estimate an average.

A subsample of UK Biobank undertook a 6 min graded submaximal fitness test on a cycle ergometer.

Cox-proportional hazard models were adjusted for BMI, social deprivation, ethnicity, employment, medications, alcohol use, diet, frequency of physical activity, and television viewing time.

Mortality status was tracked for a median of 6.3years.

❚ Results:

Self-reported walking speed was strongly related to maximal oxygen uptake in both men and women. A weaker relationship was observed for handgrip strength (kg) assessed with a dynamometer.

Male and female participants reporting a slow walking pace had a 67% greater risk of all-cause mortality, respectively, compared with participants reporting a brisk walking pace adjusting for socio-demographic factors, lifestyle factors including frequency of walking and moderate or vigorous physical activity, and body mass index (BMI). Additionally, men and women who reported slow walking showed a ~2-fold increase in cardiovascular mortality risk compared with those who reported brisk walking.

Associations of walking pace with mortality were modified by BMI. In women, the hazard ratio (HR) for all-cause mortality in slow compared with fast walkers were 2.16 and 1.31 in the bottom and top BMI tertiles, respectively; corresponding HRs for men were 2.01 and 1.41. Hazard ratios for cardiovascular mortality remained above 1.7 across all categories of BMI in men and women, with modest heterogeneity in men. Handgrip strength was associated with cardiovascular mortality in men only (HR tertile 1 v/s. tertile 3=1.38), without differences across BMI categories, while associations with all-cause mortality were only seen in men with low BMI. Associations for walking pace and handgrip strength with cancer mortality were less consistent.

Conclusion:

The study found that a slow self-reported walking pace was associated with a higher risk of all-cause and cardiovascular mortality in women and men with associations remaining robust across multiple layers of adjustment. There was a stronger association in those with low BMI. Self-reported walking pace was also an important measure of physical fitness. On the other hand, handgrip strength appeared to be a less generalizable marker of risk within the general population.

Clinical Relevance:

Cardiorespiratory (CR) fitness measurement in routine clinical practice as an optimal approach for cardiovascular risk stratification is advocated by The American Heart Association in a scientific statement. However, exercise testing that is used to test cardiovascular fitness is typically not practical to conduct on a wide spread scale. Self-reported walking pace was found to correlate well with CR fitness and could serve well as a prognosticator.

An interesting finding from the study was that the strength of the association of walking pace with all-cause (men and women), cardiovascular (men), and cancer (men) mortality was modified by BMI, with stronger associations seen in the lowest tertile of BMI, which could be due to malnutrition and higher levels of sarcopenia.

Some limitations of the study were the possibility of reverse causation, especially in low BMI population and some residual confounding due to unmeasured factors.

Various studies have shown improvement in physical fitness with exercise training, besides reducing the risk of chronic disease and improvement of cardiometabolic risk factors, including type 2 diabetes, blood pressure, and cholesterol.

Thus monitoring and improving walking speed can be a tangible and important goal to accomplish, especially in people with low BMI.

∎ Suggested Readings

1. Ross R, Blair SN, Arena R, Church TS, Després J, Franklin BA, Haskell WL, Kaminsky LA, Levine BD, Lavie CJ. Importance of assessing cardiorespiratory fitness in clinical practice: a case for fitness as a clinical vital sign: a scientific statement from the American Heart Association. Circulation 2016;134: e653-e699.

2. Authors/Task Force Members Piepoli MF, Hoes AW, Agewall S, Albus C, Brotons C, Catapano AL, Cooney MT, Corra U, Cosyns B, Deaton C, Graham I, Hall MS, Hobbs FD, Lochen ML, Lollgen H, Marques-Vidal P, Perk J, Prescott E, Redon J, Richter DJ, Sattar N, Smulders Y, Tiberi M, van der Worp HB, van Dis I, Verschuren WM Additional Contributor Simone Binno (Italy)Document Reviewers De Backer G, Roffi M, Aboyans V, Bachl N, Bueno H, Carerj S, Cho L, Cox J, De Sutter J, Egidi G, Fisher M, Fitzsimons D, Franco OH, Guenoun M, Jennings C, Jug B, Kirchhof P, Kotseva K, Lip GY, Mach F, Mancia G, Bermudo FM, Mezzani A, Niessner A, Ponikowski P, Rauch B, Ryden L, Stauder A, Turc G, Wiklund O, Windecker S, Zamorano JL. 2016 European Guidelines on cardiovascular disease prevention in clinical practice: the Sixth Joint Task Force of the European Society of Cardiology and Other Societies on Cardiovascular Disease Prevention in Clinical Practice (constituted by representatives of 10 societies and by invited experts): developed with the special contribution of the European Association for Cardiovascular Prevention & Rehabilitation (EACPR). Eur J Prev Cardiol 2016;23:NP1-NP96.

3. Chainani V, Shaharyar S, Dave K, Choksi V, Ravindranathan S, Hanno R, Jamal O, Abdo A, Rafeh NA. Objective measures of the frailty syndrome (hand grip strength and gait speed) and cardiovascular mortality: a systematic review. Int J Cardiol 2016;215:487-493.

75

Anti Inflmmatory Therapy with Canakinumab for Atherosclerotic Disease

Ref.: Paul M Ridker, M.D., Brendan M. Everett, M.D., Tom Thuren, M.D., Jean G. MacFadyen, B.A., William H. Chang, Ph.D., et al

LINK: NEJM 2017;377(12)1109-1205

Key Points:

1) In patients with high sensitivity C-Reactive Protein (CRP) with prior myocardial infarction (MI) anti inflammatory canakinumab reduces the risk of non fatal MI, non fatal stroke or cardiovascular death.

2) It is associated with reduction in the high sensitivity CRP and interleukin - 6 levels.

3) The maximum benefit was obserobserved in the high dose group.

4) No difference in all cause mortality reported

Dev Pahlajani

Introduction:

CAD and atherothrombosis is linked with inflammation and low density lipoproteins (LDL). Despite treatment with statins to reduce LDL and other risk factor modification drugs several patients have residual risk that can lead to future adverse cardiocavascular events due to atherothrombosis which could be attributed to inflammation.

Objects of the Study :

To assess whether risk of future atherothrombotic events can be reduced by decreasing inflammation by anti inflammatory drug canakinumab.

Material and Methods:

10061 patients randomized to placebo, and 3 doses of canakinumab (50mg, 150mg, and 300mg each) administered subcutaneously at 3 monthly intervals. These patients had high sensitivity CRP of 2 mg/ltr or more and had pre-existing MI.

Results:

Follow up was for 48 months. The primary efficacy end points were non fatal MI, non fatal stroke or death. There was a 41 percentage drop in the high sensitivity CRP in 300 mg group, 37 percentage in 150mg and 26 percentage in the 50 mg group as compared to placebo. There was no further reduction in lipid level from baseline. The primary end point also was lower in the 150 and 300 mg group.

a) 4.5 events / 100 person years in placebo group

b) 4.1 events / 100 person years in 50mg group

c) 3.8 events / 100 person years in 150mg group

d) 3.9 events / 100 person years in 300mg group

There was a higher incidence of fatal infection in canakinumab group and there was no significant difference in all cause mortality in all the randomized groups(Ref Fig A-D).

▎ Conclusion:

In patients with residual risk of atherothrombosis, anti inflammatory therapy targeting the interleukin-1β immunity pathway with canakinumab is associated with reduced risk of recurrent atherothrombosis events.

▎ Discussion:

Inflammation is considered as an important pathophysiological mechanism for patients developing atherothrombosis which is mediated through interleukin-1β pathway which is a cytokine important to inflammation response and link to interleukin-6 signalling pathway. Canakinumab is monoclonal antibody and targets interleukin-1β. It was also found that the effect was mediated through reducing inflammation since there was a reduction in the plasma interleukin 6 and high sensitivity CRP. Apparently residual risk after the LDL cholesterol reduction by statins is mainly due to inflammation since there was no further reduction in LDL cholesterol during the study period. The CANTOS study highlights the importance of targeting not only the lipids but also the inflammation. Best results were observed in high dose group. One of the disturbing side effect was fatal infection. However, furthet studies need to be done to evaluate the role of anti inflammatory drugs in reducing the risk of atherothrombosis and also exploring the possibility by other agents.

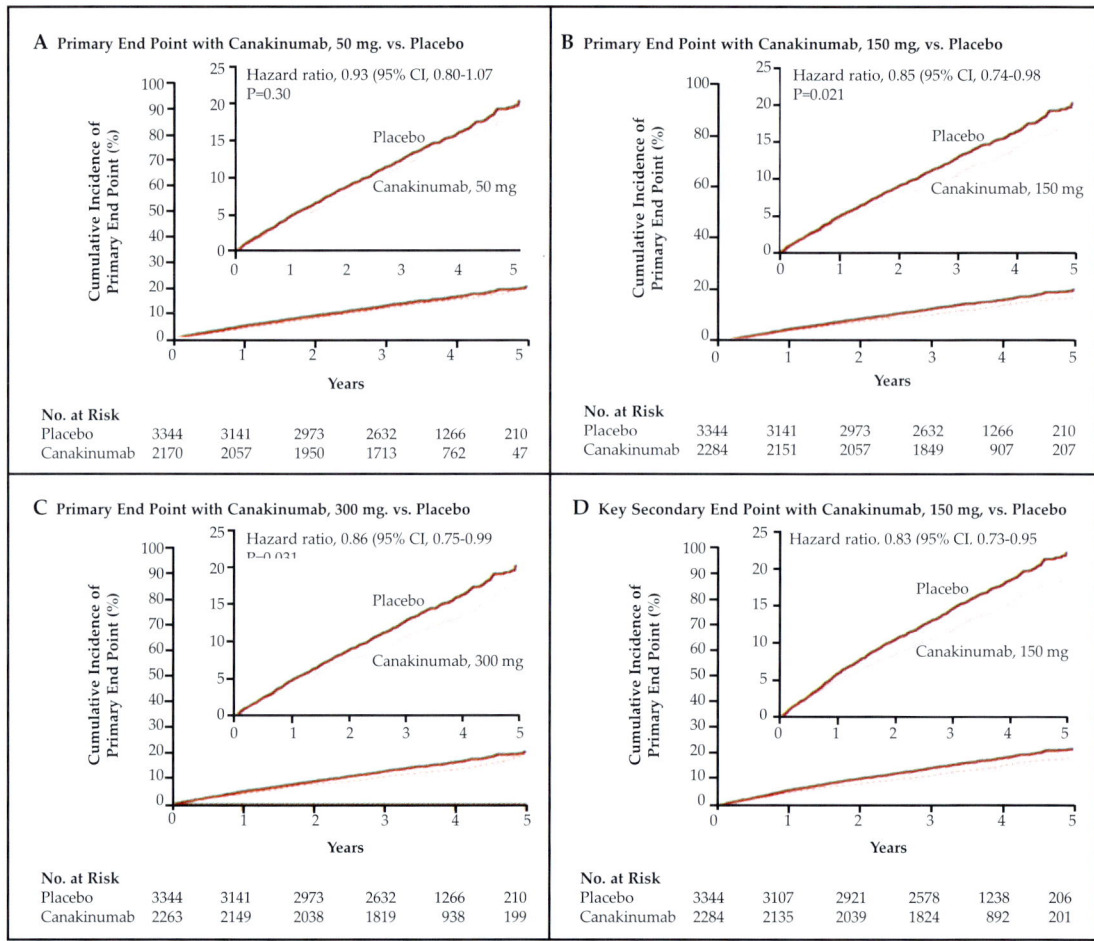

A Primary End Point with Canakinumab, 50 mg. vs. Placebo

Hazard ratio, 0.93 (95% CI, 0.80-1.07
P=0.30

No. at Risk
Placebo   3344   3141   2973   2632   1266   210
Canakinumab 2170   2057   1950   1713   762   47

B Primary End Point with Canakinumab, 150 mg, vs. Placebo

Hazard ratio, 0.85 (95% CI, 0.74-0.98
P=0.021

No. at Risk
Placebo   3344   3141   2973   2632   1266   210
Canakinumab 2284   2151   2057   1849   907   207

C Primary End Point with Canakinumab, 300 mg. vs. Placebo

Hazard ratio, 0.86 (95% CI, 0.75-0.99
P=0.031

No. at Risk
Placebo   3344   3141   2973   2632   1266   210
Canakinumab 2263   2149   2038   1819   938   199

D Key Secondary End Point with Canakinumab, 150 mg, vs. Placebo

Hazard ratio, 0.83 (95% CI, 0.73-0.95

No. at Risk
Placebo   3344   3107   2921   2578   1238   206
Canakinumab 2284   2135   2039   1824   892   201

Suggested Readings

1. Hansson GK. Inflammation, atherosclerosis, and coronary artery disease. N Engl J Med 2005;352::1685-95.

2. Libby P, Ridker PM, Hansson GK. Inflammation in atherosclerosis: from pathyphysiology to practice. J Am Coll Cardiol 2009;54:2129-38

3. Nissen SE, Tuzcu EM, Schoenhagen P, et al. Statin therapy, LDL cholesterol, C-reactive protein, and coronary artery disease. N Engl J Med 2005;352:29-38

4. Ridker PM, Danielson E, Fonseca FAH, et al. Rosuvastatin to prevent vascular events in men and women with elevated C-reactive protein. N Engl J Med 2008; 359:2195-207.

5. Lachmann HJ, Kone-Paut I, Kuemmerle-Deschner JB, et al Use of canakinumab in the cryopyrin-associated periodic syndrome. N Engl J Med 2009;360:2416-25.

6. Ridker PM, Howard CP, Walter V, etal. Effects of interleukin-1β inhibition with canakinumab on hemoglobin A1c, lipids, C-reactive protein, interleukin-6, and fibrinogen: a phase IIb randomized, placebo-controlled trial. Circulation 2012;126:2739-48.

7. Ridker PM, Thuren T, Zalewski A, Libby P. Interleukin-1β inhibition and the prevention of recurrent cardiovascular events: rationale and design of the Canakinumab Anti-inflammatory Thrombosis Outcomes Study (CANTOS). Am Heart J 2011;162:597-605.

8. Sager HB, Heidt T, Hulsmans M, et al. Targeting interleukin-1β reduces leukocyte production after acute myocardial infarction. Circulation 2015;132:1880-90.

9. Sabatine MS, Giugliano RP, Keech AC, et al. Evolocumab and clinical outcomes in patients with cardiovascular disease. N Eng J Med 2017;376:1713-22.

10. Ridker PM, Luscher TF. Anti-inflammatory therapies for cardiovascular disease. Eur Heart J 2014;35: 1782-91.

76

Catheter Interventions Not ATTRACTIVE for Preventing Post Thrombotic Syndrome in DVT !

Ref.: Suresh Vedantham, M.D., Samuel Z. Goldhaber, M.D., Jim A. Julian, M.Math., Susan R. Kahn, M.D., Michael R. Jaff, D.O., David J. Cohen, M.D., Elizabeth Magnuson, Sc.D., Mahmood K. Razavi, M.D., Anthony J. Comerota, M.D., Heather L. Gornik, M.D., Timothy P. Murphy, M.D., Lawrence Lewis, M.D., James R. Duncan, M.D., Ph.D., Patricia Nieters, B.S.N., Mary C. Derfler, M.S.N., Marc Filion, M.Sc., Chu-Shu Gu, Ph.D., Stephen Kee, M.D., Joseph Schneider, M.D., Ph.D., NaelSaad, M.D., Morey Blinder, M.D., Stephan Moll, M.D., David Sacks, M.D., Judith Lin, M.D., John Rundback, M.D., Mark Garcia, M.D., Rahul Razdan, M.D., Eric VanderWoude, M.D., Vasco Marques, M.D., and Clive Kearon, M.B., Ph.D., for the ATTRACT Trial Investigators*

N Engl J Med 2017; 377:2240-2252December 7, 2017DOI: 10.1056/NEJMoa1615066.

LINK : Pharmacomechanical Catheter-Directed Thrombolysis for Deep-Vein Thrombosis

Akshay Mehta

▌ Introduction:

Post thrombotic syndrome, occurs in about half of patients with proximal DVT despite use of standard blood-thinning drugs.

The value of pharmaco-mechanical catheter-directed thrombolysis, which entails catheter delivery of tPA to the thrombus along with thrombus aspiration or maceration in such patients is controversial.

Preliminary studies suggest that removing the clot may improve long-term outcomes but there has not been a large rigorous study to establish whether this is so.

▌ Aims:

To assess in a randomized trial whether the addition of pharmaco-mechanical catheter-directed thrombolysis to anticoagulation results in a lower risk of the post-thrombotic syndrome.

▌ Methods:

Six hundred ninety two (692) patients with acute proximal deep-vein thrombosis were randomly assigned to receive either anticoagulation alone (control group) or anticoagulation plus pharmaco-mechanical thrombolysis (catheter-mediated or device-mediated intrathrombus delivery of recombinant tissue plasminogen activator and thrombus aspiration or maceration, with or without stenting).

█ End Points:

The primary outcome was development of the post-thrombotic syndrome defined as a Villalta score of 5 or higher or an ulcer in the leg with the index deep-vein thrombosis at 6 to 24 months.

Secondary outcome was reduction in symptom severity compared with anticoagulation alone.

█ Results :

There were no significant between-group difference in the percentage of patients with the post-thrombotic syndrome or in recurrent venous thromboembolism seen over the 24-month follow-up period.(47% versus 48% with a risk ratio (RR) of 0.96 :95% CI 0.82-1.11; P=0.56).

Pharmaco-mechanical thrombolysis led to more major bleeding events within 10 days.

Moderate-to-severe post-thrombotic syndrome occurred 27% lower in the pharmaco-mechanical-thrombolysis group as compared to the control group. However there was no difference in quality of life from baseline to 24 months between the treatment groups.

█ Conclusions:

1. In patients with acute proximal deep-vein thrombosis, the addition of pharmaco-mechanical catheter-directed thrombolysis to usual anticoagulation did not result in a lower incidence of the post-thrombotic syndrome but had a higher risk of major bleeding.

2. Although improvement in quality of life from baseline to 24 months did not differ significantly between the treatment groups, the severity scores for the post-thrombotic syndrome were lower in the pharmaco-mechanical-thrombolysis group than in the control group at 6, 12, 18, and 24 months of follow-up.

█ Clinical Implications:

The main message from the ATTRACT trial is that most patients can avoid an unnecessary procedure that would confer some bleeding risk and significant cost.

Lessening of the severity of the syndrome with intervention in patients who had a higher Villalta score suggests it could be of benefit in carefully selected patients, for instance in a young patient with a very extensive high proximal DVT who is very symptomatic but who is at low risk for bleeding.

Future studies must hence be directed at particular groups of patients who may experience benefit from this therapy, such as patients with the largest blood clot and the most symptoms when they present, like worse pain and swelling.

∎ Suggested Readings

1. Tzu-TingKuoab Chun-YangHuangcChiao-PoHsuabd Chiu-YangLee

   Catheterdirectedthrombolysisandpharmacomechanicalthrombectomy improve midterm outcome in acute iliofemoral deep vein thrombosis.

   Journal of the Chinese Medical Association

   Volume 80, Issue 2, February 2017, Pages 72-79.

2. Maureen P. Kohi, Ryan Kohlbrenner, Kanti P. Kolli, Evan Lehrman, Andrew G. Taylor, and Nicholas Fidelman

   Catheter directed interventions for acute deep vein thrombosis

   CardiovascDiagnTher. 2016 Dec; 6(6): 599-611.

3. Vedantham S

   Catheter-directed thrombolysis for deep vein thrombosis.

   CurrOpinHematol.2010Sep;17(5):464-8.doi: 10.1097/MOH.0b013e32833cad98.

77

Physical Activity and Mortality in Patients with Stable Coronary Heart Disease

Ref.: Ralph A.H. Stewart, MD, Claes Hel, MD, PHD, Nermin Hadziosmanovic, MSC, Paul W. Armstrong, MD et al.

LINK: JACC 2017, 70 (14):1689-1700

Key Points:

1. Increased habitual exercise is associated with graded decrease in mortality.

2. Lower all cause mortality occurred while doubling exercise volume.

3. No difference in myocardial infarction (MI) or stroke with volume after adjusting co-variants.

4. Strong association with decrease in mortality with increased exercise with co-relation to age, smoking, diabetes, peripheral arterial disease and biomarkers.

Dev Pahlajani

■ **Introduction:**

In general population various studies have indicated that habitual exercise is associated with decreased adverse cardiovascular events. However, the data in specific population of individuals with coronary artery disease is lacking.

■ **Objectives:**

Analyze relationship of self reported exercise and mortality in patients with stable coronary heart disease (SCHD).

■ **Methods:**

The study involves 15486 patients from 39 countries who had SCHD and were enrolled in the STABILITY study which was undertaken to study the role of darapladib in SCHD. Patients were requested to complete the questionnaires on the hours spent each week taking mild, moderate and vigorous exercise. The association of risk of cardiovascular events between the volume of habitual exercise in metabolic equivalent of task hours in week was analyzed. Median follow up was for 3.7 years.

■ **Results:**

The primary end point was all cause mortality and the secondary end points were cardiovascular death, MI, stroke, non cardiovascular mortality and major adverse cardiac events defined as first occurrence of death or stroke. Active participants in the study were less likely to have chronic disease, multivessel coronary artery disease or diabetes. There was a graded lower total cardiovascular and non cardiovascular mortality with higher physical activity. However, the maximum benefit was seen in the patients who were least active. The physical activity corelates with cardiovascular death and major adverse cardiac events. Doubling of exercise volume was associated with lower all cause mortality. It was observed for both cardiovascular and non cardiovascular mortality. Increase from mild to moderate or from moderate to vigorous exercise was associated with decreased mortality. Doubling and duration of exercise was associated with lower all cause mortality. The increase of mild intensity exercise between subjects was associated with mortality sub groups who were not taking moderate or vigorous exercise. Those who were undertaking vigorous exercise, increased and more moderate intensity was associated with lower mortality. There was no clear association between increased duration of vigorous exercise in individuals who reported taking vigorous exercise. However, they had lower mortality than those who took no vigorous exercise.

Diabetes, individuals with significant renal dysfunction, peripheral vascular disease, smoking had greater benefit. Patients with limitation of exercise by dyspnea or chest pain or discomfort also had benefit of exercise (Fig.1).

▮ Conclusion:

Patients who are sedentary even smaller amount of habitual exercise, either small or moderate could provide significant and substantial reduction in cardiovascular and non cardiovascular mortality. Those who reported taking moderate or vigorous activity, by further increasing active exercise did benefit but not as much as those who were sedentary or taking mild exercise. Benefits of exercise are not linear.

▮ Comments:

The study is important that suggests even small increase in the exercise particularly in the patients who lead a sedentary life style could greatly benefit in the reduction in cardiovascular and non cardiovascular death. However, there have been earlier reports that vigorous exercise may trigger MI and sudden death especially in patients with pre existing coronary artery disease. Reverse J shape between exercise level and mortality have been reported in patients with pre existing coronary artery disease. To establish the exact role of strenuous exercise in patients with pre existing coronary artery disease should be performed under supervised exercise program. Patients with pre existing SCHD and leading sedentary life or taking mild exercise should be encouraged to increase the level of exercise.

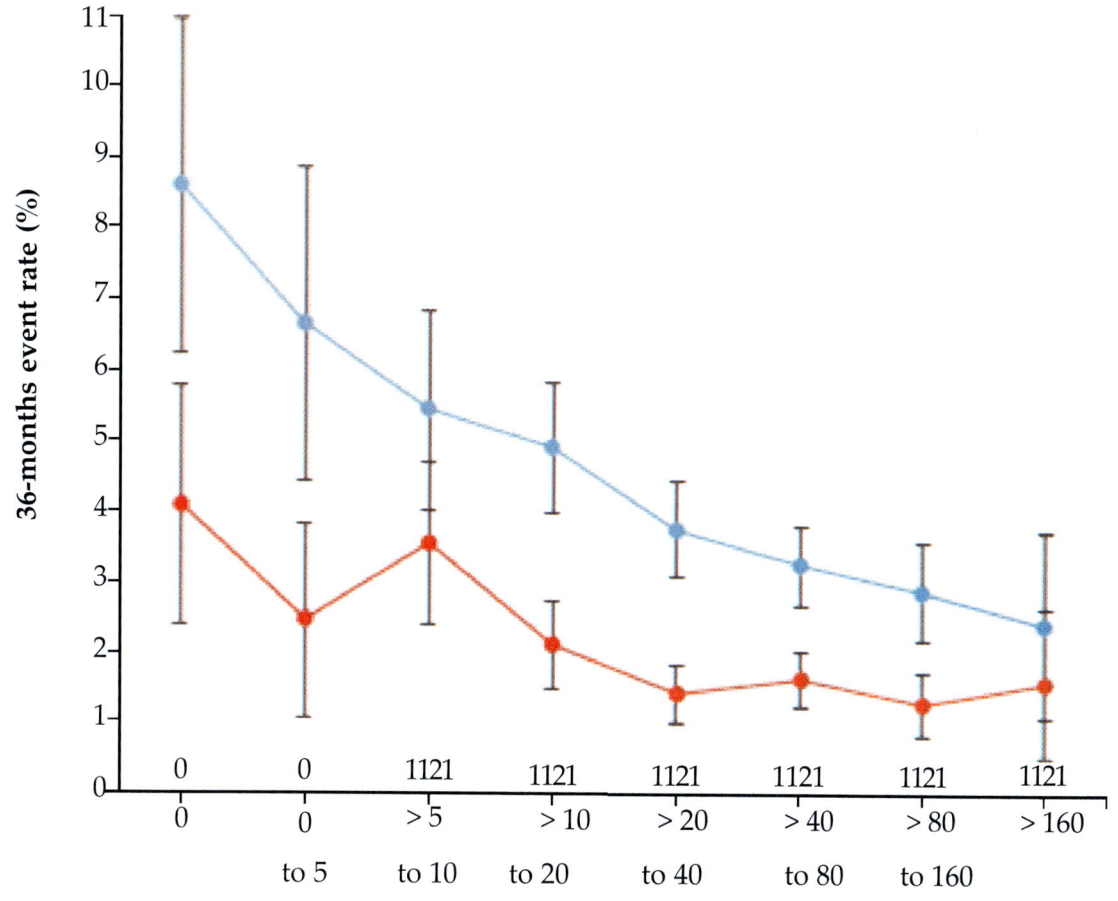

Fig. 1: *Association among the volume of mild, moderate and vigorous physical activity and CV and Non CV mortality*

Physical acitivity MET hours / week

CV mortality   Non CV mortality

▌ Suggested Readings

1. Perk J, De Backer G, Gohlke H, et al. European guidelines on cardiovascular disease prevention in clinical practice (version 2012): the Fifth Joint Task Force of the European Society of Cardiology and Other Societies on Cardiovascular Disease Prevention in Clinical Practice (constituted by representatives of nine societies and by invited experts). Eur Heart J 2012;33:1635-701.

2. Ross R, Blair SN, Arena R, et al. Importance of assessing cardiorespiratory fitness in clinical practice: a case for fitness as a clinical vital sign: a scientific statement from the American Heart Association. Circulation 2016;134: e653-99.

3. Sattelmair J, Pertman J, Ding EL, et al. Dose response between physical activity and risk of coronary heart disease: a meta-analysis. Circulation 2011;124:789-95.

4. Moore SC, Patel AV, Matthews CE, et al. Leisure time physical activity of moderate to vigorous intensity and mortality: a large pooled cohort analysis. PLoS Med 2012;9:e1001335.

5. Mons U, Hahmann H, Brenner H. A reverse J-shaped association of leisure time physical activity with prognosis in patients with stable coronary heart disease: evidence from a large cohort with repeated measurements. Heart 2014;100:1043-9.

6. Stewart R, Held C, Brown R, et al. Physical activity in patients with stable coronary heart disease: an international perspective. Eur Heart J 2013;34:3286-93.

7. White HD, Held C, Stewart R, et al. Darapladib for preventing ischemic events in stable coronary heart disease. N Engl J Med 2014;370:1702-11.

8. White HD, Held C, Stewart RA, et al. Study design and rationale for the clinical outcomes of the STABILITY Trial (STabilisation of Atherosclerotic plaque By Initiation of TherapY) comparing darapladib versus placebo in patients with clinical coronary heart disease. Am Heart J 2010;160:655-61.

78

Catheter Ablation Versus Medical Rate Control in Atrial Fibrillation and Systolic Dysfunction

The CAMERA-MRI Study

Ref.: SandeepPrabhu, Andrew J. Taylor, Ben T. Costello, David M. Kaye, Alex J.A. McLellan et al.
Link:JACC 2017;70(16):1949-1961

Key Points

1. In patients with atrial fibrillation(AF) and left ventricular systolic dysfunction (LVSD) restoration of sinus rhythm with catheter ablation results in improved ventricular function.

2. Absence of fibrosis as determined by late Gadolinium enhancement (LGE) on cardiac MRI (CMR) is a strong indicator for improvement following catheter ablation.

3. In patients with AF associated with LVSD rhythm control with catheter ablation is superior to rate control with medical treatment.

Dev Pahlajani

▋ Introduction:

Several patients of AF have associated LVSD. It becomes difficult for clinician to ascertain whether LVSD is due to AF or AF is due to left ventricular and left atrial dilatation as a result of left ventricular failure. Further there have been conflicting reports regarding the efficacy of rhythm control with catheter ablation versus rate control with drugs to improve left ventricular function in patients with AF.

▋ Objectives of the study:

To compare the efficacy of rhythm control with catheter ablation versus rate control with medical treatment and identify patients who would benefit maximum from rhythm control.

▋ Methods:

Multicentre randomized trial that enrolled patients with persistent AF and idiopathic cardiomyopathy with left ventricular ejection fraction of =<45%. After applying several exclusion criteria 33 patients were randomized to catheter ablation and 33 to medical treatment to control rate to 80 beats per minute or less. Patients were also subjected to CMR to diagnose myocardial fibrosis by LGE.

Results:

There was absolute improvement in LVEF by 18 ± 13% in catheter ablation group compared with 4.4 ± 13% in medically treated group (p=<0.0001). LVEF normalized in 58% in rhythm control versus 9% in rate control (p=0.0002). There was significant decrease in the left ventricular systolic volume and left atrial volume in the catheter ablation group while there was no change in left ventricular and left atrial volumes the rate control group. There was also a drop in the serum BNP levels in catheter ablation group.

Further there was significant improvement in the NYHA functional classification in patients subjected to catheter ablation as compared to patients in rate control group. Absence of fibrosis as determined by LGE was a strong predictor of improvement following catheter ablation (Fig. 1).

Appraisal:

Some of the earlier trials have shown mixed and varying results of left ventricular function with rhythm versus rate control. This is an important randomized control trial that has clearly shown significant superiority of rhythm control by catheter ablation versus rate control with medical treatment. The study also indicates an important role of LGE in identifying patients who will benefit from catheter ablation. Further more study confirms some of the earlier observations that AF itself can be responsible for LVSD.

Fig. 1: *LGE and change in absolute LVEF*

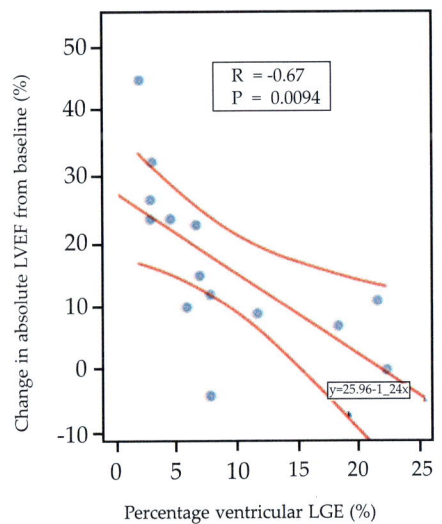

A — ALVEF stratified by LGE status in Patients following catheter ablation

B — Correlation between % of ventricular LGE and ALVEF following catheter ablation

▌ Suggested Readings

1. Roy D, Talajic M, Nattel S, et al. Rhythm control versus rate control for atrial fibrillation and heart failure. N Engl J Med 2008;358:2667-77.

2. Di Biase L, Mohanty P, Mohanty S, et al. Ablation versus amiodarone for treatment of persistent atrial fibrillation in patients with congestive heart failure and an implanted device: results from the AATAC multicenter randomized trial. Circulation 2016;133:1637-44.

3. Jones DG, Haldar SK, Hussain W, et al. A randomized trial to assess catheter ablation versus rate control in the management of persistent atrial fibrillation in heart failure. J Am CollCardiol 2013;61:1894-903.

4. Hunter RJ, Berriman TJ, Diab I, et al. A randomized controlled trial of catheter ablation versus medical treatment of atrial fibrillation in heart failure (the CAMTAF trial). CircArrhythm Electrophysiol 2014;7:318.

5. Ling LH, Taylor AJ, Ellims AH, et al. Sinus rhythm restores ventricular function in patients with cardiomyopathy and no late gadolinium enhancement on cardiac magnetic resonance imaging who undergo catheter ablation for atrial fibrillation. Heart Rhythm 2013;10:1334-9.

6. Addison D, Farhad H, Shah RV, et al. Effect of late gadolinium enhancement on the recovery of left ventricular systolic function after pulmonary vein isolation. J Am Heart Assoc 2016;5.

79

Lesion Complexity and Outcomes of Extended DAPT After PCI

Ref.: Robert W. Yeh, MD, MSC, Dean J. Kereiakes, MD, P. Gabriel Steg, MD, et al
LINK: JACC 2017;70(18):2213-2223

Key Points:

1. Patients with complex target lesion anatomy have increased risk of ischemic events in the first year after percutaneous coronary intervention (PCI).

2. Benefits of extended dual antiplatelet (DAPT) are similar in subjects with and without complex lesions.

3. However, high DAPT score could identify patients who could benefit from extended treatment with and without complex anatomy.

Dev Pahlajani

▌ Introduction:

DAPT is the standard of care for patients who undergo PCI. The current guidelines recommend 6-12 months DAPT following PCI. Extending the duration could lead to increased risk of bleeding. However, it has been suggested that patients with complex lesions could benefit from extended, duration. The current study assessed the effect of 30 months versus 12months of DAPT after PCI depending upon the presence or absence of anatomically complex target lesions.

Enrollment: Study enrolled 8381 patients with complex anatomy and 17035 patients of non-complex anatomy. Intially 25416 subjects were enrolled in the DAPT study. After several exclusions 3730 patients were included in the study as complex and 7824 as non-complexlesions. Patients were randomized at 12 months.

Primary end points: Combined myocardial infarction (MI) or stent thrombosis and major adverse cardiac and cerebrovascular events (MACCE) in all randomized subjects at 12-30 months.

▌ Results:

The primary end points were moderate or severe bleeding. Subjects with complex anatomy experienced increased rate of MACCE (5.3for complex v/s 3.5% for non complexp=<0.001) and M or stent thrombosis 3.9% for complex and 2.4% for non complex resprctivel (p=<0.001). Bleeding rates were similar in both the groups. During the subsequent 12-30 months period there was n difference in the MI or stent thrombosis (3.5 v/s 2.9% respectively p=0.07) and MACCE (5.5% v/

4.8% respectively p=0.11) and bleeding. However, there was a trend for increased adverse events with increasing number of complexity characteristics at 0-12 months after enrolment and 12-30 months after enrolment. The relative reduction of MI or stent thrombosis with continued DAPT was similar for subjects with and without complexity. There was no benefit of continuing DAPT for additional 18 months amongst the complex coronary lesions. However, there was a trend towards increased benefits amongst patients with higher complexity score (Table & Fig. 1).

▌ Conclusion:

The study indicates that amongst those patients who did not have adverse events in the first 12 months there is no benefit of extending DAPT for the additional 18 months even amongst patients with complex lesions. However, those with high score could benefit from extended treatment.

Table 1: Kaplan-Meier rates of outcomes in randomized subjects with versus without anatomic lesion complexity between 12 to 30 months after percutaneous coronary intervention

Event	Complex Anatomy (n = 3,730)	Noncomplex Anatomy (n = 7,824)	Long rank p Value
MI or stent thrombosis	127 (3.5)	219 (2.9)	0.07
MACCE	199 (5.5)	364 (4.8)	0.11
Bleeding (moderate/severe)	68 (1.9)	145 (1.9)	0.91
Stent thrombosis (definite/probable)	36 (1.0)	61 (0.8)	0.31
MI	127 (3.5)	215 (2.8)	0.051
Death	67 (1.9)	121 (1.6)	0.32

Value are n (%)

MACCE = Major Advice Cardiovascular and Events, MI = Myocardial infacts

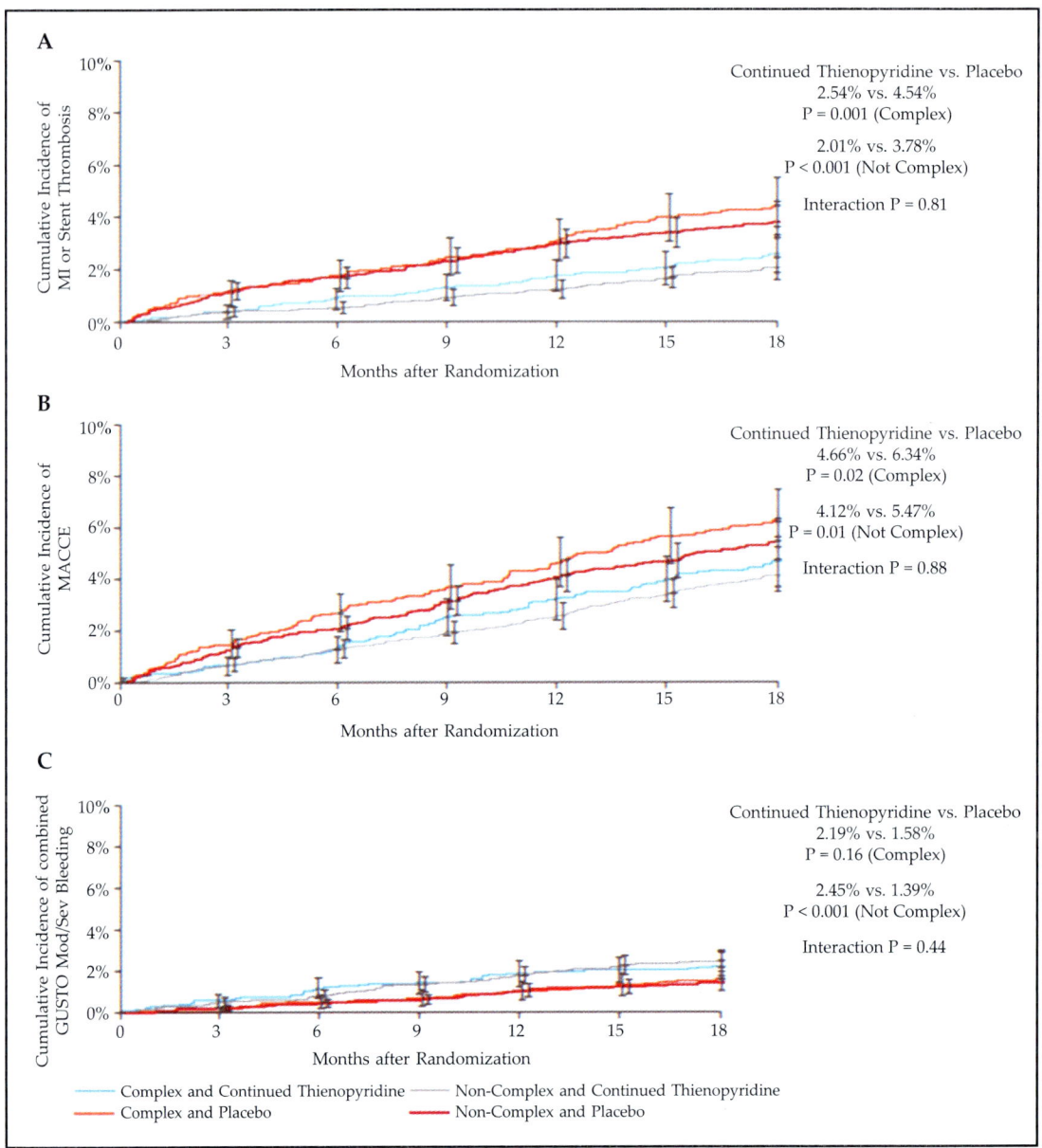

Suggested Readings

1. Mauri L, Kereiakes DJ, Yeh RW, et al. Twelve or 30 months of dual antiplatelet therapy after drug-eluting stents. N Engl J Med 2014;371: 2155-66.

2. Levine GN, Bates ER, Bittl JA, et al. 2016 ACC/AHA guideline focused update on duration of dual antiplatelet therapy in patients with coronary artery disease: a report of the American College of Cardiology/American Heart Association Task Force on Clinical Practice Guidelines. J Am Coll Cardiol 2016;68:1082-115.

3. Mauri L, Kereiakes DJ, Normand SL, et al. Rationale and design of the dual antiplatelet therapy study, a prospective, multicenter, randomized, double-blind trial to assess the effectiveness and safety of 12 versus 30 months of dual antiplatelet therapy in subjects undergoing percutaneous coronary intervention with either drug-eluting stent or bare metal stent placement for the treatment of coronary artery lesions. Am Heart J 2010;160:1035-41, 1041.e1.

4. Hermiller JB, Krucoff MW, Kereiakes DJ, et al. Benefits and risks of extended dual antiplatelet therapy after everolimus-eluting stents. J Am CollCardiolIntv 2016;9:138-47.

5. Yeh RW, Secemsky EA, Kereiakes DJ, et al. Development and validation of a prediction rule for benefit and harm of dual antiplatelet therapy beyond 1 year after percutaneous coronary intervention. JAMA 2016;315:1735-49.

6. Kereiakes DJ, Yeh RW, Massaro JM, et al. DAPT score utility for risk prediction in patients with or without previous myocardial infarction. J Am CollCardiol 2016;67:2492-502. KEY WORDS complex lesions, dual.

80

The Sabre Trial (Sirolimus PTCA Balloon for Coronary In-Stent Restenosis)
Angiographic Results and 1-Year Clinical Outcomes

Ref.: Stefan Verheye, MD, PHD, Mathias Vrolix, MD, InadulisKumsars, MD, PHD, AndrejsErglis et al
LINK:JACC 2017;10(20),:2029 - 2037

Key Points

1. Sirolimus eluting balloon (SEB) percutaneous coronary intervention (PCI) is associated with excellent success rate for patients with in-stent restenosis (ISR).

2. Late lumen loss rates over 6-months period are low and comparable to current stent free ISR treatment options.

Dev Pahlajani

■ **Introduction:**

PCI with bare metal stent (BMS) is associated with significant risk of restenosis due to late lumen loss as a result of neo intimal proliferation. First and second generation drug eluting stents (DES) have significantly reduced the chances of ISR. However, there still are number of patients who develop ISR. Strategies like brachy therapy, balloon dilatation, paclitaxel coated balloons (PCB) or deployment of new generation stents have been utilized to achieve long term event free results. However reported results are far from optimum except for treatment with everolimus eluting stents or PCI with PCB.

■ **Objective:**

To test the feasibility and initial results of SEB dilatation for ISR.

■ **Methods:**

The current study is a first in human study for the treatment of ISR with SEB.

The trial enrolled 50 patients who had documented evidence of ischemia with ISR and vessel diameter of 2.5-3 mm by visual estimate in the native coronary artery. The stents deployed in the previous PCI were BMS or DES.

The method of delivery: SirolimusVirtue balloon was used to deploy 12 mcg sirolimus per square millimeter of balloon surface delivered through micropores.

Results:

Primary safety end point was target lesion failure (TVF) which included cardiac death, target vessel MI and clinically driven revascularization at 30 days and the primary performing end point was in segment late lumen loss at 6 months.TLF occurred in 0% at 30 days while latre lumen loss at 6 months was 0.31 ± 0.52 mm in 47 patients. Binary restenosis at 6 months occurred in 19.1% patients and major adverse cardiac events in 10.2%. At 1 year the clinical outcomes were 12.2% TLF and 14.3% MACE (Fig.1 & Table 1).

Virtue balloon was expanded for 40secs at 13.9 atms. Three patients received bail out stent due to dissection.

Appraisal and clinical importance:

The study has shown safety and efficacy of the use of SEB for the treatment of ISR. The earlier approach of performing PTCA with PCB was associated with acceptable clinical benefits that could match the results of deployment of second generation everolimus stent. However, Sirolimus eluting stents in the past have shown superiority over paclitaxel eluting stents and therefore could be expected to provide better results.

Deployment of additional DES over the earlier DES for ISR has been shown to be associated with higher rates of neo atherosclerosis than deploying DES for BMS ISR. Further after deployment of additional stent, compliance and geometry of the vessel could change that could result in unfavorable long term results. Too much of metal could lead to compromise of vasomotor tone since the inner layer is covered with thick layer of two stents. With these limitations of the earlier methods it is expected that a SEB could provide better results .

Fig. 1 : *MLD at baseline, immediately after intervention, and at 6-months follow-up*

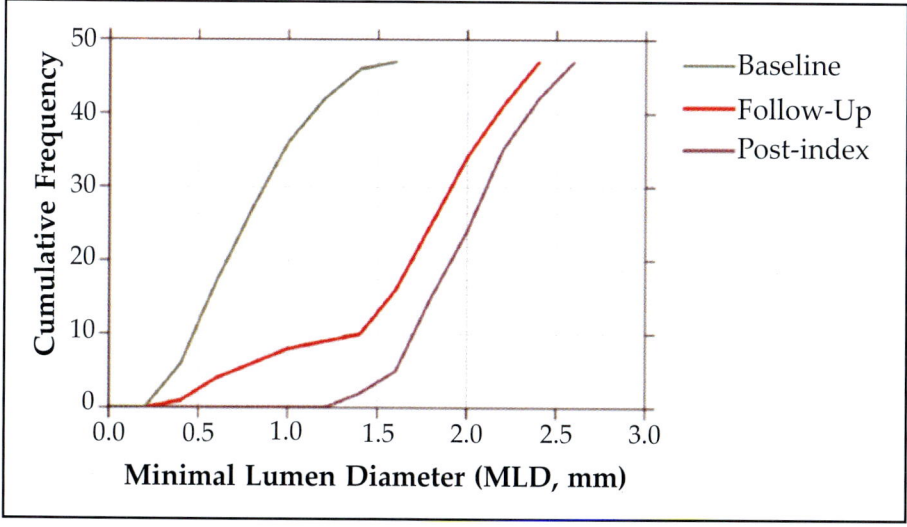

Table 1: Angiographic Results at 6 months

	ITT (n = 47)	PP (n = 36)	PP group vs. Exclusion group p Value
RVD, mm*	2.52 ± 0.38	2.52 ± 0.32	0.927
MLD, mm	1.75 ± 0.54	1.96 ± 0.32	0.0007
Diameter stenosis, %	30.27 ± 19.88	22.27 ± 9.44	0.0481
Change diameter	12.67 ± 20.64	5.22 ± 11.38	0.0020
LLL, mm	0.31 ± 0.52	0.12 ± 0.33	0.0005
Binary restenosis‡	9 (19.1)	1 (2.8)	0.0001

Values are mean ± SD or n (%). *Internormal value. Study primary performance endoint. Study secondary performance endpoint.
LLL = late lumen loss

▌ Suggested Readings

1. Kleber FX, Rittger H, Bonaventura K, et al. Drugcoated balloons for treatment of coronary artery disease: updated recommendations from a consensus group. Clin Res Cardiol 2013;102:785-97.

2. Alfonso F, Byrne RA, Rivero F, Kastrati A. Current treatment of in-stent restenosis. J Am Coll Cardiol 2014;63:2659-73.

3. Scheller B, Hehrlein C, Bocksch W, et al. Treatment of coronary in-stent restenosis with a paclitaxel-coated balloon catheter. N Engl J Med 2006;355:2113-24.

4. Alfonso F, Pérez-Vizcayno MJ, Cárdenas A, et al. A randomized comparison of drug-eluting balloon versus everolimus-eluting stent in patients with bare-metal stent-in-stent restenosis: the RIBS V Clinical Trial (Restenosis Intra-stent of Bare Metal Stents: paclitaxel-eluting balloon vs. everolimus-eluting stent). J Am CollCardiol 2014; 63:1378-86.

5. Rittger H, Brachmann J, Sinha AM, et al. A randomized, multicenter, single-blinded trial comparing paclitaxel-coated balloon angioplasty with plain balloon angioplasty in drug-eluting stent restenosis: the PEPCAD-DES study. J Am CollCardiol 2012;59:1377-82.

6. Alfonso F, Pérez-Vizcayno MJ, Cárdenas A, et al. A prospective randomized trial of drugeluting balloons versus everolimus-eluting stents in patients with in-stent restenosis of drug-eluting stents: the RIBS IV randomized clinical trial. J Am CollCardiol 2015;66:23-33.

7. Habara S, Kadota K, Shimada T, et al. Late restenosis after paclitaxel-coated balloon angioplasty occurs in patients with drug-eluting stent restenosis. J Am CollCardiol 2015;66:14-22.

8. Dangas GD, Serruys PW, Kereiakes DJ, et al. Meta-analysis of everolimus-eluting versus paclitaxel-eluting stents in coronary artery disease: final 3-year results of the SPIRIT clinical trials program (Clinical Evaluation of the Xience V Everolimus Eluting Coronary Stent System in the Treatment of Patients With De Novo Native Coronary Artery Lesions). J Am CollCardiolIntv 2013;6:914-22.

9. Clever YP, Peters D, Calisse J, et al. Novel sirolimus-coated balloon catheter: in vivo evaluation in a porcine coronary model. CircCardiovascInterv 2016;9:e003543.

10. Granada JF, Tellez A, Baumbach WR, et al. In vivo delivery and long-term tissue retention of nano encapsulated sirolimus using a novel porous balloon angioplasty system. Euro Intervention 2016;12:7407.

81

Objective Randomised Blinded Investigation with Optimal Medical Therapy of Angioplasty in Stable Angina - ORBITA

Ref.: Rasha Al-Lamee, David Thompson, Hakim-Moulay Dehbi, et al On behalf of the ORBITA Investigators, Percutaenous Coronary Intervention in stable angina (ORITA): a double-blind,randomized controlled trial.
LIINK: Lancet 2017 ; Nov 2:{Epub ahead of print}.

Dev Pahlajani

▌ Introduction:

Revascularization in obstructive coronary artery disease was expected to increase longevity, prevent myocardial infarction and reduce symptoms and thus improve quality of life. However, in patients with stable ischemic heart disease the role of percutaneous coronary artery intervention (PCI) is supposed to be limited to improving the quality of life by providing symptomatic relief. ORBITA trial was undertaken to study whether PCI indeed provides symptomatic relief by performing blinded placebo controlled procedure.

▌ Methods:

ORBITA was a randomized trial that enrolled patients with severe coronary artery obstruction (≥70% stenosis). Patients were initially treated with optimized medical treatment and underwent pre randomization assessment with exercise testing and symptom questionnaire and dobutamine stress echo. Trial enrolled 230 patients out of which 200 underwent randomization. PCI was performed in 105 patients and 95 patients were assigned to placebo shown procedure. Mean area stenosis of lesions was 84.4% with mean FFR of 0.69 . The primary end point was difference in exercise time increment between groups. The mean age of the patient was 66 years with 27% females. The patients with ACS, previous CABG, left main stem disease, CTO and valve disease were excluded. In 92% patients LVEF was normal. Majority of them had class II / III angina by Canadian Cardiovascular Society (class II or III) grading. Among enrolled patients 70% had LAD involvement. Change in the angina frequently from baseline was 14.0 v/s 9.6 (p=0.26).

▌ Results:

There was no significant difference in the primary end point in exercise time increment between groups.

Conclusion:

In patients with stable angina PCI did not offer any additional benefit over optimum medical treatment for providing symptomatic relief.

Appraisal:

It is a very important study and has confirmed results of some of the earlier large trials like COURAGE that enrolled 2300 patients with stable angina. The results of optimum medical treatment arm matched with those of PCI arm. However this study as compared to COURAGE enrolled only 203 patients. However, this study has objective strength. This is the first study in which a sham procedure has been performed. Larger number of patients would be needed to substantiate the conclusions arrived at in this particular trial.

Suggested Readings

1. William E Boden, Robert A O'Rourke, Koon K Teo et al for COURAGE Trial Research Group: Optimal Medical Treatment with or without PCI for stable coronary disease N Eng J Med 2007,356,1503-16.

Heart Failure with Preserved, Borderline, and Reduced Ejection Fraction 5-Year Outcomes

Ref.: Kevin S. Shah, HaolinXu, Roland A. Matsouaka, Deepak L. Bhatt et al
LINK: JACC 2017; 70(20): 2476-2486

Key Points:

1. Similar number of patients have heart failure with reduced ejection fraction (HFrEF) and with preserved EF (HFpEF).

2. In both groups 5 year survival is poor.

3. In patients with HFrEF, HFpEF and heart failure with borderline ejection fraction (HFbEF) 5 years mortality is 75%.

4. Readmission rates over 5 years are high end range from 80-84%.

Dev Pahlajani

■ **Introduction:**

Patients with heart failure have been known to have poor prognosis with high 5 year mortality. However, classically patients with heart failure have been thought to have reduced EF. Recently a new entity called as HFpEF has been identified. Its prognosis as compared to HFrEF is not well described. European Society of Cardiology guidelines categorize patients with heart failure to

a) EF < 40%, (HFrEF)

b) EF 40% - 49% and (HFbEF)

c) Preserved EF ≥ 50%. (HFpEF)

■ **Aims of the Study:**

To study 5 year outcomes in patients with various categories of heart failure stratified according to EF. Also to compare survival with national population according to similar age groups.

■ **Methods:**

The data was collected from the heart failure registry. The analysis involves 39982 patients with heart failure. The patients belonged to following groups of heart failure:

HFpEF : 18299 (46%)

HFbEF : 3285 (8.2%)

HFrEF : 18398 (46%)

Results:

Overall, median survival was 2.1 years. After risk adjusted analysis the composite of mortality and rehospitalization was similar for are the groups.

Five year mortality in all the 3 groups are similar

HFrEF   75.3%

HFpEF   75.7%

HFbEF   75.7%

The rehospitalization rates were higher in the HFrEF group. Cardiovascular and HF event rates were higher in patients with HFrEF and HFbEF when compared with those of HFpEF (Fig 1.A to D). As compared to national survival patients with heart failure had significantly lower age adjusted survival.

Conclusion:

The prognosis in heart failure patients over 5 year period is poor with high mortality and morbidity and high rates of readmission. There is no difference in the adverse event rates including mortality within any of the 3 groups of heart failure patients.

Fig. 1: *Cumulative incidence Plots for Mortality and Readmission outcomes by EF groups*

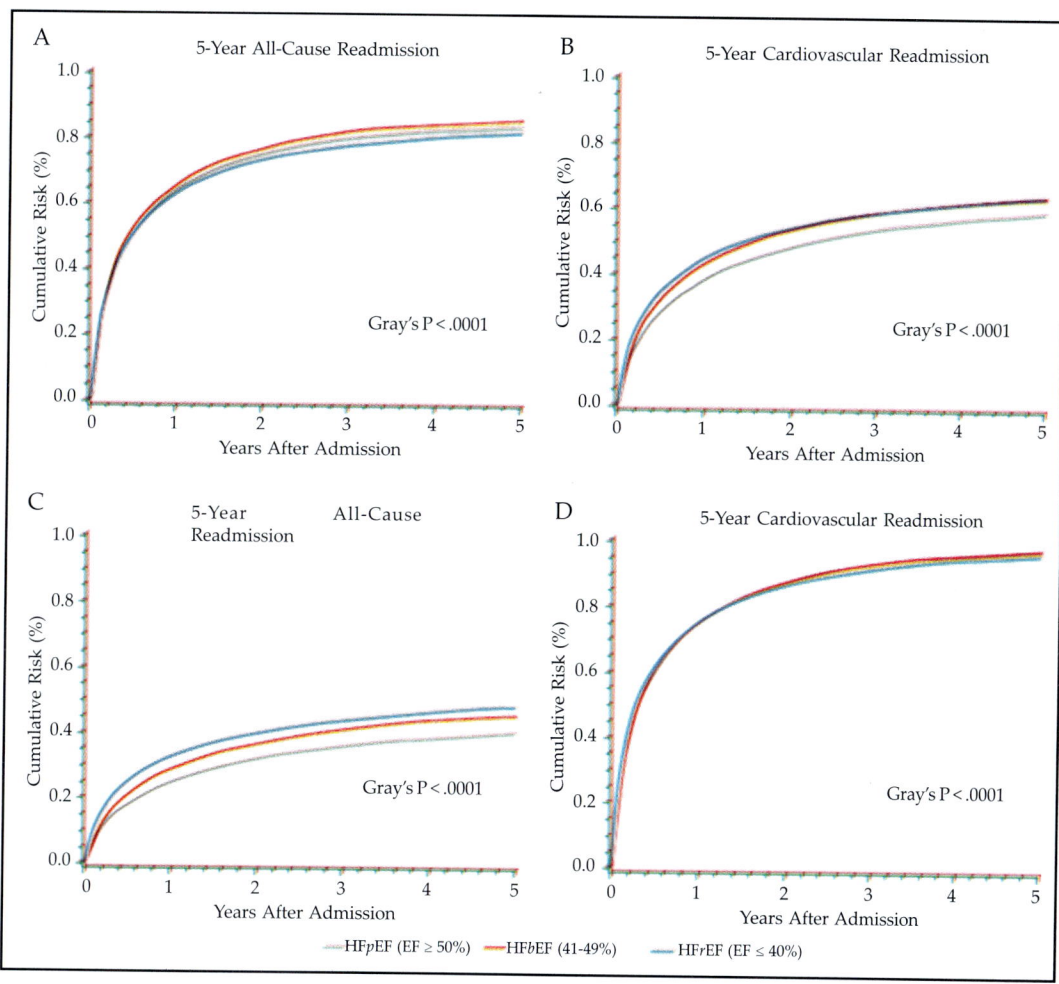

▌ Suggested Readings

1. Lekavich CL, Barksdale DJ, Neelon V, Wu JR. Heart failure preserved ejection fraction (HFpEF): an integrated and strategic review. Heart Fail Rev 2015;20:643-53.

2. Steinberg BA, Zhao X, Heidenreich PA, et al. Trends in patients hospitalized with heart failure and preserved left ventricular ejection fraction: prevalence, therapies, and outcomes. Circulation 2012;126:6575.

3. Bhatia RS, Tu JV, Lee DS, et al. Outcome of heart failure with preserved ejection fraction in a population-based study. N Engl J Med 2006;355: 260-9.

4. Ponikowski P, Voors AA, Anker SD, et al. 2016 ESC guidelines for the diagnosis and treatment of acute and chronic heart failure. Eur Heart J 2016; 37:2129-200.

5. Cheng RK, Cox M, Neely ML, et al. Outcomes in patients with heart failure with preserved, borderline, and reduced ejection fraction in the Medicare population. Am Heart J 2014;168: 721-30.e3. 12. Smaha LA. The American Heart Association Get With The Guidelines program. Am Heart J 2004; 148 Suppl 5:S46-8.

6. Borlaug BA, Paulus WJ. Heart failure with preserved ejection fraction: pathophysiology, diagnosis, and treatment. Eur Heart J 2011;32: 670-6.

83

Dual Antithrombotic Therapy with Dabigatran after PCI in Atrial Fibrillation

Ref.: Christopher P. Cannon, M.D., Deepak L. Bhatt, M.D., M.P.H., Jonas Oldgren, M.D., Ph.D., et al
LINK: N Eng J MED 2017;377(16):1513-24.

Dev Pahlajani

▮ Introduction:

Approximately 30% patients with atrial fibrillation (AF) have atherosclerotic coronary artery disease and 8 - 10% patients who undergo percutaneous coronary intervention (PCI) have AF.In such patients current standard of care includes vitamin K antagonist (VKA) with dual antiplatelet therapy (triple therapy). Such an approach carries a significant risk of bleeding and adverse cardiovascular events including mortality.

▮ Aims:

Whether replacing triple therapy with dual therapy with Dabigatran a novel oral anticoagulant (NOAC) and one P2Y12 inhibitor (clopidogrel or ticagrelor) will reduce the risk of bleeding as compared to triple theray.

▮ Methods:

REDUAL PCI is a multicenter trial that randomised 2735 patients with AF who had undergone PCI to either

a) Triple therapy with VKA + P2Y12 inhibitor (clopidogrel or Ticagrelor) and aspirin or

b) Dual therapy with Dabigatran (110 or 150 mg twice a day + P2Y12 inhibitor).

▮ Primary End Point:

Major or clinically relevant non major bleeding events with mean follow up of 14 months. Also to study non inferiority of dual therapy to triple therapy as regards to composite efficacy end point of thrombocmbolic events which included MI, stroke or systemic embolism, death, or unplanned revascularization.

▮ Results:

Primary end point of bleeding was 15.4% in 110 mg dual therapy.

26.9% in triple therapy (p < 0.001 for superiority).

20.2% in 150 mg dual therapy v/s 25.7% in the corresponding triple therapy.

The incidence of composite efficacy was similar in both the groups (Fig 1. A to C).

Conclusion:

Dual therapy with either 110 mg or 150 mg Dabigatran twice a day with P2Y12 inhibitor is superior to triple therapy with VKA and P2Y12 inhibitor with aspirin.

Clinical Implications:

It is an important trial since it provides a better strategy of preventing bleeding events in patients with AF undergoing PCI. Bleeding has been documented to be a serious complication and is associated with major adverse complications including MI, stent thrombosis and death. Moreover maintaining INR within therapeutic window is pretty cumbersome for patients and clinicians. NOACs do not need to be monitored by coagulation profile. Currently specific antidote to dabigatran-idarucizumab has been approved and is available with major institutions. The results are in conformity with

1) WOEST trial that concluded dual therapy with clopidogrel and VKA to be superior to triple therapy and that of

2) PIONEER AF trial that reported superiority of dual therapy with low dose rivaroxaban and P2Y12 inhibitor over triple therapy or a very low dose rivaroxaban with 2 antiplatelets over conventional triple therapy that included VKA.

   One wonders if we are going to watch end of VKA era soon.

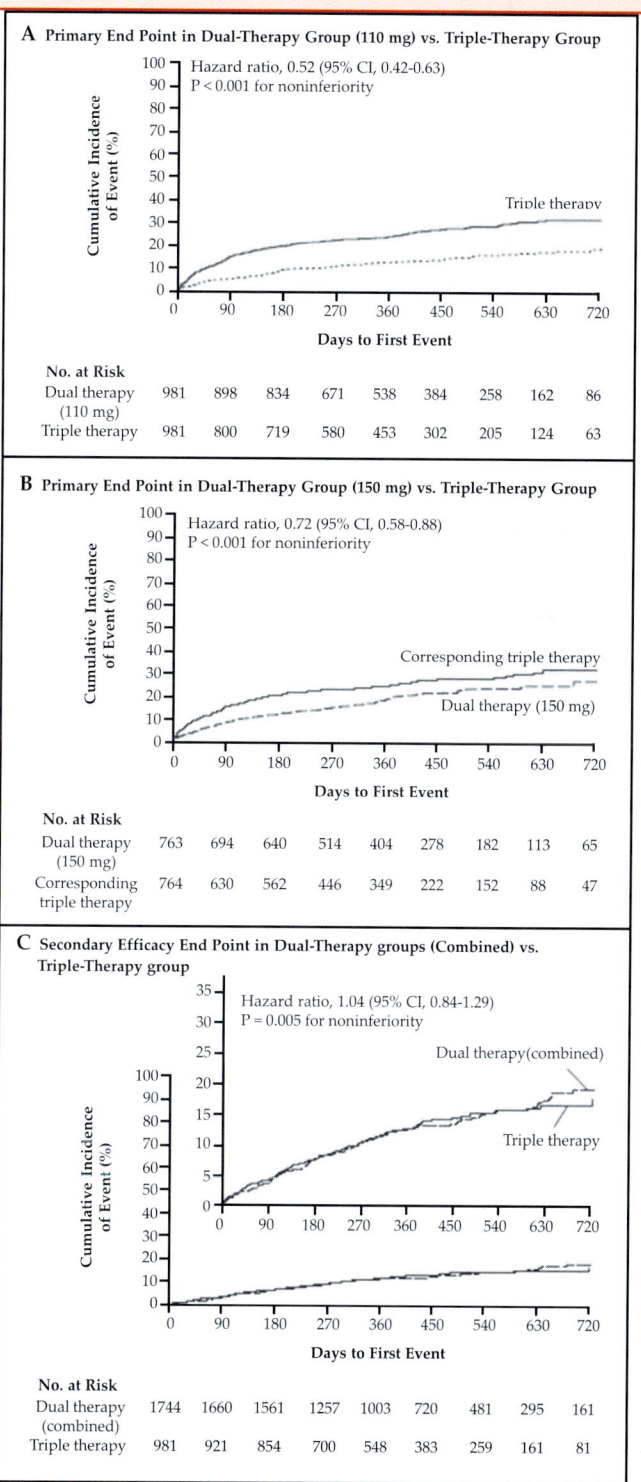

Fig. 1 :

▌ Suggested Readings

1. Lip GY, Windecker S, Huber K, et al. Management of antithrombotic therapy in atrial fibrillation patients presenting with acute coronary syndrome and/or undergoing percutaneous coronary or valve interventions: a joint consensus document of the European Society of Cardiology Working Group on Thrombosis, European Heart Rhythm Association (EHRA), European Association of Percutaneous Cardiovascular Interventions (EAPCI) and European Association of Acute Cardiac Care (ACCA) endorsed by the Heart Rhythm Society (HRS) and Asia-Pacific Heart Rhythm Society (APHRS). Eur Heart J 2014;35:3155-79.

2. January CT, Wann LS, Alpert JS, et al. 2014 AHA/ACC/HRS guideline for the management of patients with atrial fibrillation: executive summary: a report of the American College of Cardiology/American Heart Association Task Force on practice guidelines and the Heart Rhythm Society. Circulation 2014;130:2071-104.

3. Kirchhof P, Benussi S, Kotecha D, et al. 2016 ESC guidelines for the management of atrial fibrillation developed in collaboration with EACTS. Eur Heart J 2016;37: 2893-962.

4. Dewilde WJ, Oirbans T, Verheugt FW, et al. Use of clopidogrel with or without aspirin in patients taking oral anticoagulant therapy and undergoing percutaneous coronary intervention: an open-label, randomised, controlled trial. Lancet 2013; 381:1107-15.

5. Gibson CM, Mehran R, Bode C, et al. Prevention of bleeding in patients with atrial fibrillation undergoing PCI. N Engl J Med 2016;375:2423-34.

6. Gibson CM, Pinto DS, Chi G, et al. Recurrent hospitalization among patients with atrial fibrillation undergoing intracoronary stenting treated with 2 treatment strategies of rivaroxaban or a dose adjusted oral vitamin K antagonist treatment strategy. Circulation 2017;135: 323-33.

7. Bhatt DL. O PIONEERs! The beginning of the end of full-dose triple therapy with warfarin? Circulation 2017;135:334-7.

84

Renal Outcomes in Anticoagulated Patients with Atrial Fibrillation

Ref.: Xiaoxi Yao, PHD, NavdeepTangri, MD, PHD, Bernard J. Gersh, MB, CHB, DPHIL et al

LINK: JACC 2017;70(21):2621-32

Key Points:

1. Decline in renal function is commonly observed in patients with atrial fibrillation (AF) treated with oral anticoagulants

2. The risk of decline is lower in patients treated with dabigatran and rivaroxaban as compared to Vitamin K antagonists (VKA)

3. Apixaban has no significant relation withlower renal outcomes

4. High INR values are associated with greater degree of nephropathy

Dev Pahlajani

▮ Introduction:

Current guidelines recommend oral anticoagulants for patients with nonvalvular AF to prevent stroke. With the availability of novel oral anticoagulants (NOACs) most of the physicians prefer to treat them with NOACs rather than with VKA if the economics permit. In developing countries it is estimated that approximately 50% patients are treated with NOACs and rest with VKA. Physicians tend to avoid prescribing NOACs in patients with renal dysfunction. Patients with eGFR below 33 are prescribed VKA considering it to be less nephrotoxic than NOACs. The comparative risk of renal dysfunction with currently available 3 NOACs versus VKA has not been studied in great detail.

▮ Objectives:

To compare the effect of 4 oral anticoagulant agents apixaban, dabigatran, rivaroxaban and warfarin on renal functions.

▮ Methods:

The study included 9769 patients who were treated with oral anticoagulants for prevention of stroke in AF. The average on treatment follow up was 10.7 ± 9.9 months. Study evaluated 4 renal outcomes.

1) ≥ than 30% decline in eGFR

2) Rise in serum creatinine by 100%

3) Acute kidney injury

4) Kidney failure

The overall risk of adverse kidney outcome at the end of 2 years was

a) 24.4% for 30% decline in eGFR

b) 4% for doubling of serum creatinine

c) 14.8% for acute kidney failure

d) 1.7% for kidney failure

With 3 NOACs combined there was statistically significant reduction in risk of all 4 kidney injury parameters studied as compared to VKA. Individually evaluated dabigatranwas associated with lower risk of decline in eGFR and AKI and rivaroxaban carried a lower risk of fall in eGFR, doubling of creatinine and AKI as compared to VKA.

As compared to rivaroxaban and dabigatran, apixaban did not have significant relationship with adverse renal outcomes when compared to VKA (Fig.1. A - C).

▌ Clinical Implications:

Patients with renal failure and AF pose therapeutic challenge since it has been thought that use of NOACs in these patients would lead to excessive bleeding. Comparative effects of NOACs and warfarin on kidney function are lacking. Patients with AF have several co morbidities like diabetes, hypertension, pre existing renal dysfunction and coronary artery disease predisposing them to develop further kidney injury. Choice of anticoagulant is therefore of paramount importance. Warfarin inhibits Vitamin K dependent protein matrix leading to damage to the renal vessels while NOVACs because of their effect on inhibiting factor Xa or thrombin could reduce vascular inflammation.The study also highlights the evidence that very high INR values are associated with greater renal damage. The therapeutic relevance of the study is that it defies the earlier assumptions of NOVACs being more injurious to kidney as compared to Warfarin. Dabigatran and rivaroxaban could be better alternative to warfarin to reduce the chances of kidney damage.

Fig. 1 : *Cumulative Incidence of Renal Outcomes*

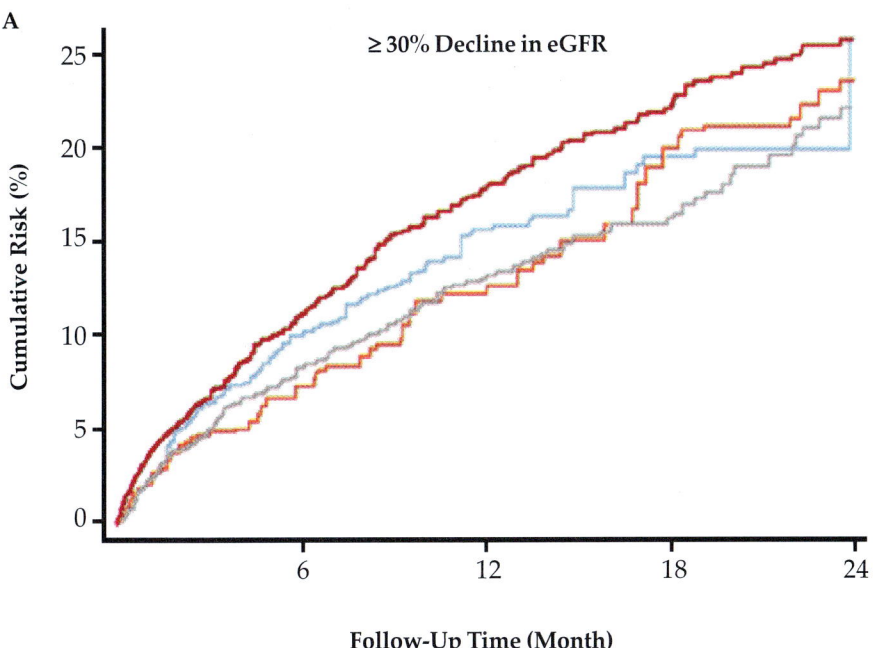

Apixaban	10.2 (9.3, 11.2)	15.6 (14.4, 17.0)	19.6 (17.9, 21.4)	25.7 (22.8, 28.9)
Dabigatran	7.2 (6.5, 8.0)	12.3 (11.3, 13.4)	20.0 (18.4, 21.8)	23.6 (21.7, 25.6)
Rivaroxaban	8.2 (7.5, 9.0)	13.2 (12.1, 14.3)	16.3 (14.9, 17.7)	22.1 (20.0, 24.4)
Warfarin	11.2 (10.4, 12.0)	17.9 (16.8, 19.2)	22.4 (20.9, 24.0)	25.8 (24.0, 27.8)

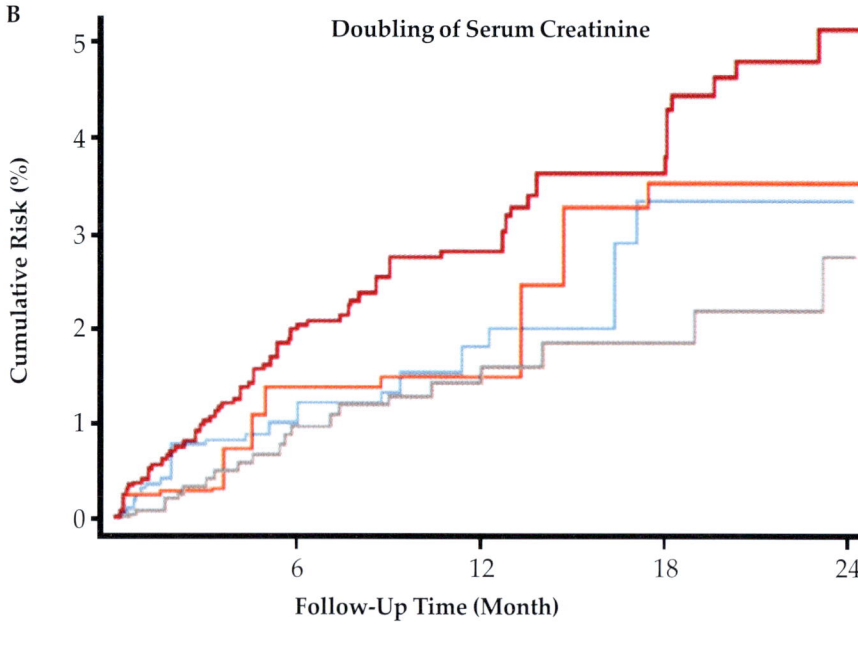

Apixaban	1.2 (0.9, 1.6)	1.8 (1.4, 2.4)	3.3 (2.4, 4.4)	3.3 (2.4, 4.4)
Dabigatran	1.4 (1.1, 1.8)	1.5 (1.2, 1.9)	3.5 (2.8, 4.4)	3.5 (2.8, 4.4)
Rivaroxaban	0.9 (0.7, 1.3)	1.6 (1.2, 2.1)	1.8 (1.4, 2.4)	2.7 (2.0, 3.8)
Warfarin	2.0 (1.7, 2.4)	2.8 (2.3, 3.3)	4.4 (3.6, 5.3)	5.1 (4.1, 6.2)

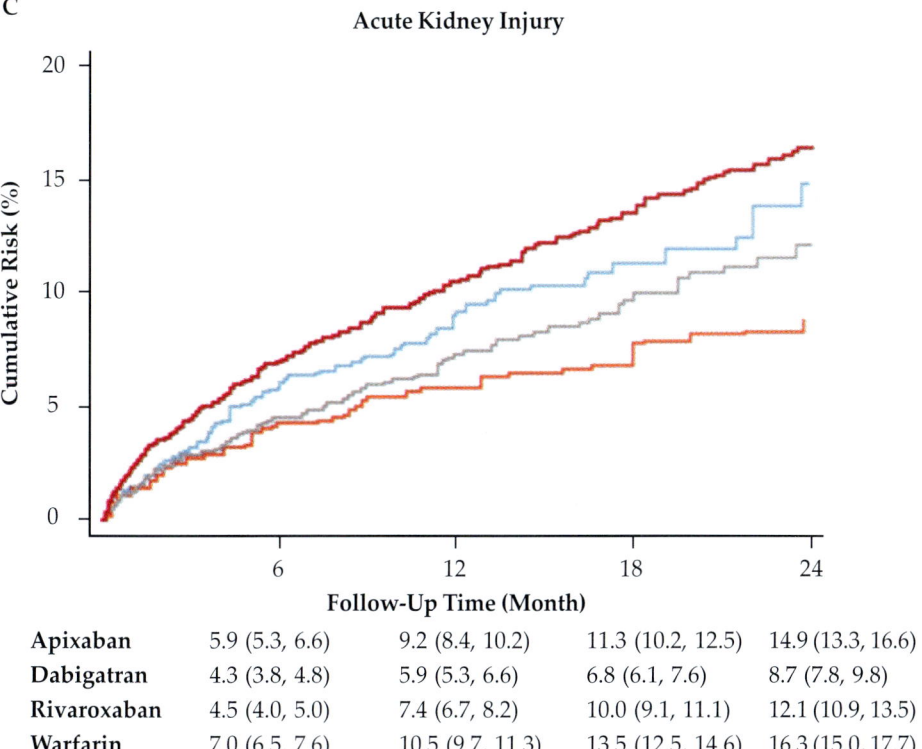

C

Acute Kidney Injury

Cumulative Risk (%) vs Follow-Up Time (Month)

	6	12	18	24
Apixaban	5.9 (5.3, 6.6)	9.2 (8.4, 10.2)	11.3 (10.2, 12.5)	14.9 (13.3, 16.6)
Dabigatran	4.3 (3.8, 4.8)	5.9 (5.3, 6.6)	6.8 (6.1, 7.6)	8.7 (7.8, 9.8)
Rivaroxaban	4.5 (4.0, 5.0)	7.4 (6.7, 8.2)	10.0 (9.1, 11.1)	12.1 (10.9, 13.5)
Warfarin	7.0 (6.5, 7.6)	10.5 (9.7, 11.3)	13.5 (12.5, 14.6)	16.3 (15.0, 17.7)

▌ Suggested Readings

1. Connolly SJ, Ezekowitz MD, Yusuf S, et al. Dabigatran versus warfarin in patients with atrial fibrillation. N Engl J Med 2009;361:1139-51.

2. Patel MR, Mahaffey KW, Garg J, et al. Rivaroxaban versus warfarin in nonvalvular atrial fibrillation. N Engl J Med 2011;365:883-91.

3. Yao X, Abraham NS, Sangaralingham LR, et al. Effectiveness and safety of dabigatran, rivaroxaban, and apixaban versus warfarin in nonvalvular atrial fibrillation. J Am Heart Assoc 2016;5: e003725.

4. Böhm M, Ezekowitz MD, Connolly SJ, et al. Changes in renal function in patients with atrial fibrillation: an analysis from the RE-LY Trial. J Am CollCardiol 2015;65:2481-93.

5. Fordyce CB, Hellkamp AS, Lokhnygina Y, et al. On-treatment outcomes in patients with worsening renal function with rivaroxaban compared with warfarin: insights from ROCKET AF. Circulation 2016;134:37-47.

6. Chatrou ML, Winckers K, Hackeng TM, Reuteling sperger CP, Schurgers LJ. Vascular calcification: the price to pay for anticoagulation therapy with vitamin K-antagonists. Blood Rev 2012;26:155-66.

7. Schurgers LJ, Joosen IA, Laufer EM, et al. Vitamin K-antagonists accelerate atherosclerotic calcification and induce a vulnerable plaque phenotype. PloS One 2012;7:e43229.

8. Chan YH, Yeh YH, See LC, et al. Acute kidney injury in Asians with atrial fibrillation treated with dabigatran or warfarin. J Am CollCardiol 2016;68: 2272-83.

85

Double Kissing Crush Versus Provisional Stenting for Left Main Distal Bifurcation Lesions

DK CRUSH-V Randomized Trial

Ref.: Shao-Liang Chen, MD, Jue-Jie Zhang, PHD, Yaling Han, MD, Jing Kan, MBBS, et al

LINK: JACC 2017;70(21):2605 - 2617

Key Points

1. In patients with true distal left main coronary artery (LMCA) bifurcation double kissing (DK) crush is associated with lower rates of target lesion failure (TLF) as compared to provisional stenting.

2. Target vessel myocardial infarction (TVMI), definite or probable stent thrombosis and target vessel revascularization (TVR) are also lower with DK Crush technique.

Dev Pahlajani

▌ Introduction:

Approximately 80% of patients with LMCA have distal bifurcation lesions. Various strategies have been deployed to treat them. In the non LMCA bifurcation lesions the preferred strategy is that of provisional stenting since it is associated with lower adverse event rates as compared to dedicated 2 stent strategy. Recently DK Crush has been reported to have more favorable outcomes as compared to the provisional stenting in non LMCA situations. Whether DK Crush will prove to be superior to provisional stenting in LMCA bifurcations lesions has not been studied so far.

▌ Objectives:

To compare outcomes of DK crush with provisional stenting in true LMCA bifurcation lesions.

▌ Methods:

Multinational multicenter randomized trial of 482 patients with true distal LMCA bifurcation lesions. Trial randomized 242 patients to provisional stenting and 240 to DK Crush.

▌ Primary End Point:

Composite of TLF: cardiac death, target vessel MI or clinically driven TLR 1 year.

▌ Results:

At the end of one year:

TLF occurred in 26 patients (10.7%) treated with provisional stenting and 12 patients (5%) assigned to DK Crush technique (p=0.02).

As compared to provisional stenting there were significantly lower rates of TVMI (2.9% versus 4% p=0.03), definite or probable stent thrombosis (3.3% versus 0.4%) (p=0.02) in patients who underwent DK Crush. TLR occurred in practically half of the patients who underwent DK Crush as compared to those who underwent provisional stenting (7.9% versus 3.8%). Angiographic restenosis was also significantly lower in patients with DK Crush as compared to provisional stenting. Cardiac death rate was similar in both the groups (Fig. 1 & 2, Table 1).

▊ Critical Analysis:

Thus the study indicates that in LMCA true bifurcation lesions DK Crush stenting significantly reduces incidence of TLF when compared with provisional stenting. The difference mainly was driven by definite or probable stent thrombosis.

EXCEL trial compared the outcome of PCI with everolimus eluting stent versus CABG in patients with LMCA disease. There were 80% patients who had distal LMCA bifurcation. Major adverse events were similar in both the groups. However PCI patients had higher risk of TVR as compared to CABG treated patients. NOBLE trial also compared outcomes of PCI performed with earlier generation stent versus CABG in LMCA disease. Large majority of these patients had bifurcation lesions. CABG proved to be superior to PCI. It is noteworthy that provisional stenting was the preferred strategy for treating bifurcation lesions in both the trials. Whether deploying DK Crush technique for LMCA bifurcation will match the results of CABG has to be seen with larger trials.

▊ Clinical Relevance:

Results of the current trial if confirmed by larger trials could provide a better strategy to treat LMCA bifurcation comparable to CABG.

Fig. 1 : *Stenting for LM bifurcations*

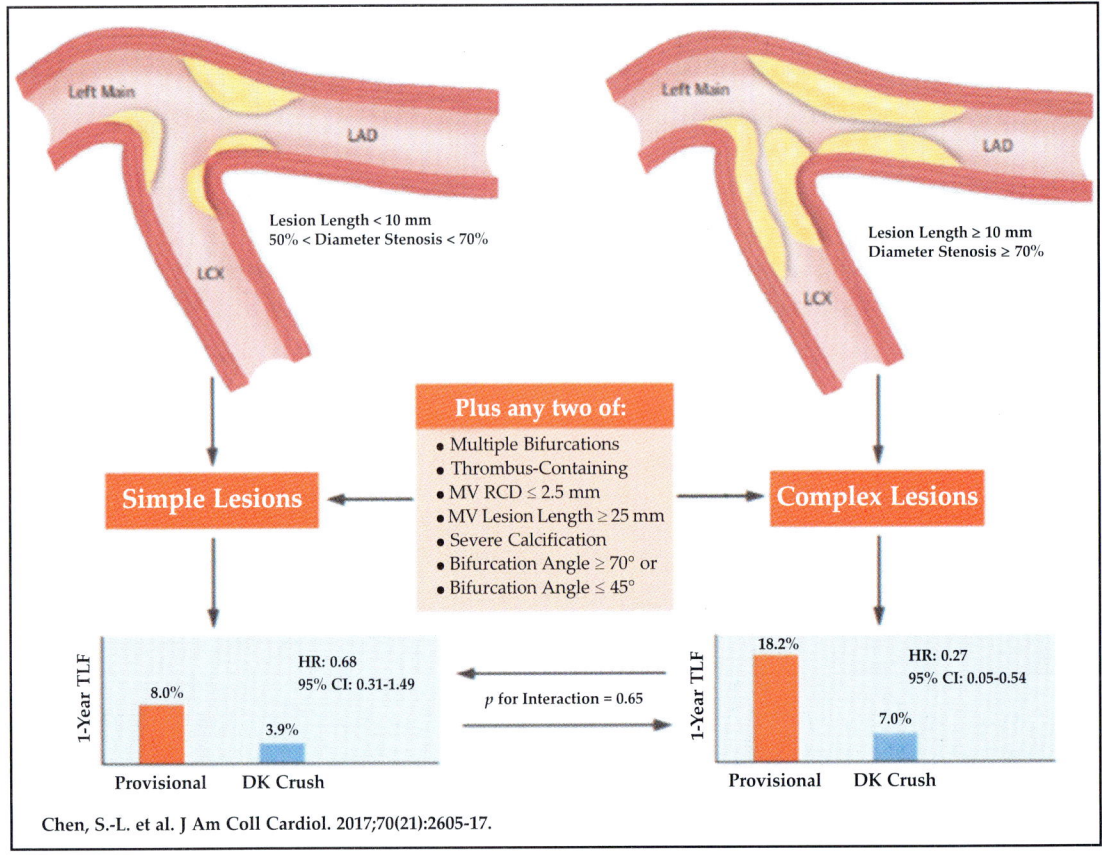

Chen, S.-L. et al. J Am Coll Cardiol. 2017;70(21):2605-17.

Fig. 2 : Kaplan-Meier Time-to-First Event Curves

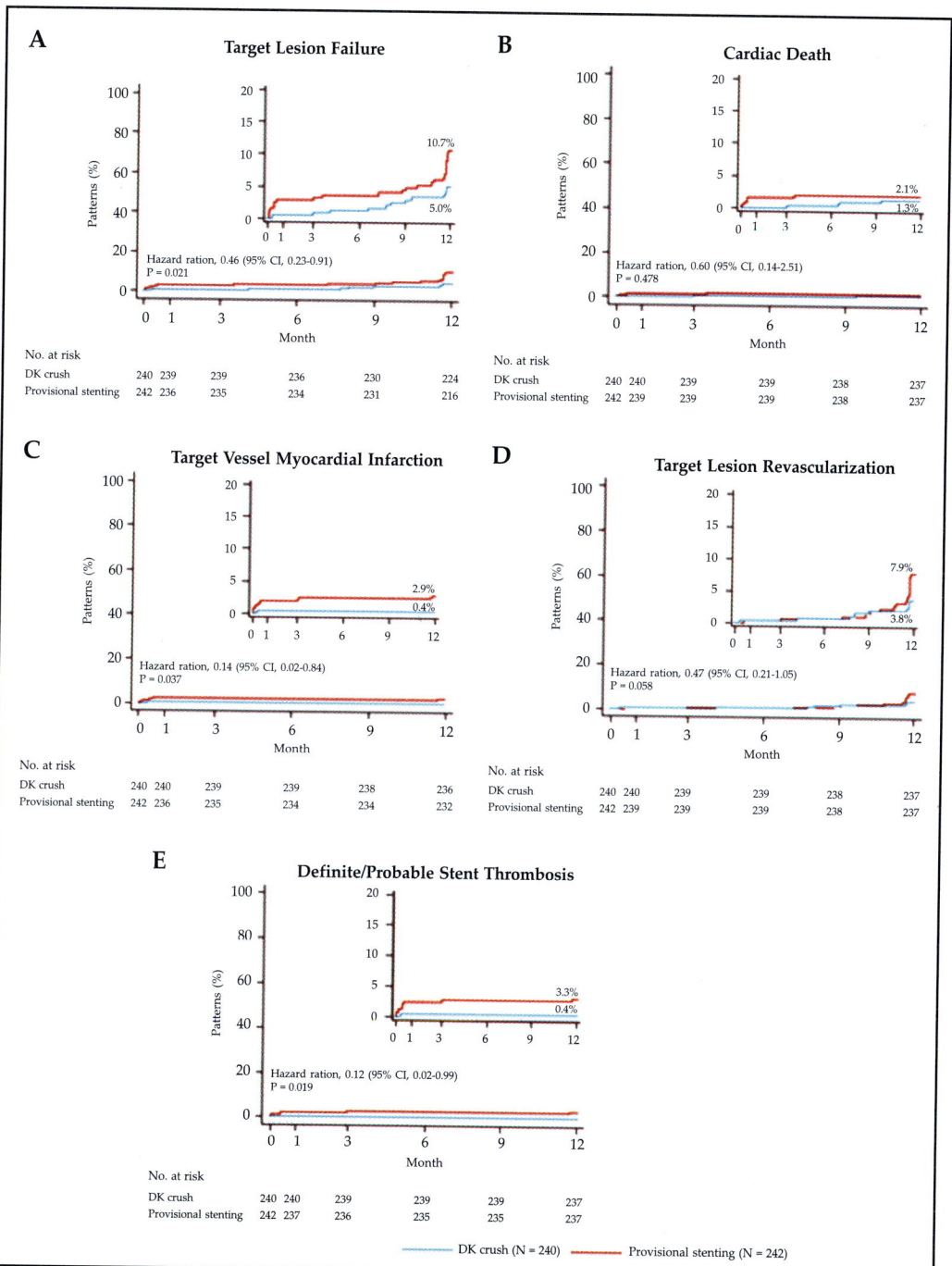

Table 1: Baseline characteristics of the rendomized groups

	Provisional stent (n = 242)	DK Crush stent (n = 240)	p Value
Demographics			
Age, years	64 ± 10	65 ± 9	0.15
Male	188 (77.7)	199 (82.9)	0.17
Height, cm	167 ± 7	168 ± 7	0.50
Weight, kg	70 ± 10	70 ± 10	0.94
Systolic blood pressure, mmHg	132 ± 19	135 ± 18	0.07
Diastolic blood pressure mmHg	79 ± 10	79 ± 10	0.85
Heart rate, beats/min	73 ± 10	74 ± 12	0.34
Risk factors			
Hyperlipidemia	115 (47.5)	114 (47.5)	1.00
Hypertension	156 (64.5)	175 (72.9)	0.051
Diabetes	62 (25.6)	69 (28.8)	0.47
Insulin-treated	18 (29.0)	19 (27.5)	0.85
Current smoker	78 (32.2)	82 (34.2)	0.64
Prior stroke	4 (1.7)	3 (1.3)	1.00
Creatinine, umol/L	78 ± 30	80 ± 25	0.40
eGFR,ml/min/1.73m^2	81.1 ± 24.1	78.5 ± 23.0	0.22
<15 ml/min/1.73m^2	1 (0.4)	0 (0.0)	
15-29 ml/min/1.73m^2	3 (1.2)	2 (0.8)	
30-60 ml/min/1.73m^2	31 (12.8)	39 (16.3)	
>60 ml/min/1.73m^2	207 (85.5)	199 (82.9)	
Peripheral artery disease	16 (6.6)	18 (7.5)	0.73
Medical history			
Prior MI	51 (21.1)	52 (21.7)	0.91
Prior PCI	43 (17.8)	33 (13.8)	0.28
Prior CABG	2 (0.8)	2 (0.8)	1.00
LVEF, %	60 ± 9	59 ± 9	0.81
LVEF <30%	7 (2.9)	11 (4.6)	0.12
Symptomatic heart failure	33 (13.6)	37 (15.4)	0.58
Clinical presentation			0.49
Silent ischemia	10 (4.1)	7 (2.9)	
Stable angina	26 (10.4)	34 (14.2)	
Unstable angina	180 (74.4)	168 (70.0)	
Recent MI (>24 h)	26 (10.7)	31 (12.9)	
Laboratory			
Red blood cell, x 10^{12}/L	4.4 ± 0.6	4.4 ± 0.7	0.52
White blood cell x 10^9/L	6.91± 2.1	6.9 ± 2.1	0.79
Hemoglobin g/L	135 ± 15	134 ± 17	0.61
Platelet count x 10^9/L	203 ± 63	194 ± 59	0.13
Total cholestrol mmoL/L	4.2 ± 1.2	4.0 ± 1.2	0.15

▌ Suggested Readings

1. Morice MC, Serruys PW, Kappetein AP, et al. Five-year outcomes in patients with left main disease treated with either percutaneous coronary intervention or coronary artery bypass grafting in the synergy between percutaneous coronary intervention with Taxus and cardiac surgery trial. Circulation 2014;129:2388-94.

2. Fihn SD, Blankenship JC, Alexander KP, et al. 2014 ACC/AHA/AATS/PCNA/SCAI/STS focused on update of the guideline for the diagnosis and management of patients with stable ischemic heart disease: a report of the American College of Cardiology/American Heart association Task Force on Practice Guidelines, and the American Association for Thoracic Surgery, Preventive Cardiovascular Nurses Association, Society for Cardiovascular Angiography and Interventions, and Society of Thoracic Surgeons. J Am Coll Cardiol 2014;64:1929-49.

3. Stone GW, Sabik JF, Serruys PW, et al. Everolimus-eluting stents or bypass surgery for left main coronary artery disease. N Engl J Med 2016;375:2223-35.

4. Steigen TK, Maeng M, Wiseth R, et al., Nordic PCI Study Group. Randomized study on simple versus complex stenting of coronary artery bifurcation lesions: the Nordic bifurcation study. Circulation 2006;114:1955-61.

5. Ferenc M, Gick M, Kienzle RP, et al. Randomized trial on routine vs. provisional T-stenting in the treatment of de novo coronary bifurcation lesions. Eur Heart J 2008;29:2859-67.

6. Chen SL, Santoso T, Zhang JJ, et al. A randomized clinical study comparing double kissing crush with provisional stenting for treatment of coronary bifurcation lesions: results from the DKCRUSH-II (Double Kissing Crush versus Provisional Stenting Technique for Treatment of Coronary Bifurcation Lesions) trial. J Am Coll Cardiol 2011;57:914-20.

Coronary Artery Calcium - Look Beyond the Agatston Score!

Akshay Mehta

Since a few decades, presence and extent of coronary artery calcium (CAC) has been found to be associated with the overall burden of coronary atherosclerosis.

CAC has been traditionally quantified by using Agatston method which uses multiplication of calcified plaque density and area (volume) giving a value called CAC score. Graded increase in the risk of cardiovascular events are seen with increasing CAC score which also provides significant improvement over traditional cardiovascular risk scores in risk discrimination and reclassification.

A couple of recent studies on CAC have revealed features of CAC besides simple scoring which can significantly improve CV risk prediction.

In one of these studies, Ferencik et al explore CAC regional distribution as an additional prognostic feature related to CAC. From amongst participants drawn from the offspring and the third-generation cohorts of the community-based Framingham Heart Study, measures of CAC distribution (number of coronary arteries with CAC and the presence of CAC in the proximal dominant coronary artery) were found to be associated with major coronary heart disease events. The association persisted after adjustment for traditional measure of CAC extent by Agatston score and cardiovascular risk factors.

The results suggest that simple measures of CAC distribution-number of coronary arteries with CAC and the presence of CAC in the proximal dominant coronary artery-may serve as an additional marker of risk for coronary heart disease events in people with CAC.

Hence not only should future studies evaluate these simple measures of regional CAC distribution, but that these measures of CAC distribution should also be considered for routine reporting in addition to the traditional Agatston score.

The second study was an analysis of MESA (Multi-Ethnic Study of Atherosclerosis), in which CAC volume was positively and CAC density inversely associated with cardiovascular disease (CVD) events.

In a recent extension of this study, Michael H. Criqui et al report that during a median 11.0 years of follow-up, with each SD increase of CAC volume (1.62), risk of CHD increased 73% ($p < 0.001$) and risk of CVD increased 61% ($p < 0.001$). Conversely, each SD increase of CAC density (0.69) was associated with 28% lower risk of CHD ($p < 0.001$) and 25% lower risk of CVD ($p < 0.001$). The inverse association of CAC density with incident CHD and CVD events was consistent across all levels of CAC volume, and across multiple strata of other risk variables.

Thus, the CAC volume score significantly improved prediction compared with the Agatston score, and the addition of CAC density to CAC volume further significantly improved the prediction of CVD events. Compared with assessment by clinical risk factors alone, the magnitude of net reclassification improvement for CVD events was 25.4% for the Agatston CAC score, 27.2% for the CAC volume score, and 34.5% for the model combining CAC volume and density score. This suggests that measurement of CAC volume and CAC density provides improved CVD risk prediction and future research should integrate density into CAC scoring and identify clinical situations where such advanced risk stratification might be most useful.

So looking for features of CAC beyond the Agatston score may be useful for better risk prediction. The important additional parameters found by the above 2 studies are :

1. Number of coronary arteries with CAC

2. Presence of CAC in the proximal dominant coronary artery

3. Volume of calcium and

4. Density of calcium

While the first three show a positive correlation with events, the last one shows an inverse correlation.

▌ Suggested Readings

1. Maros Ferencik, Karol M. Pencina, Ting Liu, Khristine Ghemigian, Kristin Baltrusaitis, Joseph M. Massaro, Ralph B. D'Agostino, Christopher J. O'Donnell, Udo Hoffmann.

   Coronary Artery Calcium Distribution Is an Independent Predictor of Incident Major Coronary Heart Disease Events. Results From the Framingham Heart Study.

   Circulation: Cardiovascular Imaging. 2017;10:e006592, Originally published September 27, 2017.

2. Michael H. Criqui, Jessica B. Knox, Julie O. Denenberg, Nketi I. Forbang, Robyn L. McClelland, Thomas E. Novotny, VeitSandfort, Jill Waalen, Michael J. Blaha and Matthew A. Allison.

   Coronary Artery Calcium Volume and Density.Potential Interactions and Overall Predictive Value: The Multi-Ethnic Study of Atherosclerosis.

   JACC: Cardiovascular ImagingVolume 10, Issue 8, August 2017.

3. Agatston AS, Janowitz WR, Hildner FJ, Zusmer NR, Viamonte M Jr., Detrano R. Quantification of coronary artery calcium using ultrafast computed tomography. J Am CollCardiol. 1990;15:827-832.

87

Valvular Heart Disease Patients on Edoxaban or Warfarin in the ENGAGE AF-TIMI 48 Trial

Dev Pahlajani

Bioresorbable stents were developed to improve outcomes in patients who undergo percutaneous coronary intervention (PCI). Metallic drug eluting stents (DES) though, reduce the risk of restenosis, there have been concerns about the loss of vasomotor tone and endothelial dysfunction after their deployment. Further, there is need for dual antiplatelet therapy (DAPT) for 6 to 12 months to reduce the risk of stent thrombosis. It was expected that bioresorbable stents will overcome some of the short comings of metallic DES. Early observations showed that the vasomotor tone and the endothelial function will be restored after the stent is completely absorbed. ABSORB from Abbot was the first absorbable stent to have been developed. Its earlier results were very promising and various trials showed it's noninferiority to the metallic Xience stent to which it was compared. It was also assumed that with the absence of metal in the arteries, the incidence of late and very late stent thrombosis and need for prolonged DAPT will be considerably reduced.

However, the current data presented at the TCT 2016 and the 3 years data published in Lancet last year from ABSORB II has proved to be disappointing. Target vessel myocardial infarction (MI) occurred in 7% of ABSORB patients as opposed to 1% in the Xience treated patients (p=0.006). What was more disturbing was the observation that there was two fold increase in stent thrombosis in the ABSORB versus Xience treated patients. About one-third of patients were on DAPT for 3 years. ABSORB was a prospective randomized multicenter study in which 501 patients were randomized to 2:1 treatment with ABSORB bioresorbable stent or Xience V metallic stent. There was no greater vasomotor responses in ABSORB treated patients as compared to those who received Xience stent. The late lumen loss was also greater in ABSORB patients than Xience patients (0.37 versus 0.25 mm). Still more disturbing was the fact that the clinical events of composite of cardiac death, target vessel MI and clinically indicated TLR occurred in twice the number of patients in ABSORB arm as compared to Xience arm.

In a recent data on the vasomotor response to nitroglycerine over 5 years follow up in ABSORB treated patients published in Journal of American College of Cardiology Cardiovascular Interventions, there was no statistically significant increase of vasomotor response to nitroglycerine after implantation of ABSORB stent. There was no increase in the mean luminal diameter response. However, ABSORB China which included 480 subjects at 24 sites there was no difference in the device oriented clinical events between the two stents.

Some workers and Abbott company has attributed the adverse events to the technique of deployment of ABSORB and patient selection with substantial number of "off lable" indications.

They advise that the patients coronary arteries be prepared, sized and to post dilate the stent. However, the faulty deployment technique cannot explain the late and very late stent thrombosis. At best it could explain acute and sub-acute thrombosis.

Currently Abbott is contemplating to withdraw the ABSORB from the Indian market on account of price. In Europe the device use is restricted to certain selection centers to monitor and report any adverse events.

What does this mean for ABSORB? Maybe ABSORB is meant for selected group of patients and not meant for off-label use. Maybe it has been over used in long, calcified, tortuous, small caliber vessels. At the same time one must not forget the fact that the strut thickness of ABSORB is 150 microns with rectangular design. Moreover the polymer is not able to sustain high pressure leading to some amount of malapposition. DAPT needs to be continued for at least 1 year. Very important is to use added imaging techniques like IVUS and OCT liberally to ensure optimum results. Until newer bioresorbable magnesium stents come to the market and results from the European centers become available it is necessary that the stent be deployed in the appropriately selected patients with properly advised technique.

▌ Suggested Readings

1. Brugaletta S, Heo JH, Garcia-Garcia HM, et al. Endothelial-dependent vasomotion in a coronary segment treated by ABSORB everolimus-eluting bioresorbable vascular scaffold system is related to plaque composition at the time of bioresorption of the polymer: indirect finding of vascular reparative therapy? Eur Heart J 2012; 33:1325-33.

2. Sarno G, Bruining N, Onuma Y, et al. Morphological and functional evaluation of the bioresorption of the bioresorbable everolimus-eluting vascular scaffold using IVUS, echogenicity and vasomotion testing at two year follow-up: a patient level insight into the ABSORB A clinical trial. Int J Cardiovasc Imaging 2012;28:51-8.

3. Serruys PW, Chevalier B, Sotomi Y, et al. Comparison of an everolimus-eluting bioresorbable scaffold with an everolimus-eluting metallic stent for the treatment of coronary artery stenosis (ABSORB II): a 3 year, randomised, controlled, single-blind, multicentre clinical trial. Lancet 2016;388:2479-91.

4. Ormiston JA, Serruys PW, Onuma Y, et al. First serial assessment at 6 months and 2 years of the second generation of absorb everolimus-eluting bioresorbable vascular scaffold: a multi-imaging modality study. Circ Cardiovasc Interv 2012;5:620-32.

5. Shin DI, Kim PJ, Seung KB, et al. Drug-eluting stent implantation could be associated with longterm coronary endothelial dysfunction. Int Heart J 2007;48:553-67.

6. Hofma SH, van der Giessen WJ, van Dalen BM, et al. Indication of long-term endothelial dysfunction after sirolimus-eluting stent implantation. Eur Heart J 2006;27:166-70.

7. Sabate M, Kay P, van der Giessen WJ, et al. Functional assessment of coronary arteries previously treated with angioplasty and intracoronary radiation. Circulation 1999;100:1623-9.

8. Serruys PW, Ormiston JA, Onuma Y, et al. A bioabsorbable everolimus-eluting coronary stent system (ABSORB): 2-year outcomes and results from multiple imaging methods. Lancet 2009;373:897.

9. Serruys PW, Onuma Y, Dudek D, et al. Evaluation of the second generation of a bioresorbable everolimus-eluting vascular scaffold for the treatment of de novo coronary artery stenosis 12-month clinical and imaging outcomes. J Am Coll Cardiol 2011;58:1578-88.

10. Onuma Y, Serruys PW, Perkins L, et al. Intracoronary Optical coherence tomography and histology at 1 month and 2, 3, and 4 years after implantation of everolimus-eluting bioresorbable vascular scaffolds in a porcine coronary artery model: an attempt to decipher the human optical coherence tomography images in the ABSORB trial. Circulation 2010;122:2288-300.

11. Otsuka F, Pacheco E, Perkins LE, et al. Long-term safety of an everolimus-eluting bioresorbable vascular scaffold and the cobalt chromium XIENCE V stent in a porcine coronary artery model. Circ Cardiovasc Interv 2014;7: 330.

12. Dariusz Dudek, MD, PHD, ukasz Rzeszutko, MD, PHD, Yoshinobu Onuma, MD, PHD, Yohei Sotomi, MD, Rafa Depukat, Susan Veldhof, RN, Divine Ediebah, MS, Peter Staehr, MD, WojciechZasada, MD, PHD, Krzysztof P. Malinowski, MS,Grzegorz L. Kaluza, MD, PHD, Patrick W. Serruys, MD, PHD. Vasomotor Response to Nitroglycerine Over 5 Years Follow-Up After Everolimus-Eluting Bioresorbable Scaffold Implantation. : JACC INTERVENTIONS 2017; 10(8): 786-795.

13. Gao R, Yang Y, Han Y, Huo Y, Chen J, Yu B, Su X, Li L, Kuo HC, Ying SW, Cheong WF, Zhang Y, Su X, Xu B, Popma JJ, Stone GW; ABSORB China Investigators. Bioresorbable Vascular Scaffolds Versus Metallic Stents in Patients With Coronary Artery Disease: ABSORB China Trial. J Am Coll Cardiol. 2015 Dec 1;66(21):2298-309.

88

Brain-Heart Connection: The Psychoneuro immunology of ACS

Akshay Mehta

From the description of Type A personality by cardiologists Meyer Friedman and Ray Rosenman in the 1950s and its ensuing criticisms and modifications, to the INTERHEART study, psychosocial factors and emotional stress have been ascribed an important role as risk factors for coronary heart disease and its outcomes.

Individuals with increased stress perception have a substantially higher prevalence of myocardial infarction than controls, as was reported by Rosengren and colleagues in 2004.

Young and middle-aged women who are recovering from acute MI have higher levels of perceived stress than men, which is associated with worse recovery, according to the results of a study by Xu X et al.(1)

The problem with emotional stress as a risk factor for coronary heart disease is that

1. It cannot be quantitated like smoking and blood pressure,
2. Nor its direct effects be separated from its effect through altered life style, like eating and physical activity behaviors.

However, a recent study in two parts (2) throw light on the direct effects of stress in the brain affecting cardiovascular outcomes.

One showed that increased resting metabolic activity in the amygdala independently and robustly predicted CVD events. Researchers at Massachusetts General Hospital in Boston, MA, in a longitudinal study of 293 patients who were injected with 18F fluorodeoxy glucose (18F-FDG) and had full-body PET/CT scans, showed simultaneous activity in the bone marrow and arterial wall with amygdalar activity which correlated with increased risk of stroke, MI, or angina during follow-up.

More specifically, the patients had a 1.6-fold increased risk of a CVD event for each one standard deviation in amygdalar signal (hazard ratio 1.59, 95% CI 1.27-1.98; $P<0.001$) after multivariable adjustment. It supported the hypothesized path of increased amygdalar activity leading to increased bone-marrow activity, leading to increased arterial inflammation, leading to cardiovascular disease events.

The second study of 13 patients with posttraumatic stress disorder (PTSD) who had 18F-FDG PET scans and who replied to a 10-item Perceived Stress Scale (PSS-10) questionnaire, showed that high levels of perceived stress correlated with increased amygdalar activity, arterial inflammation, and C-reactive protein.

Thus the studies show the downstream mechanisms linking emotional stressors to arterial inflammation the psycho-neural-hemopoietic-arterial axis.

Over the past 25 years, the science of what is now called "psychoneuroimmunology" has proven that prolonged stress and traumatic experiences change the biochemistry of our brain, our hormones and the cells and processes, including cytokines, that fuel chronic inflammation - a risk factor for cardiovascular disease and cancer. Persistent negative emotions of isolation, anxiety, depression or hostility have been shown to be the cause of immune system suppression that can lead to illness.

The silver lining is that positive emotions can bolster both immune and endocrine system responses. This was seen a study in 151 patients which showed that adding stress management to cardiac rehabilitation lowered the risk of 5-year CV-related events by 50%.(3)

Thus the messages are that

1. Patients with ACS could be routinely screened for perceived stress using the PSS-10 questionnaire, and

2. When [stress is] found, to consider advising patient to pay attention to stress and consider them for some stress-reduction management which can substantially improve their outcomes.

▌ Suggested Readings

1. Xu X, Bao H, Strait K, et al. Sex differences in perceived stress and early recovery in young and middle-aged patients with acute myocardial infarction. Circulation 2015; DOI:10.1161/circulation aha.114.012826.

2. Tawakol A, Ishai A, Takx RAP, et al. Relation between resting amygdalar activity and cardiovascular events: a longitudinal and cohort study. Lancet 2017; DOI:10.1016/S0140- 6736(16)31714-7.

3. Blumenthal JA, Sherwood A, Smith PJ, et al. Enhancing cardiac rehabilitation with stress management training: A randomized, clinical efficacy trial. Circulation 2016; 13:1341-1350.

89

LDL Controversy Put to Rest

Dev Pahlajani

Over the past few years there has been rising concerns about the definite role of cholesterol and particularly that of LDL in the causation of atherosclerotic cardiovascular disease (ASCVD). Some of the articles in the scientific journals and lay press have questioned the scientifically well documented cause and effect role of LDL. Some labele cholesterol as the greatest hoax of the century. LDL has been considered more as a marker of atherosclerosis rather than the causal factor.

However, recently a very well researched document based on the evidence gathered over the last few decades has been published in the April issue of European Heart Journal by the European Atherosclerosis Society Consensus Panel. The panel looked at the exhaustive scientific literature available till date. Several meta-analysis of over 200 prospective core studies, Mendelian randomization studies which included more than 200 million participants with over 20 million person years follow up. The consensus panel closely looked at the data of over 150000 cardiovascular events that studied whether the LDL cholesterol was associated and was indeed a causative factor for ASCVD. The consensus document looked at various aspects LDL and its relationship to ASCVD:

1. *Pathology of atherosclerosis:* Several studies have indicated that the ASCVD is initiated by the retention and accumulation of cholesterol apoB lipoprotein within the arterial intima. These lead to formation of a plaque. The progression of a plaque increases in a dose dependent manner with that of LDL.

2. *Cholesterol LDL and LDL-C:* The consensus document has highlighted the fact that in clinical practice plasma LDL is not measured directly but instead it is measured indirectly using Friedwald equation (LDL Cholesterole = Total Cholesterol-HDL Cholesterole-Triglycerides 5). Though in most of the conditions LDL-C and LDL particle numbers correlate and LDL-C is a good surrogate for LDL concentration. However in conditions like metabolic syndrome, diabetes and hyperglyceridemia LDL-C and LDL concentrate can become discordant. Friedwald equation is invalid in samples collected in non fasting state and in presence of increased triglycerides levels.

3. *Evidence of inherited disorders of lipid metabolism like familial hypercholesterolemia:* These genetic disorders are a result of genetic mutation in the LDL receptor and the affected individuals have a dose dependent increased risk of ASCVD over life time as compared to unaffected siblings. These could be considered as strong evidence that LDL indeed causes ASCVD.

4. *Evidence from prospective epidemiological studies:* These studies which included more than 300000 persons indicated that the plasma LDL cholesterol concentration was linearly associated with increased risk of non-fatal myocardial infarction (MI) or coronary heart disease death.

5. *Evidence from Mendelian randomization studies:* These studies have consistently shown that variants of over 50 genes that are associated with lower LDL-C are correspondingly associated with lower risk of coronary heart disease. Several meta-analysis of Mendelian randomization studies which included more than 300,000 participants and 80,000 coronary heart disease cases provide that LDL is an incriminating factor for development of ASCVD.

6. *Evidence from randomized control trials:* Several studies have shown that reducing LDL cholesterol decreases the risk of cardiovascular events. In several meta-analysis which included 170,000 individuals involving 26 statin trials showed that there was linear reduction by 20-22% in the risk of major cardiac vascular events per millimol/Litre reduction in LDL-C over median of 5 years treatment.

It is also known that the development of atherosclerotic ASCVD is not only dose-dependent of LDL-C but also time-dependent. Longer the exposure to higher LDL levels greater is the likelihood of developing ASCVD.

So what does this exhaustive consensus document by European Atherosclerosis Society suggest?

1. LDL definitely has a strong causal relationship to developing ASCVD.

2. The disease development is dose and time-dependent to LDL.

3. Lowering of cholesterol reduces the risk of ASCVD.

4. The document should open up the avenues for the development of new cholesterol lowering agents like PCSK 9 inhibitors, a drug which has already proved its' efficacy in the treatment particularly of familial hyercholestrolemia.

■ **Suggested Readings**

1. Brian A. Ference1 *, Henry N. Ginsberg2 , Ian Graham3 , Kausik K. Ray4, Chris J. Packard5, Eric Bruckert6, Robert A. Hegele7, Ronald M. Krauss8 , Frederick J. Raal9 , Heribert Schunkert10,11, Gerald F. Watts12, Jan Bore'n13, Sergio Fazio14, Jay D. Horton15,16, Luis Masana17, Stephen J. Nicholls18, Børge G. Nordestgaard19, 20,21, Bart van de Sluis22, Marja-Riitta Taskinen23, LaleTokgo¨ zoglu 24, Ulf Landmesser25,26, Ulrich Laufs27, Olov Wiklund28,29, Jane K. Stock30, M. John Chapman31†, and Alberico L. Catapano :European Heart Journal (2017)0:1-14.

2. Goldstein JL, Brown MS. A century of cholesterol and coronaries: from plaques to genes to statins. Cell 2015;161:161-172.

3. Ravnskov U, Diamond DM, Hama R, Hamazaki T, Hammarskjo¨ld B, Hynes N, Kendrick M, Langsjoen PH, Malhotra A, Mascitelli L, McCully KS, Ogushi Y, Okuyama H, Rosch PJ, Schersten T, Sultan S, Sundberg R. Lack of an association or an inverse association between low-density-lipoprotein cholesterol and mortality in the elderly: a systematic review. BMJ Open 2016;6:e010401.

4. Nordestgaard BG, Chapman MJ, Humphries SE, Ginsberg HN, Masana L, Descamps OS, Wiklund Hegele RA, Raal FJ, Defesche JC, Wiegman A, Santos RD, Watts GF, Parhofer KG, Hovingh GK, Kovanen PT, Boileau C, Averna M, Bore'n J, Bruckert E, Catapano AL, Kuivenhoven JA, Pajukanta P, Ray K, Stalenhoef AF, Stroes E, Taskinen MR, Tybjærg-Hansen A; European Atherosclerosis Society Consensus Panel. Familial hypercholesterolaemia is underdiagnosed and undertreated in the general population: guidance for clinicians to prevent coronary heart disease. Consensus Statement of the European Atherosclerosis Society. Eur Heart J 2013;34:3478-3490.

5. Ference BA, Yoo W, Alesh I, Mahajan N, Mirowska KK, Mewada A, Kahn J, Afonso L, Williams KA Sr, Flack JM. Effect of long-term exposure to lower low-density lipoprotein cholesterol beginning early in life on the risk of coronary heart disease: a Mendelian randomization analysis. J Am Coll Cardiol 2012;60:2631-2639.

6. Linsel-Nitschke P, Go"tz A, Erdmann J, Braenne I, Braund P, Hengstenberg C, Stark K, Fischer M, Schreiber S, El Mokhtari NE, Schaefer A, Schrezenmeier J, Rubin D, Hinney A, Reinehr T, Roth C, Ortlepp J, Hanrath P, Hall AS, Mangino M, Lieb W, Lamina C, Heid IM, Doering A, Gieger C, Peters A, Meitinger T, Wichmann HE, Ko"nig IR, Ziegler A, Kronenberg F, Samani NJ, Schunkert H. Lifelong reduction of LDL-cholesterol related to a common variant in the LDLreceptor gene decreases the risk of coronary artery disease: a MendelianRandomisation study. PLoS One 2008;3:e2986.

7. Nissen SE, Nicholls SJ, Sipahi I, Libby P, Raichlen JS, Ballantyne CM, Davignon J, Erbel R, Fruchart JC, Tardif JC, Schoenhagen P, Crowe T, Cain V, Wolski K, Goormastic M, Tuzcu EM. ASTEROID Investigators. Effect of very high-intensity statin therapy on regression of coronary atherosclerosis: the ASTEROID trial. JAMA 2006;295:1556-1565.

8. Cannon CP, Blazing MA, Giugliano RP, McCagg A, White JA, Theroux P, Darius H, Lewis BS, Ophuis TO, Jukema JW, De Ferrari GM, Ruzyllo W, De Lucca P, Im K, Bohula EA, Reist C, Wiviott SD, Tershakovec AM, Musliner TA, Braunwald E, Califf RM. IMPROVE-IT Investigators. Ezetimibe added to statin therapy after acute coronary syndromes. N Engl J Med 2015;372:2387-2397.

9. Nicholls SJ, Puri R, Anderson T, Ballantyne CM, Cho L, Kastelein JJ, Koenig W, Somaratne R, Kassahun H, Yang J, Wasserman SM, Scott R, Ungi I, Podolec J, Ophuis AO, Cornel JH, Borgman M, Brennan DM, Nissen SE. Effect of evolocumab on progression of coronary disease in statin-treated patients. The GLAGOV randomized clinical trial. JAMA 2016;316:2373-2384.

90

What is the Best Percutaneous Treatment for In-Stent Restenosis (ISR) of Drug Eluting Stents (DES)?

Akshay Mehta

Although drug-eluting stents (DES) are widely used because of their unique ability to inhibit neointimal proliferation and reduce the restenosis risk, in-stent restenosis (ISR) still occurs after their implantation. Several studies suggest that treatment of DES-ISR is more challenging than treatment of bare-metal stent (BMS) ISR.

This could be because ISR after DES may be due to a more complex pathology, greater drug resistance and hence prone to recurrences. Also neoatherosclerosis, which seems to be more prevalent in patients with DES-ISR may account for these unfavorable findings.

▮ Definition:

ISR is classically defined as recurrent diameter stenosis > 50% at the stent segment or its edges (5-mm segments adjacent to the stent). On angiography, the Mehran system permits a morphological classification of BMS-ISR lesions (pattern I, focal; pattern II, diffuse; pattern III, proliferative; and pattern IV, occlusion).

The underlying cause of ISR may be mechanical (under expansion, which may be due to stent under deployment as a result of under sizing or due to the use of low deployment pressures, or stent misplacement or stents not fully covering the underlying lesion or stent fractures). Repeat stent implantation is frequently advocated in the setting of stent fracture. Drug resistance or local hypersensitivity reactions have also been associated with DES failure.

▮ Methods of treatment:

Various methods of treating DES ISR have been tried. These are: Conventional balloon angioplasty,cutting and scoring balloon therapy debulking techniques, vascular brachytherapy, repeat stenting with BMS or DES and drug coated balloon (DCB) angioplasty.

Siontis GC, Stefanini GG, Mavridis D, et al. (1) performed a network meta-analysis of 27 trials that enrolled 5,923 patients, with angiographic follow-up 6-12 months after the index intervention in 84% of patients. Percutaneous coronary intervention with everolimus-eluting stents (EES) was the most effective treatment for percent diameter stenosis, difference -9.0% versus drug-coated balloons (DCB), -9.4% versus sirolimus-eluting stents, -10.2% versus paclitaxel-eluting stents, -19.2%, versus vascular brachytherapy, -23.4% versus bare-metal stents, -24.2% versus balloon angioplasty, and -31.8% versus rotablation. DCB were ranked as the second most effective treatment, but without significant differences from sirolimus-eluting or paclitaxel-eluting stents. Thus, The authors concluded that EES is the most effective treatment for ISR.

Currently, the use of both DES and DEB are supported by the same evidence (class I, level A) in patients with BMS-ISR and DES-ISR. The RIBS IV and V studies, however, suggest a potential additional benefit of EES, a new-generation DES, in these patients.

The RIBS V (Restenosis Intra-Stent of Bare Metal Stents: Paclitaxel-Eluting Balloon vs Everolimus-Eluting Stent) trial demonstrated that in patients with BMS-ISR, everolimus-eluting stents (EES) provided superior late angiographic findings compared with DEB.(2)

Likewise, the RIBS IV (Restenosis Intra-Stent of Drug-Eluting Stents: Paclitaxel-Eluting Balloon vs Everolimus-Eluting Stent) trial demonstrated that in patients with DES-ISR, EES obtain not only better long-term angiographic results but also superior 1-year clinical outcomes compared with DEB.(3) Accordingly, the use of EES emerges as a attractive therapeutic strategy for patients presenting with ISR.

▌ What about BVS in DES ISR?

The recent RIBS VI (4) trial showed that the acute and late angiographic findings of BVS appear to be similar to those obtained with DEB but poorer than those seen after EES implantation. However, caution is required in its interpretation as historical controls from prior RCT's were used for comparison.

▌ What about laser atherectomy?

ISR typically is basically due to intimal ingrowth within a fully expanded stent, and hence angioplasty alone will have limited value due to the "rubber band effect" that is, we acutely dehydrate the intimal hyperplasia [when treating it with PTA alone], but after time it rehydrates, and the lesion is back. So, it is important in some way, to remove some of that tissue. That is the principle behind photoablation, which actually removes the offending material and would result in better outcomes.

Although no randomized studies are available for coronaries, initial Results From the EXCITE ISR Trial (EXCImer Laser Randomized Controlled Study for Treatment of FemoropopliTEal In-Stent Restenosis) (5), the first large, prospective, randomized study to demonstrate superiority of ELA + PTA versus PTA alone for treating femoropopliteal ISR, showed that over all, ELA + PTA reduced the occurrence of TLR by over 50% compared with PTA alone, over a period of 12 months.

▌ What about combination therapy with laser atherectomy and DCB?

DCB has the advantage of not leaving another stent behind and at the same time eluting drug for a short time. Whether in femoral artery or in coronaries, its effect is much better than plain balloons and equivalent to another DES (except EES).

Since recoil is not the main cause of DES ISR, another stent within a stent does not seem mechanisticially a logical answer to DES ISR. Combining the advantages of laser atherectomy, which removes tissue ingrowth, with DCB which prevents regrowth, may be the answer to DES ISR. Only future will tell whether this logic will work.

Suggested Readings

1. Siontis GC, Stefanini GG, Mavridis D, et al. percutaneous coronary interventional strategies for treatment of in-stent restenosis: A network meta-analysis. Lancet 2015; 386:655-664.

2. RIBS V Study Investigators, under the auspices of the working group on interventional cardiology of the Spanish society of cardiology. Alfonso F, Pérez-Vizcayno MJ, Cárdenas A, García Del Blanco B, Seidelberger B, Iñiguez A, Gómez-Recio M, Masotti M, Velázquez MT, Sanchís J, García-Touchard A, Zueco J, Bethencourt A, Melgares R, Cequier A, Dominguez A, Mainar V, López-Mínguez JR, Moreu J, Martí V, Moreno R, Jiménez-Quevedo P, Gonzalo N, Fernández C, Macaya C; A randomized comparison of drug-eluting balloon versus everolimus-eluting stent in patients with bare-metal stent in-stent restenosis: the RIBS V Clinical Trial (Restenosis Intra-Stent of Bare Metal Stents: Paclitaxel-Eluting Balloon vs Everolimus-Eluting Stent). J Am Coll Cardiol. 2014;63:1378-1386. doi: 10.1016/j. jacc.2013.12.006.

3. RIBS IV study investigators (under auspices of interventional cardiology working group of spanish society of cardiology) Alfonso F, Pérez-Vizcayno MJ, Cárdenas A, García del Blanco B, García-Touchard A, López-Minguéz JR, Benedicto A, Masotti M, Zueco J, Iñiguez A, Velázquez M, Moreno R, Mainar V, Domínguez A, Pomar F, Melgares R, Rivero F, Jiménez-Quevedo P, Gonzalo N, Fernández C, Macaya C; A prospective randomized trial of drug-eluting balloons versus everolimus-eluting stents in patients with in-stent restenosis of drug-eluting stents: the RIBS IV randomized clinical trial. J Am Coll Cardiol. 2015;66:23-33. doi: 10.1016/j.jacc.2015.04.063.

4. RIBS VI : Fernando Alfonso MD, PhD, FESC Hospital Universitario "La Princesa" Madrid. Spain. On behalf of the RIBS VI investigators. A prospective, multicenter, registry of Bioresorbable vascular Scaffolds in patients with coronary artery bare-metal or drug-eluting in-stent restenosis TCT 2016.

5. Eric J. Dippel, Prakash Makam, Richard Kovach, Jon C. George, Raghotham Patlola, D. Christopher Metzger, Carlos Mena-Hurtado, Robert Beasley, Peter Soukas, Pedro J. Colon-Hernandez, Matthew A. Stark, Craig Walker, EXCITE ISR investigators. Randomized controlled study of excimer laser atherectomy for treatment of femoropopliteal in-stent restenosis. Initial results from the excite ISR trial (Excimer laser randomized controlled study for treatment of femoropopliteal in-stent restenosis). JACC: Cardiovascular interventions. Volume 8, Issue 1 Part A, January 2015 > DOI: 10.1016/j.jcin.2014.09.009.

91

Revascularisation in Multivessel Disease with Diabetes-2017: Advantage Coronary Artery Bypass Surgery?

Dev Pahlajani

More than 25% patients with coronary artery disease (CAD) have diabetes and about 75% diabetics succumb to death due to cardiovascular event. Choice and optimum treatment of CAD particularly multi vessel disease (MVD) with diabetes has been a subject of various randomized controlled trials and registries and attracted several debates during various national and international scientific conferences. Large scale data regarding the benefit and outcomes of medical versus percutaneous coronary intervention (PCI) versus coronary artery bypass graft surgery (CABGS) is available that has formed a ground work for current guidelines.

▌ Pathophysiology of diabetes and atherosclerotic coronary artery disease:

Diabetic patients usually have MVD which is diffuse in nature. Coronary arteries more often than not are of smaller diameter as compared to the non-diabetics. The disease also involves smaller arteries and several diabetics have micro vessel disease and associated cardiomyopathy. Thus the results of PCI and CABGS in diabetics are associated with unfavorable outcomes as compared to non-diabetics. CAD and diabetes are linked to altered inflammatory pathways with insulin resistance and defective free fatty acid metabolism. Both of them have endothelial dysfunction. There is an increased thrombogenicity and altered smooth muscle cell migration. Plaque burden in patients with diabetes and MVD is larger than in non diabetics. There is an increased platelet activity and decreased nitric oxide production. In diabetes there is an increased production of pro inflammatory cytokines and there is altered monocyte and leucocyte binding on the platelets and increased platelet reactivity that predisposes diabetes to thrombosis (1,2). All these factors combined predispose diabetic with CAD to new adverse cardiac events following revascularization procedure - be it CABG or PCI. Diabetics are prone to develop restenosis, stent thrombosis and increased risk of death following PCI.

With such unfavorable pathology it can be anticipated that revascularization procedure would be achieved with sub optimal results.

▌ Revascularization in diabetics and MVD:

Several large scale randomized control trials have been undertaken in last 30 years to assess the efficacy and safety of CABG versus PCI. One of the earliest trial, BARI compared the results of PTCA versus CABG in patients with CAD. The trial enrolled 1829 patients and randomized them to PTCA versus CABGS. The initial results of trial reported that patients with diabetes who underwent PTCA had increased risk of death, myocardial infarction (MI) and target vessel revascularization (TVR) than those treated with CABGS(3). Ten years follow up data has further strengthened the initial results of the trial (4). However, the trial has attracted criticism since majority of PCI procedures were performed with balloon angioplasty.

Arterial Revascularization Therapy Study-1 (ARTS I) trial compared the outcomes of PCI with bare metal stent (BMS) versus CABGS in patients with CAD and diabetes. Results of trial also demonstrated superiority of CABGS over PCI in diabetics even after stent deployment. Subsequently ARTS I and II reported the safety and efficacy of PCI with sirolimus eluting stent (SES) versus CABGS in patients with and without DM. This was a historical comparison and showed the superiority of SES over BMS. In ARTS I and II studies, 367 diabetic patients were included. Five year follow up showed that the major adverse cardiac and cerebrovascular events (MACCE) were higher in the BMS treated patients versus SES treated patients. However, the rate of TVR was significantly higher in the SES treated patients as compared to those subjected to CABGS (SES 32.2% versus CABG 10.7%) (p=<0.001). In both these trials CABGS was associated with decreased rate of TVR as compared to PCI treated patients (5).

CARDia trial enrolled 510 patients with complex CAD or MVD with diabetes. Out of these 71% patients in PCI treated group received SES and 29% received BMS. The trial was anon inferiority trial. The primary end point of death was 14% for PCI and 12.6% for CABG. However, non fatal MI and repeat revascularization were significantly higher for PCI group as compared to CABG at 5 years (6).

Subsequently a large scale FREEDOM trial was conducted (7). The trial was a prospective randomized multicenter trial. It was a superiority trial that compared PCI to CABGS patients on optimum medical therapy. The trial enrolled 1900 patients at 140 international centers to ascertain whether aggressive medical therapy and the use of DES could alter the revascularization approach for patients with diabetes and CAD.

The primary outcome was composite of death, non-fatal MI from any cause and non-fatal stroke. The primary outcome occurred in 26.6% in PCI group and 18.7% in CABGS group. The CABGS benefit was mainly driven by difference in death and MI and death from any cause. Incidence of stroke was higher in CABGS group at 5 years. CABGS proved to be superior to PCI by reduction of all cause mortality, non fatal MI.

SYNTAX trial has been one of the landmark trial that enrolled 1800 patients to see if PCI performed with paclitaxel coated stent was not inferior to CABGS (8). Amongst the patients enrolled in the study 30% had diabetes. At the end of 5 years the overall rates were lower with the CABG patients (27%) than PCI treated patients (37%) (p=<0.01). While all cause mortality did not differ significantly between the two groups the rates of MI and repeat revascularization were higher with PCI than CABG (9.7% versus 3.8% and 26% versus 14%) respectively. The advantage of CABG was mainly driven by patients with higher SYNTAX score of greater than 33 and anatomical complexity. Patients with low and intermediate SYNTAX score of < 33 fared equally well when compared with CABGS. In the patients with high SYNTAX score CABGS had distinct advantage over PCI with overall event rate of 27% in CABG arm versus 44% in the PCI arm. In the subgroup analysis of 452 medically treated diabetics patients treated with paclitaxel coated stent had higher 1 year major adverse cardiac and cerebrovascular events as compared those who underwent CABGS. The higher event rate was mainly driven by increased repeat revascularization rate (6.4%vs20.3%). Diabetics with higher SYNTAX score and highly complex lesions had higher mortality with PCI as compared to CABGS (4.1% vs 13.5%).

All these earlier trials involved patients who underwent PCI with balloon angioplasty or BMS or first generation DES. Also current antiplatelet therapy consists of more potent P2Y12 inhibitors as compared to the earlier ones. One could expect that the results of PCI would be comparable to CABGS with new second generation stents and more potent antiplatelets (9,10,11).

A recent meta-analysis of 6 randomized control trials compared the results of CABGS to PCI in patients with insulin treated type 2 diabetes mellitus. Patients who underwent CABGS had lower major adverse cardiac events (MACE) as compared to PCI. CABGS was associated with a significantly lower mortality compared to PCI (OR 0.59 p=0.004). Repeat revascularization was significantly lower in the CABGS group (OR 0.34 p<0.00001). In another recently published review and meta-regression to assess the difference in mortality between PCI and CABGS in patients with CAD and diabetes, Peter Herbison analyzed the data from 14 studies involving 4686 diabetic patients reported over 3 decades. Meta regression showed no relationship between the year of publication and difference in long term all cause mortality between PCI and CABG. There was a persistent and continuous maintenance of reduced difference of mortality of 30% in favor of CABG as compared to PCI. The difference was not affected by the fact that whether the patients were treated by insulin or non insulin requiring diabetics.

Thus despite improvement in PCI technology CABGS continues to be a better choice for revascularization in MVD with diabetes. The advantage could be due to the generalized endothelial dysfunction, platelet reactivity, small vessel size, diffuse disease and associated comorbidities in diabetics. May be it will need better control of diabetes, treatment of endothelial dysfunction, preventing comorbidities that would help PCI to match the results of CABGS.

▌ Suggested Readings

1. Hartge MM, Unger T, Kintscher U. The endothelium and vascular inflammation in diabetes. Diabetes and Vascular Disease Research. 2007;4:84-88.

2. Vinik AI, Erbas T, Park TS, Nolan R, Pittenger GL. Platelet dysfunction in type 2 diabetes. Diabetes Care. 2001;24:1476-1485.

3. W.J. Rogers. W.A. Baxley, L.S. Dean, G.S. Roubin, J.K. Kirklin, J.W. Kirklin, A. Pacifico, G.L. Zorn, E. Charles, T.D. Paine, S. Brewer, L.C. Carr, G. Duke, L.E. Maske, T.E. Morgan, K. Doss, J.A. Trobaugh, K.W. Anderson, M. Brunner-Scott, D. Bunn, F. Harris. Former participants: T. Bulle, J.B. Cavender, P.J. Garrahy. Influence of diabetes on 5-year mortality and morbidity in a randomized trial comparing CABG and PTCA in patients with multivessel disease: the Bypass Angioplasty Revascularization Investigation (BARI). Circulation. 1997;96(6):1761-1769.

4. The final 10-year follow-up results from the BARI randomized trial. J Am CollCardiol. 2007;49: 1600-1606.

5. Onuma Y, Wykrzykowska JJ, Garg S, Vranckx P, Serruys PW, Arts I, Investigators II. 5-year follow-up of coronary revascularization in diabetic patients with multivessel coronary artery disease: Insights from ARTS (arterial revascularization therapy study)-II and ARTS-I trials. JACC: CardiovascInterv. 2011;4:317-323.

6. Kapur A, Hall RJ, Malik IS, et al. Randomized comparison of percutaneous coronary intervention with coronary artery bypass grafting in diabetic patients. 1-year results of the CARDia (Coronary Artery Revascularization in Diabetes) trial. J Am CollCardiol. 2010;55:432-40.

7. Farkouh ME, Domanski M, Sleeper LA, Siami FS, Dangas G, Mack M, Yang M, Cohen DJ, Rosenberg Y, Solomon SD, Desai AS, Gersh BJ, Magnuson EA, Lansky A, Boineau R, Weinberger J, Ramanathan K, Sousa JE, Rankin J, Bhargava B, Buse J, Hueb W, Smith CR, Muratov V, Bansilal S, King S 3rd, Bertrand M, Fuster V, FREEDOM Trial Investigators. Strategies for multivessel revascularization in patients with diabetes. N Engl J Med. 2012;367(25):2375-84.

8. Kappetein AP, Head SJ, Morice MC, Banning AP, Serruys PW, Mohr FW, Dawkins KD, Mack MJ. Treatment of complex coronary artery disease in patients with diabetes: 5-year results comparing outcomes of bypass surgery and percutaneous coronary intervention in the syntax trial. Eur J Cardiothorac Surg. 2013;43:1006-1013.

9. Stone GW, Kedhi E, Kereiakes DJ, et al. Differential clinical responses to everolimus-eluting and paclitaxel-eluting coronary stents in patients with and without diabetes mellitus. Circulation. 2011;124(8):893-900.

10. Kim WJ, Lee SW, Park SW, Kim YH, Yun SC, Lee JY, Park DW, Kang SJ, Lee CW, Lee JH, Choi SW, Seong IW, Lee BK, Lee NH, Cho YH, Shin WY, Lee SJ, Lee SW, Hyon MS, Bang DW, Park WJ, Kim HS, Chae JK, Lee K, Park HK, Park CB, Lee SG, Kim MK, Park KH, Choi YJ, Cheong SS, Yang TH, Jang JS, Her SH, Park SJ, Investigators E-DS. Randomized comparison of everolimus-eluting stent versus sirolimus-eluting stent implantation for de novo coronary artery disease in patients with diabetes mellitus (essence-diabetes): Results from the essence-diabetes trial. Circulation. 2011;124:886-892.

11. Park S-J, Ahn J-M, Kim Y-H, et al. Trial of everolimus-eluting stents or bypass surgery for coronary disease. N Eng J Med 2015;372:1204-12.

12. ParveshkumarBundhun, ZiJia Wu and Meng-Hua Chen. Coronary artery bypass surgery compared with percutaneous coronary interventions in patients with insulin-treated type 2 diabetes mellitus: a systematic review and meta-analysis of 6 randomized controlled trials. CardiovascDiabetol 2016:15:2.

13. Herbison P, Wong C-K. BMJ Open 2015;5:e010055.Has the difference in mortality between percutaneous coronary intervention and coronary artery bypass grafting in people with heart disease and diabetes changed over the years? A systematic review and meta-regression.

92

The Value of Vaccines for CVD Prevention

Akshay Mehta

Influenza is an important cause of deaths and hospitalizations, the world over. The risk of death and serious complications from influenza is especially high for persons with underlying CVD or diabetes (1) and cardiovascular-related death is the leading cause of mortality during influenza season, (2,3,4)

There is a peak of both influenza and cardiac deaths in winter (2,5) and evidence for the association between influenza infection and acute myocardial infarction (AMI). For example, observational studies have shown that recent influenza infection was about two times more likely in patients with myocardial infarction than those without (6). Patients with heart failure are also at a high risk for influenza-related complications (7) including hospitalizations, which occur more frequently during the winter months, often in conjunction with influenza infection (8).

▌ How does influenza increase CV risk ?

A severe upper respiratory infection can initiate a cascade of physiological events that ultimately lead to acute worsening or exacerbation of underlying heart disease. A number of mechanisms support a causal association between influenza infection and CV events.

Influenza infection can result in increased metabolic demand, adrenergic surge, endothelial dysfunction, hypercoagulability, and hypoxia. Systemic immune stimulation and inflammation in the setting of influenza infection can trigger acute plaque rupture. Influenza predisposes patients to develop other infections such as pneumonia, which may itself be associated with increased CV risk due to prolonged elevation in cytokine levels and a pro-coagulant state. Moreover, influenza is known to cause myocardial depression directly, possibly mediated through increases in pro-inflammatory cytokines, and histological evidence of myocardial injury, myocarditis, and myocyte necrosis has been demonstrated from patients following influenza-related deaths.

▌ Can vaccination reduce the risk of CV events?

Influenza vaccination has been accepted as an effective, well-established strategy to reduce influenza-related illness, and additional potential benefit in high-risk CV populations is reflected in several meta-analyses and observational analyses that have demonstrated lower rates of CV outcomes in patients who received influenza vaccination.(9-11) In one meta-analysis of nearly 300 000 patients in five randomized trials, vaccination was associated with a 27% reduction in myocardial infarction, and a 40% reduction in all-cause mortality. In another meta-analysis of 6735 patients from six randomized controlled trials, influenza vaccine was associated with a 36% reduced risk of major adverse CV events. This benefit was most robust in patients with recent acute coronary syndrome.

Observational studies have shown that the protective effectiveness of influenza vaccine against AMI is between 19% and 45% (13,14,). A meta-analysis of case-control studies showed that influenza vaccine has a summary vaccine effectiveness of 29% against AMI (15).

In contrast to the above meta- analyses, observational and small randomized studies, a very recent study (16) by Mohseni and colleagues using patients as their own controls, examined the association between influenza vaccination and the risk for CV hospitalization in patients with heart failure using health records in England between 1990 and 2013.

In this largest investigation of its kind in 59,202 heart failure patients, rates of CV, respiratory, and all-cause hospitalizations on an individual patient level were compared from two years-one year during which the patient was vaccinated, and an adjacent year during which the patient was not vaccinated. The authors found a lower risk for CV hospitalizations, including hospitalizations for heart failure, during the vaccinated year compared with the risk during the unvaccinated year.

They found the uptake of vaccination to be varied and generally low (49% in 2013). Influenza vaccination was associated with a lower risk of hospitalization due to cardiovascular disease (0.73 [0.71, 0.76]), with more modest effects for hospitalization due to respiratory infections (0.83 [0.77, 0.90]), and all-cause hospitalizations (0.96 [0.95, 0.98]). Hence in HF patients, influenza vaccination is associated with reduced risk of hospitalizations.

All the above evidence is similar to the extent of benefits that accrue with the accepted routine coronary prevention measures such as smoking cessation (32-43%), statins (19-30%) and antihypertensive therapy (17-25%).

▮ Mechanism of CV protection:

Influenza vaccine protects against AMI by preventing influenza, thereby preventing the possibility of AMI triggered by the mechanisms discussed above. An additional possible mechanism could be that vaccine-induced antibody cross-reacts with a human bradykinin receptor. It is postulated that this interaction could lead to increased levels of nitric oxide, which increases the efficiency of myocardial oxygen use, as well as improvement in endothelial function.

▮ Dual Influenza and pneumococcal vaccination:

Although there are no randomized trials that have studied the effects of both vaccines administered together, a cohort study has suggested that dual influenza and pneumococcal vaccination is superior to either vaccine alone for preventing complications in older adults with chronic illnesses [17]. In adults ≥ 65 years of age with chronic illnesses, dual vaccination with the inactivated influenza vaccine and the pneumococcal polysaccharide vaccine resulted in lower rates of death (hazard ratio [HR] 0.65, 95% CI 0.55-0.77), pneumonia (HR 0.57, 95% CI 0.51-0.64), ischemic stroke (HR 0.67, 95% CI 0.54-0.83), and acute myocardial infarction (HR 0.52, 95% CI 0.38-0.71) compared with unvaccinated individuals. Dual vaccination also resulted in fewer coronary (HR 0.59, 95% CI, 0.44-0.79) and intensive care unit admissions (HR 0.45, 95% CI 0.22-0.94) compared with unvaccinated individuals.

Despite this large body of evidence showing the benefits of vaccination being as robust as other secondary prevention measures such lifestyle changes, statins and smoking cessation, and despite guidelines recommendations, rates of influenza vaccination in patients with heart diseases are low, and vaccination is not seen as a priority.

It is time it is rejuvenated and receives a "booster" dose from practitioners for CVD management and prevention.

▮ Suggested Readings

1. Glezen WP, Decker M, Perrotta DM. Survey of underlying conditions of persons hospitalized with acute respiratory disease during influenza epidemics in Houston, 1978-1981. Am Rev Respir Dis. 1987;136(3):550-555.

2. Collins SD. Excess mortality from causes other than influenza and pneumonia during influenza epidemics. Public Health Reports (1896-1970) 1932;47:2159-79.

3. Madjid M, Miller CC, Zarubaev VV, et al. Influenza epidemics and acute respiratory disease activity are associated with a surge in autopsy-confirmed coronary heart disease death: results from 8 years of autopsies in 34,892 subjects. Eur Heart J 2007;28:1205-10.

4. Yap FH, Ho PL, Lam KF, et al. Excess hospital admissions for pneumonia, chronic obstructive pulmonary disease, and heart failure during influenza seasons in Hong Kong. J Med Virol 2004;73:617-23.

5. Warren-Gash C, Smeeth L, Hayward AC. Influenza as a trigger for acute myocardial infarction or death from cardiovascular disease: a systematic review. Lancet Infect Dis 2009;9:601-10.

6. Barnes M, Heywood AE, Mahimbo A, Rahman B, Newall AT, Macintyre CR.
   Acute myocardial infarction and influenza: a meta-analysis of case-control studies. Heart 2015;101:1738-1747.

7. Reichert TA Simonsen L Sharma A Pardo SAFedson DSMiller MA. Influenza and the winter increase in mortality in the United States, 1959-1999. Am J Epidemiol 2004;160:492-502.

8. Sandoval C Walter S D Krueger P Smieja M Smith A Yusuf S Loeb MB. Risk of hospitalization during influenza season among a cohort of patients with congestive heart failure. EpidemiolInfect 2007;135:574-82.

9. Sandoval CWalter SD Krueger P Smieja M Smith A Yusuf S Loeb MB. Risk of hospitalization during influenza season among a cohort of patients with congestive heart failure. EpidemiolInfect 2007;135:574-82.

10. Ciszewski A Bilinska ZT Brydak LB Kepka CKruk MR omanowska MK siezycka E Przyluski J Piotrowski WMaczynska RRuzyllo W. Influenza vaccination in secondary prevention from coronary ischaemic events in coronary artery disease: FLUCAD study. Eur Heart J 2008;29:1350-1358.

11. Gurfinkel EPLeondela Fuente RMendizOMautner B. Flu vaccination in acute coronary syndromes and planned percutaneous coronary interventions (FLUVACS) Study. Eur Heart J 2004;25:25-31.

12. Johnstone J Loeb M Teo KK Gao P Dyal L LiuL Avezum A Cardona-Munoz E Sleight P Fagard RYusuf S; Ongoing Telmisartan Alone and in Combination With Ramipril Global EndPoint Trial (ON TARGET);

Telmisartan Randomized Assessment Study in ACE Intolerant Subjects With Cardiovascular Disease (TRANSCEND) investigators. Influenza vaccination and major adverse vascular events in high-risk patients. Circulation 2012;126:278-286.e.

13. Vardeny O Claggett BU dell JA Packer M Zile M Rouleau J Swedberg K Desai AS Lefkowitz M ShiV McMurray J J Solomon SD; PARADIGM-HF Investigators. Influenza vaccination in patients with chronic heart failure: the PARADIGM-HF trial. JACC Heart Fail 2016;4:152-158.

14. Hsu SY, Chen FL, Liaw YP, et al. A matched influenza vaccine strain was effective in reducing the risk of acute myocardial infarction in elderly persons: a population-based study. Medicine (Baltimore) 2016;95:e2869.

15. Siriwardena AN, Gwini SM, Coupland CAC. Influenza vaccination, pneumococcal vaccination and risk of acute myocardial infarction: matched case-control study. CMAJ 2010;182:1617-23.

16. Barnes M, Heywood AE, Mahimbo A, et al. Acute myocardial infarction and influenza: a meta-analysis of case-control studies. Heart 2015;101:1738-47.

17. Hamid Mohseni Amit Kiran Reza Khorshidi Kazem Rahimi. Influenza vaccination and risk of hospitalization in patients with heart failure: a self-controlled case series study. Eur Heart J (2016) Published: 21 September 2016.

18. Hung IF, Leung AY, Chu DW, Leung D, Cheung T, Chan CK, Lam CL, Liu SH, Chu CM, Ho PL, Chan S, Lam TH, Liang R, Yuen KY. Prevention of acute myocardial infarction and stroke among elderly persons by dual pneumococcal and influenza vaccination: a prospective cohort study. Clin Infect Dis. 2010;51(9):1007.

It is noteworthy that the 2016 AHA/ACC Guideline on the management of patients with lower extremity peripheral artery disease gives a class I recommendation, to annual influenza vaccination as a component of medical therapy for patients with PAD, on the basis of evidence on patients with CVD. Also, the 2011 AHA/ACCF guideline on secondary prevention, recommends that all patients with CVD should receive an annual influenza vaccination.

Each year, currently circulating influenza strains are tested to determine the three or four strains that will be included in the vaccine, most commonly made from embryonated chicken eggs. Usually, one to two strains covered by the vaccine change each year.

The influenza vaccine (using inactivated influenza virus) is approved for use among healthy people six months of age or older and those with chronic medical conditions (such as asthma, diabetes, or heart disease).

The choice of vaccine formulation depends upon several factors, including age, comorbidities, and risk of adverse reactions:

For individuals between 18 and 64 years of age, a standard-dose of intramuscular quadrivalent formulation of the inactivated vaccine is recommended.

For individuals ≥ 65 years of age, the high-dose intramuscular inactivated influenza vaccine when available is recommended.

93

Optimizing Anticoagulation and Antiplatelets in PCI with Atrial Fibrillation

Dev Pahlajani

Approximately 30% patients with atrial fibrillation (AF) have concomitant ischemic heart disease and several of them will need to undergo percutaneous coronary intervention (PCI) during their life.

It is estimated that 8-10% patients who undergo PCI have AF. The current guidelines suggest triple drug therapy with two antiplatelet agents and warfarin so as to prevent stroke and stent thrombosis. However such a strategy is associated with high risk of bleeding. Currently at least 3 well controlled randomised trials - WOEST, PIONEER-AF, and RE-DUAL - PCI have provided data that indicates use of one antiplatelet drug with either warfarin or NOAC could reduce the risk of bleeding as compared to triple therapy.

In WOEST trial 279 were randomized to clopidogrel with Vitamin K antagonist (VKA) - dual therapy, whereas 284 patients received triple drug therapy with aspirin, clopidogrel and VKA. Primary end point was occurrence of all bleeding events while secondary end points were combination of death, stroke myocardial infarction (MI), stent thrombosis and target vessel revascularization (TVR) and all individual components of primary and secondary end points. Follow up was for one year. Antiplatelet therapy was continued for a minimum of one month after BMS and one year after DES in both the arms. Primary end point of TIMI bleeding events occurred in 44.9% in triple drug therapy group and 19.5% in double therapy group. Secondary end points of death, MI, TVR, stroke and stent thrombosis occurred in 17.7% for triple drug therapy and 11.3% in double therapy group. All cause mortality was also significantly higher in tripple drug therapy group (6.4% in triple versus 2.6% in double therapy group).

This was the first randomised trial to test the hypothesis that combination of VKA with single antiplatelet clopidogrel was superior to triple therapy in reducing the bleeding events. It is a well known fact that increased bleeding following PCI is associated with higher mortality and adverse cardiovascular event rates. This reduction in the mortality could be attributed to reduce the risk of bleeding.

In the PIONEER AF trial 2124 patients with non valvular AF who had undergone PCI were randomised in a 1:1:1 ratio of

a) Low dose Rivaroxaban (15 mg once daily) with P2Y12 inhibitor for 12 months-group 1.

b) Very low dose Rivaroxaban (2.5 mg twice daily) with dual antiplatelet therapy (DAPT) for 1, 6, 12 months-group 2.

c) Standard therapy with dose adjusted VKA + DAPT for 1, 6 or 12 months - group 3.

Primary safety outcome was clinically significant bleeding. Two arms who received Rivaroxaban low dose with either single antiplatelet or very low dose Rivaroxaban with DAPT had significantly lower bleeding rates as compared to the group of patients who received standard therapy with VKA and DAPT (16.8% in group 1, 18% in group 2 and 26.7% in group 3). The rates of death from cardiovascular causes, MI or stroke were similar in 3 groups.

Thus the study concluded that either low dose Rivaroxaban with single anti platelet P2Y12 inhibitor or very low dose Rivaroxaban + DAPT was superior in reducing risk of significant bleeding as compared to standard therapy with VKA and DAPT.

Recently in the RESIDUAL PCI trial the safety of Dabigatran in the doses of 110 mg or 150 mg twice daily with P2Y12 inhibitor was tested against the standard triple drug therapy with VKA plus P2Y12 inhibitor and aspirin. The primary end point was major or clinically relevant non major bleeding up to mean follow up of 14 months. The trial also tested non inferiority of double therapy to triple therapy in respect to incidence of composite of thrombo-embolic event (MI or systemic embolism), death or unplanned revascularization).

Incidence of primary end point of bleeding was 15.4% in the 110mg double drug therapy group versus 26.9% in the triple drug therapy group and 20.2% in the 150 mg double drug therapy group as compared to 25.7% in the triple drug therapy group. However the double drug therapy was non inferior to triple drug therapy with respect to thrombo-embolic events.

Thus these current trials have provided new strategies to cardiologists to treat a complex clinical situation in patients with AF who undergo PCI. Bleeding is a serious issue complicating PCI that is associated with increased risk of major adverse events. Efforts have been on to reduce the risk of bleeding. Apparently data from these 3 trials suggests:

1) Double therapy with P2Y12 inhibitor and VKA is superior to triple therapy.

2) Double therapy with reduced dose Rivaroxaban and P2Y12 inhibitor is superior to triple therapy.

3) Double therapy with dabigatron in 110 0r 150 BID dose and P2Y12 inhibitor is superior to triple therapy.

There is need for large scale trials to substantiate these useful conclusions from these 3 trials.

Suggested Readings

1. Levine GN, Bates ER, Bittl JA, et al. 2016 ACC/AHA guideline focused update on duration of dual antiplatelet therapy in patients with coronary artery disease: a report of the American College of Cardiology/American Heart Association Task Force on Clinical Practice Guidelines: an update of the 2011 ACCF/AHA/SCAI guideline for percutaneous coronary intervention, 2011 ACCF/AHA guideline for coronary artery bypass graft Surgery, 2012 ACC/AHA/ACP/AATS/PCNA/SCAI/ STS guideline for the diagnosis and management of patients with stable ischemic heart disease, 2013 ACCF/AHA guideline for the management of ST-elevation myocardial infarction, 2014 AHA/ACC guideline for the management of patients with non-ST-elevation acute coronary syndromes, and 2014 ACC/AHA guideline on perioperative cardiovascular evaluation and management of patients undergoing noncardiac surgery. Circulation 2016;134(10): e123-e155.

2. Andrade JG, Deyell MW, Khoo C, Lee M, Humphries K, Cairns JA. Risk of bleeding on triple antithrombotic therapy after percutaneous coronary intervention/stenting: a systematic review and meta-analysis. Can J Cardiol 2013;29:204-12.

3. Lamberts M, Gislason GH, Olesen JB, et al. Oral anticoagulation and antiplatelets in atrial fibrillation patients after myocardial infarction and coronary intervention. J Am Coll Cardiol 2013;62:981-9.

4. Dans AL, Connolly SJ, Wallentin L, et al. Concomitant use of antiplatelet therapy with dabigatran or warfarin in the Randomized Evaluation of Long-Term Anticoagulation Therapy (RE-LY) trial. Circulation 2013;127:634-40.

5. Gibson CM, Mehran R, Bode C, et al. Prevention of bleeding in patients with atrial fibrillation undergoing PCI. N Engl J Med 2016;375:2423-34.

6. Gibson CM, Pinto DS, Chi G, et al. Recurrent hospitalization among patients with atrial fibrillation undergoing intracoronary stenting treated with 2 treatment strategies of rivaroxaban or a doseadjusted oral vitamin K antagonist treatment strategy. Circulation 2017;135: 323-33.

7. Bhatt DL. O PIONEERs! The beginning of the end of full-dose triple therapy with warfarin? Circulation 2017;135:334-7.

8. Dewilde WJ, Oirbans T, Verheugt FW, et al. Use of clopidogrel with or without aspirin in patients taking oral anticoagulant therapy and undergoing percutaneous coronary intervention: an open-label, randomised, controlled trial. Lancet 2013; 381:1107-15.

9. Christopher P. Cannon, M.D., Deepak L. Bhatt, M.D. M.P.H. Jonas Oldgren M.D., Ph.D., et al. Dual Antithrombotic Therapy with Dabigatran after PCI in Atrial Fibrillation N Engl J Med 2017;377: 1513-1524.

Is there a Poor Man's Dobutamine Stress Echo for Aortic Valve Evaluation?

Akshay Mehta

After Bhave et al (1) reported a case in which the increase in transaortic gradient during post extra systolic beats (PESP), matched that found on dobutamine echocardiography (DSE) in a patient with low flow, low gradient, low EF aortic stenosis (AS), Brandon M. Wiley et al (2) now report a study of 249 transthoracic DSEs from January 1, 2011 to April 30, 2015 with aortic stenosis and impaired left ventricular systolic function (left ventricular ejection fraction [LVEF] < 55%).

A review of 212 echocardiograms that yielded 43 PESP events in 32 studies (29 patients) showed excellent correlation between PESP and dobutamine derived maximum velocities and mean gradients.

The mean transaortic PESP and dobutamine derived Vmax were 3.62 ± 0.56 m/s and 3.66 ± 0.59 m/s, respectively (p = 0.53). The average mean pressure gradients for PESP and dobutamine were 28.50 ± 8.56 mm Hg and 30.20 ± 10.10 mm Hg, respectively (p = 0.46).

Of the 16 DSE studies that demonstrated dobutamine Vmax ≥ 4.0 m/s (true AS), the corresponding PESP was Vmax > 3.9 m/s in 14 (87.5%) and ≥ 3.7 m/s in the 2 outliers.

A few limitations of the study were 1. An independent method to validate the severity of stenosis was not used. 2. The study was limited to those patients with PESP gradients that could be analyzed and 3. A statistically significant correlation with PESP and contractile reserve could not be demonstrated.

Yet, the excellent correlation between PESP and dobutamine transaortic gradients suggests that PESP could be used to identify true severe LFLG-AS.

More prospective studies can confirm the value of PESP for assessment of contractive reserve and true severity of AS. This study provides excellent validation of PESP as a substitute for dobutamine echo for evaluation of low gradient, low flow aortic stenosis with low EF and can be used for economically disadvantaged patients, that saves time too.

▮ Suggested Readings

1. Bhave N.M., Patel A.R., Shah A.P., Lang R.M. (2013) Post extrasystolic potentiation in low-gradient, severe aortic stenosis: a poor man's stress echo? Echocardiography 30:E148-E151.

2. Brandon M. Wiley, Ari Pollack, Ajay S. Vaidya, Sunil K. Agarwal, Partho P. Sengupta, Farooq A. Chaudhry. Post-Extrasystolic Transaortic Valve Gradients Differentiate "Pseudo" and "True" Low-Flow, Low-Gradient Severe AS During Dobutamine Stress Echocardiography. JACC: Cardiovascular Imaging January 2017, DOI: 10.1016/j.jcmg.2016.09.024.

For NOACS, only significant Mitral Stenosis and Mechanical Valves Comprise "Valvular AF"

Akshay Mehta

The definition of the term 'valvular' in relation to atrial fibrillation (AF) is inconsistent in the literature. Many clinicians are hesitant to prescribe the newer oral anticoagulants (NOACS) in patients with some degree of VHD, although some forms of valvular heart disease (VHD) were included in the trials comparing NOACS with Vitamin K antagonists.

What type of VHD can be considered for NOAC treatment?

To answer this question without the benefit of a prospective, large randomized trial (RCT), a recent meta-analysis of published data from 4 large RCTs, showed that NOACs were more effective than warfarin for thromboembolic prophylaxis in patients with AF with and without VHD and were not associated with overall differences in risks of major bleeding. No evidence was found of differential effects of DOACs versus warfarin based on VHD status for either outcome. The analysis was of 4 multicenter, international RCTs comparing apixaban, dabigatran, edoxaban, and rivaroxaban to warfarin. The eligible studies included the following valve lesions: aortic stenosis/regurgitation, mild mitral stenosis, mitral regurgitation, tricuspid stenosis/regurgitation in all studies; bioprosthetic valves in 2 studies; and annuloplasty or valvuloplasty in 3 studies. Lesions had to be of at least moderate severity to qualify for the VHD groups in the main analyses, except for the RE-LY trial (Randomized Evaluation of Long-Term Anticoagulant Therapy), which also included mild severity lesions in the VHD group.

In comparison to warfarin, bleeding rates were more in the rivaroxaban-treated VHD subgroup and less in the apixaban-treated patients in the non-VHD subgroup.

A recent exploratory analysis of the rivaroxaban clinical trial data demonstrated that the bleeding risk was highest in aortic stenosis, followed by mitral or aortic regurgitation, which could be related to an acquired coagulopathy and bleeding from intestinal angiodysplasia (Heyde's syndrome) in some patients with aortic valve disease.

Although this meta-analysis was of summarized published data, rather than individual patient data, it provides evidence in support of the notion that only hemodynamically significant mitral stenosis and mechanical valves, should preclude the use of DOACs. For all other VHD patients with AF, NOACS may be considered as first-line agents.

Suggested Readings

1. Konstantinos C. Siontis, Xiaoxi Yao, Bernard J. Gersh, Peter A. Noseworthy. Direct Oral Anticoagulants in Patients With Atrial Fibrillation and Valvular Heart Disease Other Than Significant Mitral Stenosis and Mechanical Valves. A Meta-Analysis. Circulation. 2017;135:714-716. Originally published February 13, 2017.

Radial Access? Appropriate; PCI for CTO? May be Appropriate; CTO PCI through Radial Access? Rarely Appropriate!

Akshay Mehta

If one can apply appropriate use criteria (the way they are used for coronary revascularization) to radial access and CTO PCI, they may look like what is mentioned in the title. For that is what two recent trials seem to convey.

One was a comparison of radial versus femoral access for PCI procedures.

Registry and randomized trial data have indicated the superiority of radial access for reduced mortality, less frequent access site bleeding complications, and possibly earlier hospital discharge. But what about radiation safety?

Operator and patient radiation exposure during femoral versus radial access during percutaneous coronary procedures for acute coronary syndromes was evaluated for 18 skilled operators participating in the RAD MATRIX trial. Among 777 procedures in 767 patients, the radiation dose at operator's thorax was significantly (88%) higher with radial than femoral access (77 µSv [IQR: 40-112] vs. 41 µSv [IQR:23-59], p=0.02). After normalization of operator radiation dose by fluoroscopy time or dose area product (DAP), the difference remained significant. For patients, fluoroscopy time and dose area product were significantly higher with radial as compared to femoral access.

So this robust trial raises a red alert for radial procedures and implores utilizing radiation safety measures.

DECISION CTO, the much awaited first randomized trial comparing PCI versus optimal medical treatment as an initial strategy for CTO's was presented by lead investigator Seung-Jung Park, MD, PhD, of the Asan Medical Center in Seoul, at the American College of Cardiology (ACC), 66th annual meeting.

In this prospective, open-label trial that enrolled patients with silent ischemia, stable angina, or acute coronary syndrome, the investigators enrolled 815 patients with CTO at 19 cardiac centers in Asia, randomly assigning 417 patients to receive PCI plus drugs and 398 patients to receive drugs alone. After tracking outcomes for 3 years, the results showed no significant differences in the composite primary endpoint and no differences in rates of death, heart attack, stroke, and subsequent revascularization procedures considered separately. Measures of health-related quality of life, assessed by the Seattle Angina Questionnaire, also did not differ significantly between the two groups throughout the follow-up period. Three-quarters of the study cohort presented with stable angina and another three-quarters had multivessel disease.

Thus, as per the investigators the findings suggest that it is not always necessary to open blocked arteries using PCI, which can substantially increase costs, complications and radiation exposure.

Thus if one combines the results of these two studies : doing a long procedure (CTO PCI) with doubtful benefit and that too through a route (radial) which increases the radiation hazard suggests the inadvisability of doing both together, namely CTO PCI through radial route.

Hence, till more light is thrown with more data, it may be advisable to do PCI for CTO only in appropriately selected cases maximally treated with medications, and that too through the femoral route.

97

Varieties of Morning Hypertension: Do they matter ?

Akshay Mehta

Current guidelines recommend the use of ambulatory BP measurement (ABPM) in routine clinical practice of hypertension, because of the evidence that it provides the average 24-hour BP, daytime and nighttime BP, and circadian variability, which are all superior to clinical BP for the diagnosis and prognostic evaluation of hypertensive individuals.

Recently, in the Home Blood Pressure Measurement With Olmesartan Naive Patients to Establish Standard Target Blood Pressure (HONEST) registry(1), in a cohort of 21 591 patients with essential hypertension, morning hypertension (morning home BP $\geq$ 145 mmHg) was associated with adverse cardiovascular outcomes, even among patients with well-controlled clinical BP.

Patients with morning hypertension can be those with nocturnal hypertension who have sustained hypertension upon awakening or those without nocturnal hypertension who have morning hypertension upon awakening.

Do they differ in terms of their effects on cardiovascular target organ damage and clinical outcomes?

In a recent study(2), vascular target organ damage and central hemodynamics were studied in a prospective cohort of patients at high risk for CVD having these 2 types of morning hypertension.

The researchers divided 1070 consecutive patients with high cardiovascular risk into the following 3 subtypes: (I) morning normotension; (II) morning hypertension without nocturnal hypertension; and (III) morning hypertension with nocturnal hypertension.

Besides a high prevalence of morning hypertension and nocturnal hypertension with morning hypertension, the study found that morning hypertension subtype III was independently associated with central hypertension, increased arterial stiffness and coronary artery calcium score.

Of course, in a cross sectional study such as this it is difficult to know whether increased aortic stiffness and central hemodynamic loads are responsible for elevated nocturnal hypertension and morning hypertension in these patients or they are the result. In other words one cannot distinguish the cause-effect relationship.

Nevertheless, the message is that type III morning hypertension, that is the one associated with nocturnal hypertension has greater risk and implies proper treatment with chronotherapy.

This is specially so because there are divergent experiences with regard to the clinical implications of morning hypertension, the type II morning hypertension (without nocturnal hypertension), with some studies (26,27) not finding adverse implications of this type of morning hypertension.

On the other hand, nocturnal hypertension has consistently been found to have adverse prognosis.

Outcomes in terms of events will in future throw more light on these types of morning hypertension, but for the present it is important to distinguish between these two types of morning hypertension and tailor our therapy for the same.

▋ Suggested Readings

1. Kario K, Saito I, Kushiro T, Teramukai S, Tomono Y, Okuda Y, Shimada K. Morning home blood pressure is a strong predictor of coronary artery disease: the HONEST Study. J Am CollCardiol. 2016;67: 1519-1527.

2. Jaewon Oh, Chan Joo Lee, In-Cheol Kim, Sang-Hak Lee, Seok-Min Kang, Donghoon Choi, Sungha Park, Kazuomi Kario. Association of Morning Hypertension Subtype with Vascular Target Organ Damage and Central Hemodynamics. Journal of the American Heart Association. 2017;6:e005424, originally published February 14, 2017.

3. Verdecchia P, Angeli F, Mazzotta G, Garofoli M, Ramundo E, Gentile G, Ambrosio G, Reboldi G. Day-night dip and early-morning surge in blood pressure in hypertension: prognostic implications. Hypertension. 2012;60:34-42.

4. Bombelli M, Fodri D, Toso E, Macchiarulo M, Cairo M, Facchetti R, Dell'Oro R, Grassi G, Mancia G. Relationship among morning blood pressure surge, 24-hour blood pressure variability and cardiovascular outcomes in a white population. Hypertension. 2014;64:943-950.

98

Is LDL Cholesterol 'The' Cause of Atherosclerotic Cardiovascular Disease?

Akshay Mehta

In a recent issue (1) of European Heart Journal, European Atherosclerosis Society Consensus Panel presents evidence from genetic studies, prospective epidemiologic cohort studies, Mendelian randomization studies, and randomized trials of LDL-lowering therapies to affirm that low-density lipoproteins cause atherosclerotic cardiovascular disease.

This also addresses the scepticism prevalent in the lay and scientific press about the causal nature of the relationship between LDL and the development of ASCVD.

Regardless of the underlying genetic defect, familial hypercholesterolaemia (FH) is an autosomal co-dominant disorder that is characterized by markedly elevated levels of LDL-C and premature atherosclerosis, particularly coronary artery disease.

Several large meta-analyses of prospective observational epidemiologic studies using individual participant data have consistently reported a continuous log-linear association between the absolute magnitude of exposure to plasma LDL-C levels and the risk of ASCVD.

Albeit these studies are not randomized and are therefore unavoidably vulnerable to confounding, reverse causation, and other forms of bias. Mendelian randomization studies introduce a natural way of randomization to assess whether an observed association between an exposure and an outcome is likely to be causal. For example numerous variants in multiple genes have been reported to be associated with lower LDL-C levels. Inheriting an LDL-C lowering allele in one of these genes is analogous to being randomly allocated to treatment with an LDL-C-lowering therapy, while inheriting the other allele is analogous to being randomly allocated to 'usual care'. Variants in over 50 genes that are associated purely with lower LDL-C levels are also associated with a correspondingly lower risk of CHD thus providing powerful evidence that LDL is causally associated with the risk of CHD.

Finally, evidence from randomized controlled drug trials: in a meta-analysis of individual-participant data from 26 statin trials including almost 170 000 individuals, treatment with a statin was associated with a log-linear 22% proportional reduction in the risk of major cardiovascular events per about 40 mg% reduction in LDL-C over a median of 5 years of treatment.

This effect is seen with all drugs which substantially lower LDLC. Exceptions are those trials in which the drug did not produce a substantial difference in LDL-C concentration between treatment arms, and those with short-term follow-up (2 years or less). Also, some therapies that lower LDL-C (e.g. oestrogen, CETP inhibitors) also have adverse effects that increase the risk of ASCVD which can attenuate or erase the clinical benefit of lowering LDL-C.

The causal effect of LDL on the risk of ASCVD is determined by both the absolute magnitude and the cumulative duration of exposure to LDL-C. This has therapeutic implications with regards to the initiation and duration of therapy in persons at high risk.

■ The problem of residual risk:

Two assumptions made with regards to the causality of lipids are: to equate LDLC with LDL particle number and LDL particle number with apoB, which represents all atherogenic particles.

Neither may be true for all people.

For example, in people with small dense LDL particles, the same amount of Cholesterol (C) is carried by a large number of small LDL particles, increasing its atherogenicity due to the large number (and small size, besides other properties). Thus absolute amount of C and the number of LDL particles carrying it may not always be concordant.

In others, other lipoprotein particles besides LDL may play a part like Lp(a), VLDL, IDL and remnants.

Thus although LDLC is a measure of LDL particle number, it may not always be concordant and although LDL particle number represents 90% of all atherogenic particles, it may not always be so.

Hence, although testing LDLC is convenient and cheap, it may not capture the full atherogenic potential.

■ What about HDL?

A recent analysis from the JUPITER Trial (Justification for the Use of Statins in Prevention: An Intervention Trial Evaluating Rosuvastatin) showed that cholesterol efflux capacity was associated with residual CVD in individuals on potent statin therapy but not at baseline. Among HDL-related biomarkers, HDL particle number demonstrated the strongest inverse association with incident cardiovascular events when assessed both at baseline and on potent rosuvastatin therapy. HDL-cholesterol or apolipoprotein A-I, by themselves were poor independent predictors of residual risk.

Hence, HDL particle number was a better risk predictor than the best-validated metric of HDL functionality, cholesterol efflux capacity, in primary prevention and it was the strongest HDL-related biomarker of residual risk in participants treated with potent statin therapy.

Thus atherogenecity may depend on various lipid factors.

LDLC may not be 'the' cause of atherosclerotic disease, but 'a' cause of it, the most important one.

▮ Suggested Readings

1. Brian A. Ference Henry N. Ginsberg Ian Graham Kausik K. Ray Chris J. Packard Eric Bruckert Robert A. Hegele Ronald M. Krauss Frederick J. Raal Heribert Schunkert.

   Low-density lipoproteins cause atherosclerotic cardiovascular disease. 1. Evidence from genetic, epidemiologic, and clinical studies. A consensus statement from the European Atherosclerosis Society Consensus Panel.

   Eur Heart J 2017 ehx144.doi: 10.1093/eurheartj/ehx144 Published: 24 April 2017.

2. Amit V. Khera, Olga Demler, Steve J. Adelman, Heidi L. Collins, Robert J. Glynn, Paul M. Ridker, Daniel J. Rader and Samia Mora.

   Cholesterol Efflux Capacity, HDL Particle Number, and Incident Cardiovascular Events. An Analysis from the JUPITER Trial (Justification for the Use of Statins in Prevention: An Intervention Trial Evaluating Rosuvastatin).

   Circulation. 2017; CIRCULATIONAHA.116.025678, originally published April 27, 2017.

Rapid Aspirin Desensitization - How and Why?

Akshay Mehta

Aspirin or acetyl salicylic acid forms a cornerstone of coronary artery disease (CAD) therapy and can lead to a 33% overall reduction in CAD outcomes.

Studies have shown that for acute CAD, before or shortly after coronary artery bypass grafting, and for drug-eluting stenting, aspirin nonadherence/withdrawal was associated with a 3-fold higher risk of major adverse cardiac events, which was magnified to ≈90-fold higher risk in patients with intracoronary stents.

However, aspirin hypersensitivity occurs in 0.5 to 1.9% of general population and more in patients with CAD (1.5%-2.6%) which may be a deterrent to therapy and may increase the risk of recurrent ischemic events. Aspirin sensitivity is most often manifested as rhinitis and asthma or urticaria/angio edema induced by cross-reacting nonsteroidal anti-inflammatory drugs that inhibit cyclooxygenase1.

Whatever the mechanism of sensitivity, most patients with acetylsalicylic acid sensitivity are able to undergo desensitization therapy safely and successfully. However, experience with acetylsalicylic acid desensitization in patients with CAD is very limited, especially unstable CAD, which requires rapid desensitization. Many desensitization protocols require several days to be completed.

In a recent paper, Rossini et al describe conducting the largest prospective observational study of a rapid aspirin desensitization protocol, which was highly successful and durable.

The study was carried out in 330 patients with a history of aspirin sensitivity and with known/suspected CAD or presenting with an acute coronary syndrome (in 70% of them) and undergoing PCI.

All patients underwent a rapid desensitization protocol before PCI (either in the outpatient unit or in hospital) including 24% of ST-segment-elevation myocardial infarction patients, in whom it was performed after primary PCI.

The protocol (see table) consisted of 6 sequential doses of aspirin (1, 5, 10, 20, 40, and 100 mg) administered orally over 5.5 hours. The patients were monitored closely for adverse reactions for 4 hours after the end of the protocol, and steroids, antihistamines, and antileukotrienes were discontinued 7 days before desensitization in all elective cases.

The desensitization procedure was highly successful-95.4% of patients had no reaction. Among the failures, 10 patients had an urticarial and angioedema reaction, and 5 patients had asthma, dyspnea, or bronchospasm. Out of all 330 patients enrolled, 71% underwent PCI with stenting, 3% underwent coronary bypass grafting, and 26% were managed medically. All patients who successfully completed the desensitization protocol were discharged on 100-mg aspirin per day, and 69.4% were on dual antiplatelet therapy. The overall major cardiovascular event occurrence rate was 11.8%; 4.2% in hospital and 7.6% postdischarge. There were no long-term adverse reactions reported because of aspirin desensitization procedure.

The strength of the study was the large number, especially of unstable patients needing rapid desensitization and the success of the procedure.

Chief limitations were :

1. The definition of ASA hypersensitivity by was by self-reported history of urticaria (53.6%), angioedema (20.9%), asthma (19.7%), and anaphylactic reaction (5.8%).

2. The sample size for patients with a history of anaphylaxis was limited, precluding thegeneralizable of the result to all patients with a history of anaphylactic reactions.

The other issue is the possibility of doing away with aspirin altogether in future and using newer P2Y12 inhibitors like ticagrelor or prasugrel with or without a new oral anticoagulant, for which studies are under way.

Yet, for the present, the described rapid aspirin desensitization method is simple and useful for many of our aspirin sensitive patients requiring dual antiplatelet therapy in urgent situations.

It should be born in mind that after successful desensitization, acetylsalicylic acid therapy must be indefinitely continued to prevent resensitization.

Reactions	↓ 0 min	↓ 30 min	↓ 60 min	↓ 90 min	↓ 10 min	↓ 330 min
	1mg	5 mg	10mg	20mg	40mg	100mg
Mucocutaneous						
Naso-ocular						
Pulmonary						
Pulse						
BP						
SaO$_2$						

(Adapted from Roberta Rossini et al, Aspirin Desensitization in Patients With Coronary Artery Disease: Results of the Multicentre ADAPTED registry. Circulation: Cardiovascular Interventions. 2017;10:e004368, originally published February 13, 2017)

Suggested Readings

1. Biondi-Zoccai GG, Lotrionte M, Agostoni P, Abbate A, Fusaro M, Burzotta F, Testa L, Sheiban I, Sangiorgi G. A systematic review and meta-analysis on the hazards of discontinuing or not adhering to aspirin among 50,279 patients at risk for coronary artery disease. Eur Heart J. 2006;27:2667-2674.

2. Roberta Rossini, AnnamariaIorio, Roberto Pozzi, Matteo Bianco, Giuseppe Musumeci, Sergio Leonardi, CorradoLettieri, Irene Bossi, Paola Colombo, Stefano Rigattieri, Cinzia Dossena, Angelo Anzuini, DavideCapodanno, Michele Senni and Dominick J. Angiolillo Aspirin Desensitization in Patients With Coronary Artery Disease. Results of the Multicenter ADAPTED Registry. Circulation: Cardiovascular Interventions. 2017;10:e004368, originally published February 13,2017.

3. Udaya S. Tantry and Paul A. Gurbel Rapid Desensitization of the Patients With Aspirin Hypersensitivity and Coronary Artery Disease. Circulation: Cardiovascular Interventions. 2017;10:e004881, originally published February 13, 2017.

100

Heart Failure Patients with Low Systolic Blood Pressure
- The Impact of Modern Pharmacotherapy

Akshay Mehta

Heart failure patients with reduced ejection fraction (HFrEF) and with low systolic blood pressure are an enigma. Compared to heart failure patients with higher systolic blood pressure (SBP), those with lower SBP have a worse prognosis- whether the low SBP is a marker of more advanced disease, or whether low SBP is by itself harmful below a certain threshold.

To make matters worse, these patients often are required to receive treatment with life-saving therapies that might lower blood pressure further.

Is this harmful or beneficial?

This is an extremely important issue, since low BP might limit the use of life-saving drugs exactly in those patients in which their use might be more beneficial.

In the Prospective Comparison of angiotensin-receptor blocker neprilysin inhibitor with an angiotensin converting enzyme inhibitor to Determine Impact on Global Mortality and Morbidity in Heart Failure (PARADIGM-HF) trial, treatment with sacubitril/valsartan reduced the primary composite endpoint of cardiovascular death or HF hospitalization by 20% in comparison with enalapril, on top of optimal treatment, in patients with HF with reduced ejection fraction.

Because sacubitril/valsartan acts by both inhibiting the renin-angiotensin system and enhancing the activity of natriuretic peptides and bradykinin, the BP reduction achieved in the PARADIGM study was ~5 mmHg greater in the sacubitril/valsartan arm than in the enalapril, regardless of BP at enrolment. Did this cause harm?

In a recently published post-hoc, exploratory analysis of the PARADIGM-HF trial, Bohm et al showed the effect of treatment on SBP and on the primary composite outcome (cardiovascular death or heart failure hospitalization), its components and all-cause death. Baseline SBP as a categorical (< 110, 110 to < 120, 120 to < 130, 130 to < 140 and ≥ 140mmHg) and continuous variable, as well as average in-trial SBP and time-updated SBP were examined.

Although all-cause and cardiovascular mortality rates were highest in patients with the lowest SBP, the benefit of sacubitril/valsartan over enalapril was consistent across all baseline SBP categories for all outcomes. For example, the sacubitril/valsartan versus enalapril hazard ratio for the primary endpoint was 0.88 (95% CI 0.74-1.06) in patients with a baseline SBP < 110 mmHg and 0.81 (0.65-1.02) for those with a SBP ≥ 140 mmHg. This conclusion was confirmed by an additive analysis performed by Böhm and co-authors, utilizing time-updated BP (which is the last systolic BP at the time point closest to an event or at the end of the study) and BP changes over time instead of baseline BP alone. Symptomatic hypotension, study drug dose-reduction and discontinuation were more frequent in patients with a lower SBP in both groups.

Thus patients with lower SBP at randomization, were at higher risk but maintained the same relative benefit with sacubitril/valsartan over enalapril as patients with higher baseline SBP. This was despite greater lowering of BP by sacubitril/valsartan as compared to enalapril.

Beta blocker trials in HFrEF have shown that greatest benefit was derived in patients at greatest risk, that is those with low blood pressure.

▌ How can one optimize therapy in HFrEF patients with low SBP so as to minimize drug withdrawal?

Firstly, by adding drugs rather than increasing the dose of a single drug like sacubitril/valsartan. Trials of ACEI in HF have shown that even moderate doses show benefit and it is not necessary to jack up doses if there are adverse effects.

Secondly by screening for conditions that contribute to hypotension, such as dehydration, acute coronary syndrome, ischemia, arrhythmia, autonomic dysfunction, gastrointestinal bleeding, or infection.

Thirdly by adjusting or weeding out drugs which may lower BP like nitrates, hydralazine, centrally acting agents for psychiatric disorders or Parkinson's disease, and phosphodiesterase-5 inhibitors such as sildenafil.

Fourthly by modifying doses of other drugs contributing to hypotension. For example if hypotension is associated with bradycardia, beta blockers may be a cause. Beta blockers with vasodilatory or α-blocking properties, such as carvedilol, may have slightly more BP lowering effect than metoprolol and can be replaced if required. If there is postural hypotension, or rapid weight loss, then diuresis may have to be curtailed.

Finally, spacing and adjusting the timing of required drugs so that additive hypotensive effects are avoided.

Thus, in patients with HF, a careful balance needs to be made between therapies that might lower BP, but improve survival and symptoms, while taking care to avoid hypoperfusion symptoms, azotemia and hyperkalemia. We as physicians should not be shy of prescribing life-saving treatments in HF patients because of the worry of drug-induced lowering of BP, if it can be tolerated. This is achievable even if the systolic BP (SBP) is < 100 mm Hg, but > 90 mm Hg.

▌ Suggested Readings

1. Michael Bohm, Robin Young et al. Systolic blood pressure, cardiovascular outcomes and efficacy and safety of sacubitril/valsartan (LCZ696) in patients with chronic heart failure and reduced ejection fraction: results from PARADIGM-HF. European Heart Journal (2017) 38, 1132-1143

2. Bozkurt, Biykem. "Response to Ryan and Parwani: Heart Failure Patients With Low Blood Pressure: How Should We Manage Neurohormonal Blocking Drugs?" Circulation: Heart Failure 5.6 (2012): 820-821.

101

Should we stop Aspirin before Surgery, in Patients on Secondary Prevention?

Akshay Mehta

The role of aspirin in secondary prevention of cardiovascular disease is well established and widely used in clinical practice. However, at the time of surgery (cardiac or non cardiac), the bleeding risk of continued aspirin needs to be balanced against a protective effect for thrombotic events, especially in patients who have undergone revascularization before.

For example a patient who had a coronary stent placed 7 years ago for an episode of acute coronary syndrome (ACS) at that time, is now on aspirin and requires knee replacement surgery under spinal anesthesia. Should we with-hold aspirin before surgery and for how many days before?

Clinically significant bleeding is an important consideration in surgical patients as it is an important determinant of the outcome of surgery. This also has implications for CAD outcomes.

Hence, discontinuation of aspirin before surgery may decrease clinically significant bleeding. But would that increase coronary events in patients with CAD on secondary prevention with aspirin?

Currently there is lack of evidence-based guideline recommendation regarding discontinuation of aspirin in patients with CAD requiring surgical interventions and invasive procedures.

The Thrombosis working group of the European Society of Cardiology advocates that in the absence of clear guidelines decisions should be tailored according to the patient needs.

The peri-operative ischemic evaluation (POISE II) study, was a large phase 3 randomized trial that investigated the effect of aspirin therapy (either initiation or continued treatment) and the risk of postoperative cardiac eventsin patients at risk of vascular complications(elderly, smokers, hypertensives, diabetics, those undergoing major surgery defined as intraperitoneal, intrathoracic, retroperitoneal, or major orthopedic surgery or emergency surgery or those with any evidence of cardio vascular disease). Less than 10% of the patients in POISE II had undergone revascularization procedure (either percutaneous coronary intervention or coronary artery bypass grafting).

The study showed that the administration of aspirin before noncardiac surgery (whether de novo or continued) and throughout the early postsurgical period had no significant effect on the rate of death or nonfatal myocardial infarction but increased the risk of major bleeding.

A recently published analysis by Faraz Khan Luni included patients at even higher risk (post revascularization).

From multiple databases that were searched from inception of these databases until March 2015 to identify studies that reported discontinuation of aspirin before surgery, a total of 1,018 titles were screened, after which six observational studies met the inclusion criteria. The outcomes measured were all cause mortality, nonfatal myocardial infarction and other relevant thrombotic events (MACE) which also may include, fatal and nonfatal MI, stent thrombosis and restenosis, stroke, perioperative cardiovascular complications (heart failure, MI, VTE, acute stroke) and perioperative bleeding during the perioperative period to up to 30 days after surgery.

It showed the same results as POISE II, i.e. no increase in MACE with planned discontinuation of aspirin and a decreased risk of peri-operative bleeding.

Some limitations of the study were that firstly it was an analysis of observational studies. Secondly it excluded patients on dual antiplatelet therapy, so that the results cannot be applied to patients on DAPT. Thirdly, we do not know when aspirin was restarted after surgery.

Nevertheless, when taken together with the POISE II study, it suggests that short-term discontinuation appears to be safe with no increased risk of thrombotic events and with a decreased risk of bleeding, especially important in patients undergoing neurological or posterior chamber of eye or spinal surgery.

Although one cannot determine the most effective time to stop aspirin to minimize bleeding risk, studies have suggested that hemostasis is unimpaired if at least 20% of the platelets have normal COX-1 activity and 12% of circulating platelets are replaced every 24 hours. Therefore, stopping aspirin 72 or more hours before surgery may be adequate to minimize the risk of perioperative bleeding.

Thus for surgeries such as knee replacement, in stable patients on secondary prevention with aspirin, it may be safe to stop it 3 days before surgery with the provision that it is re-started as soon as possible after surgery, which in most cases is 2 days after surgery.

▌ Suggested Readings

1. P.J. Devereaux, M.D., Ph.D., et al. for the POISE-2 Investigators. Aspirin in Patients Undergoing Noncardiac Surgery N Engl J Med 2014; 370:1494-1503 April 17, 2014.

2. Faraz Khan Luni MD, Haris Riaz MD, Abdur Rahman Khan MD, TalhaRiaz MD, Muhammad Husnain MD, Irbaz Bin Riaz MD, Muhammad Shahzeb Khan MBBS, Mohammed Taleb MD, Yusuf Kanjwal MD, Christopher J. Cooper MD, Sadik A. Khuder PhD.

   Clinical outcomes associated with per-operative discontinuation of aspirin in patients with coronary artery disease: A systematic review and meta-analysis.

   Catheterization and Cardiovascular Interventions. Volume 89, Issue 7 June 1, 2017 Pages 1168-1175.

102

What if you Find Atherosclerotic Coronary Artery Disease in a Patient with Takotsubo Cardiomyopathy ?

Akshay Mehta

Typically, Takotsubo cardiomyopathy (TC) can be differentiated from atherosclerotic ACS on the basis of epidemiological, clinical, electrocardiographic, echocardiographic and angiographic features. The classical definition of Takotsubo cardiomyopathy (TC) excludes presence of atherosclerotic coronary artery disease (CAD).

However, CAD is seen in 10% to 61% of patients with TC, as reported in literature with 29% having luminal stenosis severity greater than 50% in at least 1 epicardial vessel, raising the doubt of atherosclerotic CAD as a cause in some patients.

Indeed, a small case series of patients with TC assessed with intravascular ultrasound (IVUS) demonstrated a single, ruptured, atherosclerotic plaque in the mid left anterior descending coronary artery. Hence, acute plaque rupture leading to transient ischemia/injury and stunning of the myocardium has been proposed as the pathogenic mechanism underlying at least some cases of TC. However, other small studies have excluded plaque rupture as a cause of TC.

Since the clinical picture of TC and acute STEMI due to LAD lesion may have many similarities, it would be difficult to rule out the role of CAD in patients of TC with severe LAD disease. This may also have therapeutic implications.

Recent work of Eitel et al, for the first time, describe the optical coherence tomography (OCT) findings in a patient population with TC. OCT is more accurate than IVUS in showing plaque rupture or erosion and thrombus.

In a total of 23 consecutive TC patients, atherosclerotic plaques were seen in the left anterior descending coronary artery or both the left anterior descending coronary artery and the left main coronary artery in 16 patients (69.6%). Thin-cap fibroatheromas were also found in 6 patients (26.1%). Vessel stenosis > 50% was found in 3 patients (13.0%). However, ruptured plaques or intracoronary thrombi were not observed in any.

Most of the patients (69.6%) in the study also underwent cardiac magnetic resonance imaging (CMR), which confirmed TC by showing edema of the left ventricular (LV) myocardium as high signal intensity, with a diffuse or transmural distribution consistent with the wall motion abnormality and absence of late gadolinium enhancement which is an important distinguishing feature from myocardial infarction.

Thus, although thin cap atherosclerotic plaques are common in patients of TC with CAD, evidence of plaque rupture such as thrombus formation are lacking in these patients and this combination of OCT and MRI is extremely important to nail CT as an entity independent of CAD as the underlying etio-pathology. Other smaller studies of IVUS in patients of TC with CAD also show absence of plaque rupture or thrombus.

Although there are small case reports of spontaneous coronary artery dissection in some patients with TC, the most recent evidence supports the concept that CT is due to acatecholamine surge that might induce direct myocardial injury and coronary spasm, mostly at the microvascular level, together with an increased cardiac workload that contributes to an acute situation of supply-demand mismatch followed by postischemic stunning.

What if intracoronary imaging with OCT to exclude plaque rupture and CMR to eliminate the possibility of myocardial infarction are not available in a patient with co existingTC and CAD?

Well, a comparison with past cine angiogram if available, showing lack of CAD progression may help rule out CAD as the cause. Of course, regression of LV function over time clinches the diagnosis finally.

Hence, although CAD may be seen in patients with TC, it does not have an etiologic role and may be an association, not a causation. The incidental finding of CAD would merit its own independent management, usually after the acute phase of TC is over.

▌ Suggested Readings

1. Ingo Eitel, Thomas Stiermaier, Tobias Graf, Christian Möller, Karl-Philipp Rommel, Charlotte Eitel, Gerhard Schuler, Holger Thiele, Steffen Desch. Optical Coherence Tomography to Evaluate Plaque Burden and Morphology in Patients with Takotsubo Syndrome. Journal of the American Heart Association. 2016;5:e004474. Originally published December 22, 2016.

2. Bybee KA, Kara T, Prasad A, Lerman A, Barsness GW, Wright RS, Rihal CS. Systematic review: transient left ventricular apical ballooning: a syndrome that mimics ST-segment elevation myocardial infarction. Ann Intern Med. 2004;141:858-865.

3. Templin C, Ghadri JR, Diekmann J, Napp LC, Bataiosu DR, Jaguszewski M, Cammann VL, Sarcon A, Geyer V, Neumann CA, Seifert B, Hellermann J, Schwyzer M, Eisenhardt K, Jenewein J, Franke J, Katus HA, Burgdorf C, Schunkert H, Moeller C, Thiele H, Bauersachs J, Tschöpe C, Schultheiss HP, Laney CA, Rajan L, Michels G, Pfister R, Ukena C, Böhm M, Erbel R, Cuneo A, Kuck KH, Jacobshagen C, Hasenfuss G, Karakas M, Koenig W, Rottbauer W, Said SM, Braun-Dullaeus RC, Cuculi F, Banning A, Fischer TA, Vasankari T, Airaksinen KE, Fijalkowski M, Rynkiewicz A, Pawlak M, Opolski G, Dworakowski R, MacCarthy P, Kaiser C, Osswald S, Galiuto L, Crea F, Dichtl W, Franz WM, Empen K, Felix SB, Delmas C, Lairez O, Erne P, Bax JJ, Ford I, Ruschitzka F, Prasad A, Lüscher TF. Clinical features and outcomes of Takotsubo (stress) cardiomyopathy. N Engl J Med. 2015;373:929-938.

4. Lyon AR, Bossone E, Schneider B, Sechtem U, Citro R, Underwood SR,Sheppard MN, Figtree GA, Parodi G, Akashi YJ, Ruschitzka F, Filippatos G,Mebazaa A, Omerovic E. Current state of knowledge on Takotsubo syndrome: a position statement from the Taskforce on Takotsubo Syndrome of the Heart Failure Association of the European Society of Cardiology. Eur J Heart Fail. 2016;18:8-27.

5. Francesco Pelliccia, Juan Carlos Kaski, Filippo Crea, Paolo G. Camici. Pathophysiology of Takotsubo Syndrome. Circulation. 2017;135:2426-2441, originally published June 12, 2017.

6. Haghi D1, Papavassiliu T, Hamm K, Kaden JJ, Borggrefe M, Suselbeck T. Coronary artery disease in takotsubo cardiomyopathy.Circ J. 2007 Jul;71(7):1092-4.

103

Is it Safe to Initiate Disopyramide for Patients with Obstructive Hypertrophic Cardiomyopathy on an Outpatient Basis?

Akshay Mehta

Although drugs with a negative inotropic effect are most commonly used as first line agents in patients with obstructive hypertrophic cardiomyopathy (HCM) and include beta-blockers (BB) and/or nondihydropyridine calcium?channel blockers (primarily verapamil), a significant number of patients are refractory to these agents. In such patients, a third drug - disopyramide can be considered.

Because of its negative inotropic properties, it is effective in reducing the pressure gradient created by left ventricular outflow tract obstruction (LVOTO) and related symptoms. The European Society of Cardiology and American Heart Association/American College of cardiology guidelines hence rate disopyramide with a class I and IIa recommendation, respectively for this indication. However, disopyramide has a significant QT-prolonging effect and, as a corollary, may induce torsades de pointes (TdP), which is the reason why some (such as American Guidelines) recommend it to be started in the hospital setting. On the other hand, some (like the European Guidelines) do not give this recommendation.

Although the US Food and Drug Administration drug information package regarding disopyramide includes the following sentence: "Initiation of Disopyramide treatment, as with other antiarrhythmic agents used to treat life-threatening arrhythmias, should be carried out in the hospital", the indication discussed here for disopyramide is not antiarrhythmic and hence not directly pertinent for this patient group.

Nevertheless, to resolve this dilemma whether it is safe to initiate disopyramide treatment in the outpatient setting for HCM patients, Arnon Adler et al recently reviewed charts of patients seen in their outpatient hypertrophic cardiomyopathy clinic between 2010 and 2014.

Out of a total of 2015 patients that were seen in the clinic, 168 were started on disopyramide. There were no cardiac events within 3 months of disopyramide initiation. During long-term follow-up (averaging 447 day), only 2 patients developed cardiac events (syncope of unknown cause in both). Thirty-eight patients (23%) developed side effects of disopyramide and 18 (11%) stopped the drug because of these side effects. Disopyramide was able to keep 63% of patients off septal reduction interventions. At a starting divided dose of 300 mg it prolonged the mean QTc interval by 19 ± 23 ms; but increasing the dose to 600 mg had no further significant effect.

Hence it can be surmised from this review of cases that Initiation of disopyramide in the outpatient setting is safe and the risk of subsequent sudden cardiac death is low.

However, due to its QT-prolonging effect, precautions may be necessary in patients at higher risk of torsades de pointes.

Hence absolute contraindications for disopyramideare: reduced left ventricular (LV) systolic function, congenital long QT syndrome or history of TdP and pregnancy. Relative contraindications for disopyramide include urinary retention, prostatism, glaucoma, and myasthenia gravis, which may be exacerbated by the anticholinergic effect of disopyramide.

The drug should be used with caution in patients with a prolonged QT at baseline, in patients with renal or hepatic impairment and in patients with atrial fibrillation and atrial flutter because of the potential for disopyramide-induced augmentation of atrio ventricular conduction and increased ventricular rate and because of increased risk of TdP postconversion to sinus rhythm or after a long pause. Care is also due in elderly patients, those with cardiac conduction abnormalities, and those with history of electrolyte abnormalities or taking potassium?depleting diuretics.

Thus, with frequent outpatient ECG and electrolyte monitoring, diasopyramide can be safely initiated in the outpatient for HCM. Ofcourse, one should check if QTc prolongation of more than 525ms (or 550 ms in the presence of a baseline wide QRS) occurs, when it should be discontinued.

▌ Suggested Readings

1. Arnon Adler, Dana Fourey, Adaya Weissler-Snir, Waseem Hindieh, Raymond H. Chan, Michael H. Gollob and Harry Rakowski. Safety of Outpatient Initiation of Disopyramide for Obstructive Hypertrophic Cardiomyopathy Patients. Journal of the American Heart Association. 2017;6:e005152, originally published May 26, 2017

2. Elliott PM, Anastasakis A, Borger MA, Borggrefe M, Cecchi F, Charron P, Hagege AA, Lafont A, Limongelli G, Mahrholdt H, McKenna WJ, Mogensen J, Nihoyannopoulos P, Nistri S, Pieper PG, Pieske B, Rapezzi C, Rutten FH, Tillmanns C, Watkins H. 2014 ESC guidelines on diagnosis and management of hypertrophic cardiomyopathy: the Task Force for the Diagnosis and Management of Hypertrophic Cardiomyopathy of the European Society of Cardiology (ESC). Eur Heart J. 2014;35: 2733-2779.

3. Gersh BJ, Maron BJ, Bonow RO, Dearani JA, Fifer MA, Link MS, Naidu SS, Nishimura RA, Ommen SR, Rakowski H, Seidman CE, Towbin JA, Udelson JE, Yancy CW. 2011 ACCF/AHA guideline for the diagnosis and treatment of hypertrophic cardiomyopathy: a report of the American College of Cardiology Foundation/American Heart Association Task Force on Practice Guidelines. Developed in collaboration with the American Association for Thoracic Surgery, American Society of Echocardiography, American Society of Nuclear Cardiology, Heart Failure Society of America, Heart Rhythm Society, Society for Cardiovascular Angiography and Interventions, and Society of Thoracic Surgeons. J Am CollCardiol. 2011;58:e212-e260.

4. Sherrid MV, Arabadjian M. A primer of disopyramide treatment of obstructive hypertrophic cardiomyopathy. Prog Cardiovasc Dis. 2012;54:483-492.

104

Stimulating Extracardiac Collaterals by Distal Right Internal Mammary Artery Occlusion:

A New Option in "No Option" Patients !

Akshay Mehta

About 30 % of patients with stable coronary artery disease (CAD) needing revascularization cannot have complete revascularization, thus increasing their chances of mortality in comparison to those with complete revascularization (3-year cumulative mortality rate of 14.8% versus 6.6%).

The numerous treatment options aiming at alleviating myocardial ischemia in such 'no option' patients are: Using angiogenic therapeutic approaches (by the so-called myocardial laser revascularization, external shock wave therapy, and myocardial stem cell application), diastolic coronary pressure augmentation by external counter pulsation, coronary arteriogenesis with induction of large collateral artery remodeling, coronary sinus venous backpressure augmentation, and ischemic preconditioning. Most of these modalities require repetitive applications for a lasting effect.

The presence of a functional inter coronary collateral circulation in chronic stable CAD has been shown to confer survival benefit.

■ **What about extra cardiac collateral supply ?**

Till now there have been seven case reports documenting the existence of naturally occurring angiographic anastomoses between one of the IMAs and the human coronary circulation

In 1932 Hudson et al at postmortem examination of cardiac patients, injected India ink into the occluded native vessels and traced the opacified microvessels over the aorta, pericardiophrenic connectors, and other vascular networks in proximity to the heart.

During angiography of internal mammary arteries, the only branch moving with the heart is the pericardiaophrenic artery, which arises at approximately the second intercostal space and supplies the pericardium, the atria and the epicardial coronary circulation. This anatomic knowledge was utilized in the first surgical attempt of myocardial revascularization, more than 20 years before the first clinical coronary artery bypass grafting in 1960, by ligating the IMAs to redirect blood flow to the pericardiophrenic branch.

However, because of several factors and equivocal results, these experiments failed.

It was only in 2014 that Stoller et al by using temporary balloon occlusion of the ipsilateral IMA and inducing temporary ischemia in the native coronary also by balloon occlusion while quantitating the collateral flow index (CFI), found that RIMA occlusion increased RCA CFI while LIMA occlusion increased left anterior descending artery CFI.

Now, very recently Stoller and Seiler show the beneficial effects of permanent percutaneous right internal mammary artery (RIMA) occlusion.

In this prospective, open-label, longitudinal interventional clinical trial, 50 patients with coronary disease underwent 1-minute serial right and left coronary artery balloon occlusion at baseline and then again 6 weeks after placement of a distal RIMA vascular occluding device (Amplatzer vascular plug 4). The primary end point was the change in collateral flow index (CFI) using a pressure sensor guidewire distal to the balloon occlusion. Secondary end points included fractional flow reserve, degree of ST-segment elevation from an intracoronary electrogram, and anginal symptoms during the 1 minute of ischemia with coronary occlusion.

After 6 weeks of follow-up, CFI increased in the right coronary artery (RCA) after RIMA occlusion (from 0.071 ± 0.08 to 0.132 ± 0.12; $P < 0.0001$), whereas the left anterior descending coronary artery CFI was unchanged (0.11 ± 0.09 to 0.08 ± 0.08; $P=NS$). Concomitant with the increased RCA CFI was a decrease in the intracoronary ST-segment elevation during RCA occlusion, a response not demonstrated in the left anterior descending artery. Likewise, angina tended to be less in the follow-up 1 minute coronary occlusion.

The study shows for the first time that permanent RIMA distal occlusion can augment extra cardiac pericardiophrenic collateral anastomoses to ipsilateral native coronary arteries and reduce signs of ischemia in adjacent myocardial territories.

Although this is a non randomized, open label study, it does raise hopes of providing a solution to patients with severe diffuse atherosclerosis and those with chronic arterial occlusions who are refractory to maximal anti-ischemic medical therapy or interventions. The relative freedom of IMA's from atherosclerosis may be an additional boon.

▮ Suggested Readings

1. Stoller M, de Marchi SF, Seiler C. Function of natural internal mammary-to-coronary artery bypasses and its effect on myocardial ischemia. Circulation. 2014;129:2645-2652.

2. Stoller M, Seiler C. Effect of permanent right internal mammary artery closure on coronary collateral function and myocardial ischemia. CircCardiovascInterv. 2017;10:e004990. doi: 10.1161/CIRCINTERVENTIONS.116.004990.

3. Williams B, Menon M, Satran D, Hayward D, Hodges JS, Burke MN, Johnson RK, Poulose AK, Traverse JH, Henry TD. Patients with coronary artery disease not amenable to traditional revascularization: prevalence and 3-year mortality. Catheter CardiovascInterv. 2010;75:886-891.

4. Meier P, Hemingway H, Lansky AJ, Knapp G, Pitt B, Seiler C. The impact of the coronary collateral circulation on mortality: a meta-analysis. Eur Heart J. 2012;33:614-621.

105

Ivabradine Use Today

Akshay Mehta

1. For Coronary artery disease:

- Not approved by US FDA

- Approved by European Medicines Agency (EMA) for the symptomatic treatment of chronic stable angina pectoris in coronary artery disease with normal sinus rhythm and heart rate ≥ 70 beats/min in adults unable to tolerate or with a contraindication to the use of beta-blockers, or in combination with beta-blockers in patients inadequately controlled with an optimal beta-blocker dose

- A Class IIa recommendation by ESC as second-line treatment for angina/ischemia in those patients already treated with short-acting nitrates and beta-blockers or calcium-channel blockers

The above recommendations are based on

1. BEAUTIFUL trial, which was a randomized, double-blind, placebo-controlled, parallel-group trial that enrolled 10,917 patients with coronary artery disease and a left ventricular ejection fraction (LVEF) < 40%. The study demonstrated that despite reducing the mean heart rate, there was no improvement in the primary endpoint, a composite of cardiovascular death, admission for acute myocardial infarction (MI), or new or worsening HF (hazard ratio [HR]: 1.00; 95% confidence interval [CI]: 0.91 to 1.10; $p = 0.94$). The vast majority of patients (87%) were already on beta-blocker therapy at baseline. In a pre-specified subgroup with heart rates ≥ 70 beats/min, although there was no difference in the composite primary endpoint, admission rates for fatal and nonfatal MI (HR: 0.64; 95% CI: 0.49 to 0.84; $p = 0.001$), as well rates of coronary revascularization (HR: 0.70; 95% CI: 0.52 to 0.93; $p = 0.016$), were reduced. In a post hoc analysis of patients with activity-limiting angina at baseline, ivabradine was shown to reduce the composite primary endpoint by 24%, largely driven by a 42% reduction in hospitalization for MI. Within this analysis, a further subgroup with heart rates ≥ 70 beats/min demonstrated an even greater reduction in the rate of hospitalization for MI (73% reduction), and also a 59% reduction in rate of coronary revascularization.

2. SIGNIFY which was a randomized, double-blind, placebo-controlled trial of ivabradine added to standard background antianginal therapy in which 19,102 patients with coronary artery disease (63% with activity-limiting angina at baseline), LVEF > 40%, and heart rate ≥ 70 beats/min were randomized. Despite a reduction in heart rate by 10 beats/min at ~28 months of follow-up, ivabradine failed to reduce the composite primary endpoint of cardiovascular

death or nonfatal MI (HR: 1.08; 95% CI: 0.96 to 1.20; p = 0.20). In a pre-specified patient subgroup with activity-limiting angina, ivabradine was associated with an increase in the incidence of the primary endpoint (HR: 1.18: 95% CI: 1.03 to 1.35; p = 0.02). Patients in the ivabradine arm had an increase in the incidence of atrial fibrillation (AF) (2.2%/year) compared with placebo (1.5%/year).

2. For Heart Failure with Reduced Ejection Fraction:

- Approved by US FDA to reduce the risk of hospitalization in patients with stable, symptomatic HFrEF (LVEF ≤ 35%) and heart rate ≥ 70 beats/min on maximally tolerated beta-blockers or have a contraindication to their use

- Approved by EMA for chronic HF NYHA functional class II-IV with systolic dysfunction, in patients in sinus rhythm and whose heart rate is ≥ 75 beats/min, in combination with standard therapy, including beta-blocker therapy or when beta-blocker therapy is contraindicated or not tolerated

- Class IIa recommendation by ACC/AHA: may be beneficial to reduce HF hospitalizations in patients with stable NYHA functional class II-III symptoms, chronic HFrEF (LVEF ≤ 35%) receiving GMT or unable to tolerate or having contraindications for a beta-blocker with sinus rates ≥ 70 beats/min at rest

- Class IIa recommendation by ESC: may be considered to reduce the risk of HF hospitalization or cardiovascular death in patients with stable symptomatic HFrEF (LVEF ≤ 35%) with resting heart rate ≥ 70 beats/min despite maximal beta-blocker therapy, or when they are contraindicated or not tolerated

These recommendations are based on:

The SHIFT trial, which randomized 6,505 patients with New York Heart Association functional class II to IV symptoms, LVEF ≤ 35%, and sinus rates ≥ 70 beats/min to ivabradine versus placebo and followed them for a median of 23 months. The primary composite outcome of cardiovascular death or hospital admission for worsening HF was reduced by 18% in the ivabradine group (HR: 0.82; 95% CI: 0.75 to 0.90; p < 0.0001), and was driven primarily by a 26% reduction in hospitalizations for HF. Although there was no difference in all-cause mortality, there was also a 26% reduction in HF deaths, an 11% reduction in all-cause hospitalization, and a 15% reduction in any cardiovascular hospitalization.

A statistically significant reduction in the primary composite endpoint was seen in the subgroup with baseline heart rate greater than the median of 77 beats/min.

3. For Acute HF:

No recommendation as yet, await results of ongoing studies.

In a trial of 71 patients with acute HFrEF (LVEF < 40%) and heart rate > 70 beats/min (30). randomized within 24 hr of hospitalization to beta-blocker alone or to a combination of beta-blocker and ivabradine, there were significant reductions in heart rate at 28 days and at 4 months with ivabradine, along with the observation of a higher LVEF (44.8 ± 14.4% vs. 38.1 ± 6.1%; p = 0.039) and lower B-type natriuretic peptide (259 ± 78 pg/ml vs. 554 ± 192 pg/ml; p = 0.02). However, despite these effects, no differences in mortality or HF hospitalizations were observed.

4. **For Heart failure with preserved ejection fraction:**

No recommendation as of now. Contradictory or negative study results.

5. **For Inappropriate sinus tachycardia:**
   - Not approved by US FDA or EMA
   - Class IIa ACC/AHA/HRS recommendation for treatment of symptoms based on expert consensus statement based on:

Several case reports and small nonrandomized studies. In one 1 small randomized, double-blind, placebo-controlled, crossover trial, with 21 patients, ivabradine was associated with significant reductions in heart rate at rest (-12 beats/min), after standing (-16 beats/min), during 24 h (-11 beats/min), and during effort (-18 beats/min). Overall, ivabradine eliminated more than 70% of baseline symptoms compared with placebo.

6. **For effects on collaterals:**

Chronic bradycardia has been shown to stimulate formation of collateral vessels in experimental models.

Retrospective studies in patients with different heart rates have shown that bradycardia is associated with development of coronary collateral vessels.

Lowering of the heart rate causes increase in diastolic perfusion time and, hence, an increase in shear stress. Shear stress initiates the cascade of endothelial activation, macrophage accumulation and outward vessel remodelling in coronary vessels. Thus, a lower heart rate leads to increased formation of a collateral circulation.

Both ivabradine and beta blockers can have this effect on collaterals.

However, unlike beta blockers, ivabradine does not unmask alpha-adrenergic vasoconstriction andmaintains coronary dilation during exercise. In comparison with beta-blockers, ivabradinealso increases coronary flow reserve and collateral perfusion.

In a clinical study by Gloekler et al patients were randomised in a single-blinded fashion to ivabradine or placebo. The collateral flow index (CFI), the gold standard method to measure the capacity of the collateral circulation, was determined invasively during a 1 min balloon occlusion at baseline and repeated at 6 months follow-up. Furthermore, intracoronary ECG ST-segment shifts and the presence of angina (AP) were assessed. At follow-up, CFI was significantly increased in the ivabradine group pointing to a proarteriogenic effect of ivabradine in CAD patients.

▌ Conclusion:

Thus at present time, Ivabradine can best be described as a second-line drug for systolic HF and chronic stable angina. Its role in the treatment of IST and for development of coronary collaterals is promising but lacks the support of large studies.

The danger of initiation of AF as shown in SIGNIFY trial must be noted.

Suggested Readings

1. Fox K., Ford I., Steg P.G., Tendera M., Ferrari R., BEAUTIFUL Investigators (2008) Ivabradine for patients with stable coronary artery disease and left-ventricular systolic dysfunction (BEAUTIFUL): a randomised, double-blind, placebo-controlled trial. Lancet 372:807-816

2. Fox K., Ford I., Steg P.G., Tardif J.C., Tendera M., Ferrari R., SIGNIFY Investigators (2014) Ivabradine in stable coronary artery disease without clinical heart failure. N Engl J Med 371:1091-1099

3. Swedberg K., Komajda M., Böhm M., et al., SHIFT Investigators (2010) Ivabradine and outcomes in chronic heart failure (SHIFT): a randomised placebo-controlled study. Lancet 376:875-885.

4. Gloekler S, Traupe T, Stoller M, Schild D, Steck H, Khattab A, Vogel R, Seiler C. The effect of heart rate reduction by ivabradine on collateral function in patients with chronic stable coronary artery disease.Heart. 2014 Jan;100(2):160-6. doi: 10.1136/heartjnl-2013-304880. Epub 2013 Nov 1.

5. Patel SR, Breall JA, Diver DJ, et al. Bradycardia is associated with development of coronary collateral vessels in humans. Coron Artery Dis 2000;11:467-72.

6. Cappato R., Castelvecchio S., Ricci C., et al. (2012) Clinical efficacy of ivabradine in patients with inappropriate sinus tachycardia: a prospective, randomized, placebo-controlled, double-blind, crossover evaluation. J Am CollCardiol 60:1323-1329.

106

The HDLC Conundrum - The Carriage and the Cargo !

Akshay Mehta

Observational studies have shown an inverse relationship of HDL Cholesterol (HDLC) values with incidence of cardio vascular disease (CVD). They have shown that each 1 mg/dl decrease in HDL-C concentration is associated with a 2% to 3% increased risk of CVD.

Does this imply a causal relationship of HDLC with CVD?

In other words :

1. Does low HDLC 'cause' CVD?

2. Does high HDLC value 'prevent' CVD?

3. Would raising HDLC levels reduce chances of having CVD?

The answer that emanates from 2 sets of data is that although HDLC, an easily measurable parameter, may be epidemiologically related to CVD, it is not causally related.

1. **Mendelian Randomization Studies :** This is a method of using known genetic differences in large populations to try to establish (or refute) causal relationship between levels of a biomarker in blood with the disease. Mendelian randomization studies have shown us that single nucleotide polymorphismsin loci only affecting plasma HDL-C levels do not associate with CHD risk.

    For example, such studies in which functional genetic variants of a polipoprotein AI (apoAI), lecithin cholesterol acyltransferase (LCAT)(1), and endothelial lipase apparently exhibited isolated effects on HDL-C level, failed to show a causal relationship between genetically determined HDL-C level and predicted CVD risk, even when HDL-C level and risk were strongly related in the background population.

    Thus, any genetic polymorphism that seems to raise HDL-C does not seem to protect from heart disease. That is, patients with higher HDL-C due to a known genetic alteration did not seem to have protection from heart disease as a result of that gene.

    An extreme example is the study by Madsen et al (see below) showing that extremely high level of HDL cholesterol is an independent predictor of increased mortality.

    Conversely, the studies also show that genotypes that are associated with lifelong reductions in HDL cholesterol are not associated with an increased risk of ischemic cardiovascular disease and in particular myocardial infarction (MI). Although low plasma HDL cholesterol levels were robustly associated with increased risk of MI, genetically decreased HDL cholesterol did not. This may suggest that low HDL cholesterol levels per se do not 'cause' MI.

2. Therapeutic trials like studies on niacin, torcetrapib and dalcetrapib, are another set of evidence that show failure of clinical benefit of raising HDLC levels.

These findings contradict a direct causality of THE AMOUNT of HDL CHOLESTEROL in blood with CVD and that people with high or low HDL-C who get coronary artery disease may well have something else at play.

Why this contrast between findings from observational studies on the one hand and randomized trials and Mendelian studies on the other?

In other words, why is HDLC level or content not causally related to CVD?

Quality of HDL particle:

First of all, it should be understood that HD Lipoprotein particles are distinct from the cholesterol they carry. Human HDLs comprise multiple discrete subpopulations of particles that differ in size, shape, charge, and in composition of both lipids and proteins. They are structurally and metabolically heterogeneous and subclasses exist with differential effects on coronary heart disease.

HDLs are subject to continuous remodelling by multiple plasma factors entering and leaving the HDL particles. The potential to protect against atherosclerosis is a function of HDLs and not the cholesterol carried by them.

HDL's show diverse protective effects such as eliciting cholesterol efflux from cholesterol ester-enriched macrophage foam cells in atheromata, and antiinflammatory, antithrombotic, and antioxidant effects resulting in improved endothelial function contributing to reduction in atherosclerosis.

However, for these functions, the "quality" of HDL particle matters more than the "quantity" of the cholesterol it carries. The HDL-C blood levels do not necessarily capture the diverse atheroprotective functions of the heterogeneous HDL populations and may not be a reliable proxy for the "HDLC effect" which protects against atherosclerotic plaque development.

For example studies show that cholesterol-overloaded HDL particles are independently associated with the progression of carotid atherosclerosis, whereas small to medium-sized HDL particles seem to confer greater protection.

In addition to apoAIandapoAII, HDL carries more than 30 other proteins ,and some of them are involved in lipid metabolism and vascular inflammation, including apoCIII, apoLI, and paraoxonase 1.

Apolipoprotein (apo) C-III, a small proinflammatory protein that resides on the surface of lipoproteins, enhances the atherogenicity of lipoprotein particles. Presence or absence of apoC-III differentiates HDL into subtypes with nonprotective or protective associations with risk of future CHD.

Studies (2) show that separating HDL-C according to apoC-III identified two types of HDL with opposing associations with risk of CHD. Thus the proatherogenic effects of apoC-III, as a component of VLDL and LDL, extends to HDL.

Two HDL-associated proteins (phospholipid transfer protein [PLTP] and paroxonase [PON]) modify CV risk.

The PLTP single nucleotide polymorphism causing lower hepatic PLTP transcription and plasma activity result in increased number of small HDL particles, and lower CVD risk.

PON1 and PON3 are calcium-dependent HDL-associated enzymes that impede the peroxidation of LDL particles thus being protective against CVD.

Sphingosine-1-phosphate (S1P) is a component of high-density lipoprotein (HDL) that is derived from the ubiquitous membrane lipid sphingomyelin. Sphingosine kinase is responsible for S1P synthesis, whereas S1P-lyase accounts for S1P irreversible degradation.

S1P has recently been found to have beneficial antiatherosclerotic effects. Inhibition of sphingosine kinase results in lower S1P levels and increased atherosclerosis. Conversely, deficiency of S1P-lyase resulted in higher S1P levels and reduced atherosclerosis.

Recent studies have shown convincing demonstration of the mechanistic role of reduced S1P as a cause of HDL dysfunction which could be corrected by S1P-loading.

Function of HDL : Cholesterol efflux capacity (CEC) : The ability of HDLs to promote efflux of cholesterol from macrophages in the artery wall- calculated from ex vivo cultured macrophages, has a strong association with regression of coronary artery disease independent of plasma HDL-C levels as shown in a in a CVD imaging trial (3).

There is also evidence that the cholesterol efflux capacity of HDLs (as measured ex vivo) is an inverse predictor of the risk of having a clinical ASCVD event, independent of the plasma concentrations of HDL cholesterol and apoA-I(4).

HDLs from patients with manifest atherosclerotic disease display several functional defects, such as impairment of antioxidative and anti-inflammatory properties. This has been attributed to alterations of the HDL proteome and lipidome.

In a study reported by Madsen et al.(5) from data of the Copenhagen City Heart Study and the Copenhagen General Population Study has shown that the presence of an extremely high concentration of HDL cholesterol is predictive of an increase in all-cause mortality in both men and women. It may indicate that in people with extreme high levels of HDL cholesterol, the functionality of HDLs may be compromised, with the concentration of HDL cholesterol no longer reflecting HDL function.

Size and number of HDL particles:

Several prospective studies and clinical trials of lipid-modifying therapies show that total HDL particle concentration is a more robust biomarker of cardiovascular risk than HDL cholesterol. (6-8). The same amount of cholesterol can be present in larger number of small HDL particles as in a smaller number of large HDL particles, the former conferring greater protection against CVD. Akin to LDL particle number, HDL particle number may be more important than the content of cholesterol in HDL particles.

Prior to the statin era, The Veterans Administration High-Density Lipoprotein Intervention Trial (VA-HIT) investigated the effect of gemfibrozil therapy in CHD patients with low levels of HDL cholesterol. Gemfibrozil-treated participants had higher concentrations of small, medium, and total HDL particle numbers and on-trial increases in small HDL particle numbers were predictive of 33% lower multivariate-adjusted riskof CHD events.

Niacin increases levels of HDL cholesterol, but it has a marginal effect on HDL particles.

Since some CETP inhibitors have shown improved HDL particle numbers and size along with efflux capacity function, future studies on clinical outcomes are keenly awaited. Till now, increasing HDL cholesterol levels by inhibiting CETP in statin-treated patients has not reduced ASCVD risk. The explanation is not known but may be because inhibition of CETP somehow impairs reverse cholesterol transport and may thus have the potential not to decrease ASCVD risk in statin-treated patients.

▌ Conclision:

The Carriage and the Cargo.

It is thus highly unlikely, that the cholesterol contained in HDL plays any protective role. The distinction between HDL particle and the cholesterol it carries should be understood. The protective function of HDLC resides in the former and not in the latter, although they work as a team.

Summarizing,

HDL and HDLC are different

HDL (ipoprotein) is the Carriage.

HDLC is Cholesterol Content, the Cargo

The cargo (HDL-C) does not necessarily reflect the cardio protective effects of the carriage (HDL)

We have concentrated on the cargo (HDL C) because:

i)   It is easy to measure

ii)   Observational studies show its robust inverse relationship with CVD

Which is because in most cases HDLC is linearly related to HDL number and function

But genetic and therapeutic studies have shown exceptions to above, that HDLC is not causally related to CVD and the futility of manipulating it.

In other words, the cargo is not the cause and "loading" it alone will not help.

The cause lies in the carriage - the quality, size, function and number of HDL PARTICLES

Our future lies in modifying these aspects of HDL.

Suggested Readings

1. Christiane L. Haase Anne Tybjærg-Hansen Abbas Ali Qayyum Jesper Schou Børge G. Nordestgaard Ruth Frikke-Schmidt.

    LCAT, HDL Cholesterol and Ischemic Cardiovascular Disease: A Mendelian Randomization Study of HDL Cholesterol in 54,500 Individuals.

    The Journal of Clinical Endocrinology & Metabolism, Volume 97, Issue 2, 1 February 2012, Pages E248-E256

2. Majken K. Jensen, Eric B. Rimm, Jeremy D. Furtado, Frank M. Sacks.

    Apolipoprotein C-III as a Potential Modulator of the Association Between HDL-Cholesterol and Incident Coronary Heart Disease. J Am Heart Assoc. 2012;1:jah3-e000232 doi: 10.1161/JAHA.111.000232.

3. Khera AV, Cuchel M, de la Llera-Moya M, et al. Cholesterol efflux capacity, high-density lipoprotein function, and atherosclerosis. N Engl J Med 2011;364:127-35.

4. Rohatgi A, Khera A, Berry JD, Givens EG, Ayers CR, Wedin KE, Neeland IJ, Yuhanna IS, Rader DR, de Lemos JA, Shaul PW. HDL cholesterol efflux capacity and incident cardiovascular events. N Engl J Med 2014;371:2383-2393.

5. Madsen CM, Varbo A, Nordestgaard BG. Extreme high high-density lipoprotein cholesterol is paradoxically associated with high mortality in men and women: two prospective cohort studies. Eur Heart J 2017;38:2478-2486.

6. Mackey RH, Greenland P, Goff DC Jr, Lloyd-Jones D, Sibley CT, Mora S. High-density lipoprotein cholesterol and particle concentrations, carotid atherosclerosis, and coronary events: MESA (multi-ethnic studyof atherosclerosis). J Am Coll Cardiol. 2012;60:508-516. doi: 10.1016/j. jacc.2012.03.060.

7. Mora S, Glynn RJ, Ridker PM. High-density lipoprotein cholesterol, size, particle number, and residual vascular risk after potent statin therapy. Circulation. 2013;128:1189-1197. doi: 10.1161/ CIRCULATIONAHA.113.002671.

8. Chandra A, Neeland IJ, Das SR, Khera A, Turer AT, Ayers CR, McGuire DK, Rohatgi A. Relation of black race between high density lipoprotein Cholesterol content, high density lipoprotein particles and coronary events (from the Dallas Heart Study). Am J Cardiol. 2015;115:890-894. doi: 10.1016/ j.amjcard.2015.01.015.

107

Air Pollution - A Not-to-be-overlooked Risk Factor for CVD

Akshay Mehta

Delhi is now the world's most polluted capital according to the World Health Organization, with pollution levels that regularly exceed those of Beijing. Other cities in the country are not far behind.

Recently, the Pune-based System of Air Quality And Weather Forecasting And Research (SAFAR) has identified a West Asian dust storm as the chief trigger behind the recent smog episode in the Delhi region. On November 8, 2017, the contribution of the dust storm was 40%, eclipsing the role of emissions from stubble burning, which stood at 25%, the monitoring agency said. That was the day pollution levels peaked with PM 2.5 concentration reaching 640 micrograms per cubic metre ($\mu g/m^3$), according to the SAFAR.

The above reports are of great import given the increasing volumes of data in recent literature linking air pollution to cardio vascular disease (CVD).

In a large-scale population-based study among residents of Seoul, Korea linking the location of outdoor monitors to the ZIP code of each participant's residence, crude and adjusted analyses were performed using Cox regression models to evaluate the risk for composite cardiovascular events including cardiovascular mortality, acute myocardial infarction, congestive heart failure, and stroke. A total of 136 094 participants were followed for a median of 7 years (900 845 person-years).

The study showed that every 1-$\mu g/m^3$ increase of long-term exposure to fine particulate matter ≤ 2.5 μm in aerodynamic diameter was associated with a 36% increased risk of cardiovascular events among healthy participants with no history cardiovascular diseases.

Air pollutants including PM 2.5, PM 2.5-10, CO, SO 2, and NO 2, but not O3, demonstrated positive relationships with cardiovascular risks, and the effects were consistent after adjusting for baseline risk factors and other pollutants.

The effects were consistent for all cardiovascular events including cardiovascular mortality, acute myocardial infarction, congestive heart failure, and stroke. Although most previous studies on the long term effects evaluated mortality risks, the interesting and novel finding of this study is the association of air pollution with specific major cardiovascular diseases.

This study also demonstrated that the burden from air pollution was as large as that of conventional cardiovascular risk factors such as hypertension and diabetes mellitus in this study population.

In a recent issue of the *European Heart Journal,* Kojima and colleagues report a significant association between Asian dust events originating in the deserts of China and East Asia, and the odds of acute myocardial infarction (AMI) in neighboring south-western Japan. Use of a time-stratified case-crossover design, comparing dust storm exposure on AMI of 3713 consecutive patients on three to four control dates in the same month, to examine if AMI is more likely to occur in the setting of a dust storm event, had the strength of removingwithin-person and time-varying confounding.

There were 41 Asian dust storm events, with visibility of less than 10 km, over the 5 year study period. It was found that dust storms were associated with a 1.46 times higher risk of AMI the day following a dust storm, compared to days without a preceding dust storm event.

The World Health Organization estimates that 7 million deaths were attributable to air pollution exposure worldwide in 2012.

The Global Burden of Disease Study 2015 ranked ambient exposure to fine particulate matter with an aerodynamic diameter of < 2.5μm (PM 2.5) as the fifth most important risk factor for mortality worldwide.

The cardiovascular health consequences of air pollution exceed all its other health effects such as pulmonary diseases.

Deaths from cardiovascular causes account for more than two thirds of the premature deaths attributable to ambient PM 2.5 air pollution.

Interestingly, most previous studies were conducted in the United States or Europe, with pollution levels much less than those in developing countries where PM 2.5 levels are 10 times higher.

▌ Mechanism of effect on CVD :

Both gaseous air pollutants (i.e. ozone, sulfur and nitric oxides, carbon monoxide) and particulate matter (PM) cause adverse effects on health. However, the most serious effects are related to PM.

Epidemiologic data suggest that air pollution can promote both chronic atherogenesis and acute atherothrombosis through oxidative stress and inflammation causing atheroma plaque progression and rupture, vasomotor dysfunction, fibrinolytic imbalance, platelet activation and aggregation and arrhythmogenic effect through autonomic imbalance.

These effects could be indirectly through inhaled particles provoking an inflammatory response in the lungs, with consequent release of prothrombotic and inflammatory cytokines into the circulation.

An alternate possibility is that inhaled, insoluble, fine PM or nanoparticles could rapidly translocate into the circulation, with the potential for direct effects on hemostasis and cardiovascular integrity. Once in the circulation, nanoparticles could interact with the vascular endothelium or have direct effects on atherosclerotic plaques and cause local oxidative stress and proinflammatory effects similar to those seen in the lungs.

Acceleration of atherosclerosis and vascular inflammation in response to long-term air pollution exposure was suggested in an animal model. Recently, studies from the MESA Air (Multi-Ethnic

Study of Atherosclerosis and Air Pollution) cohort have demonstrated that long-term PM 2.5 concentrations are associated with the progression of intima-media thickness on ultrasound examination and coronary calcification measured by cardiac computed tomography.

❚ Clinical Implications:

Long-term exposure to ambient air pollutants is a major risk factor for cardiovascular diseases as strong as other established risk factors like smoking, diabetes and hypertension.

Besides controlling the source such as stubble burning, vehicular and industrial emissions, behavioral interventions to lower indoor or outdoor air pollution exposure, such as advising people to stay at home, close their windows, or wearing masks may be advisable. This is especially for people at higher risk such as those elder citizens with hypertension, diabetes, non-smokers, and/or those with chronic kidney disease. A small number of studies suggest that air filters hold promise in improving cardiovascular health.

Artificial rain by cloud seeding has been used by China, Indonesia and Malaysia to curb air pollution. An MIT study in 2015 found that rain water can attract pollutants through coagulation, but if unfiltered, such water can cause secondary water pollution and infections. Helicopter aerial sprinkling may be useful for localized pollution.

Ambient air pollution is a public health issue, and measures to control the level of air pollution or its effects are urgently required to reduce the burden of cardiovascular disease.

❚ Suggested Readings

1. Hyeanji Kim, MD;* Joonghee Kim, MD;* Sunhwa Kim, PhD; Si-Hyuck Kang, MD; Hee-Jun Kim, MD; Ho Kim, PhD; JongbaeHeo, PhD; Seung-Muk Yi, PhD; Kyuseok Kim, MD; Tae-JinYoun, MD; In-Ho Chae, MD.

   Cardiovascular Effects of Long-Term Exposure to Air Pollution: APopulation-Based Study With 900 845 Person-Years of Follow-up.

   J Am Heart Assoc. 2017;6: e007170. DOI: 10.1161/JAHA.117.007170 originally published November 8, 2017.

2. SunaoKojima Takehiro Michikawa Kayo Ueda Tetsuo Sakamoto Kunihiko Matsui Tomoko Kojima Kenichi Tsujita Hisao Ogawa Hiroshi Nitta Akinori Takami.

   Asian dust exposure triggers acute myocardial infarction.

   European Heart Journal, Volume 38, Issue 43, 14 November 2017, Pages 3202-3208,https://doi.org/10.1093/eurheartj/ehx509.

3. C. Arden Pope, Joseph B. Muhlestein, Jeffrey L. Anderson, John B. Cannon, Nicholas M. Hales, Kent G. Meredith, Viet Le, Benjamin D. Horne

   Short?Term Exposure to Fine Particulate Matter Air Pollution Is Preferentially Associated With the Risk of ST-Segment Elevation Acute Coronary Events

   Journal of the American Heart Association. 2015;4: e002506, originally published December 8, 2015.

4.   Adar SD, Sheppard L, Vedal S, Polak JF, Sampson PD, Diez Roux AV, Budoff M, Jacobs DR Jr, Barr RG, Watson K, Kaufman JD.

    Fine particulate air pollution and the progression of carotid intima-medial thickness: a prospective cohort study from the Multi-Ethnic Study of Atherosclerosis and air pollution.

    PLoS Med. 2013;10:e1001430.

5.   Kaufman JD, Adar SD, Barr RG, Budoff M, Burke GL, Curl CL, Daviglus ML, Diez Roux AV, Gassett AJ, Jacobs DR Jr, Kronmal R, Larson TV, Navas-Acien A, Olives C, Sampson PD, Sheppard L, Siscovick DS, Stein JH, Szpiro AA, Watson KE.

    Association between air pollution and coronary artery calcification within six metropolitan areas in the USA (the Multi-Ethnic Study of Atherosclerosis and air pollution): a longitudinal cohort study.

    Lancet. 2016;388:696-704.